Drug Action in the Central Nervous System

Drug Action
in the
Central Nervous System

PAUL M. CARVEY

Rush-Presbyterian St. Luke's Medical Center
Rush Medical College of Rush University

New York   Oxford
OXFORD UNIVERSITY PRESS
1998

Oxford University Press

Oxford   New York
Athens   Auckland   Bangkok   Bogota
Bombay   Buenos Aires   Calcutta   Cape Town
Dar es Salaam   Delhi   Florence   Hong Kong
Istanbul   Karachi   Kuala Lumpur   Madras
Madrid   Melbourne   Mexico City   Nairobi
Paris   Singapore   Taipei   Tokyo
Toronto   Warsaw
and associated companies in
Berlin   Ibadan

Copyright © 1998 by Oxford University Press, Inc.

Published by Oxford University Press, Inc.
198 Madison Avenue, New York, New York 10016

Oxford is a registered trademark of Oxford University Press

Library of Congress Cataloging-in-Publication Data
Carvey, Paul M.
Drug action in the central nervous system / Paul M. Carvey.
p.   cm.   Includes bibliographical references and index.
ISBN 0-19-509333-X (cloth). — ISBN 0-19-509334-8 (paper)
1. Neuropharmacology.   2. Neuropsychopharmacology.
3. Central nervous system—Effect of drugs on.
I. Title.
[DNLM: 1. Central Nervous System Agents—pharmacology.
2. Central Nervous System—drug effects.
QV 77.5 C331d 1998]
RM315.C376 1998   615'.78—dc21   DNLM/DLC   for Library of Congress   97-14183

1 2 3 4 5 6 7 8 9
Printed in the United States of America
on acid-free paper

to
Harold L. Klawans
mentor and friend

Preface

The primary focus of this book is pharmacodynamics, the study of the mechanisms by which drugs exert their effects on biological systems. Treating the symptoms of Parkinson's disease with levodopa, for example, raises the level of the neurotransmitter dopamine (DA) in a region of the brain called the striatum where DA is lost during the disease process: The rigidity and inability to move that are among the clinical hallmarks of this disease are reduced as a result. Overly aggressive levodopa therapy, however, often leads to psychotic symptoms thought to result from increased DA in limbic and frontal cortical regions of the brain. Thus, the induction of psychotic side effects is also a consequence of levodopa's pharmacodynamic action. Pharmacodynamics therefore encompasses not only the desired actions of a drug, but its side effects as well.

Much of what we currently know about brain function comes from studying the pharmacodynamics of centrally acting drugs. For decades these drugs have been used as "functional probes" to study complex brain function. Our current working theories of epilepsy, depression, anxiety, schizophrenia, Parkinson's disease, and other (neurological or psychiatric) disorders rely heavily on such observations. This approach is referred to as pharmacocentric and the hypotheses that emerge are called pharmacocentric hypotheses. Establishing the pharmacodynamics of centrally acting drugs provides the therapeutic rationale needed to treat patients and understand side effects. It also stimulates basic research into central nervous system (CNS) function and dysfunction.

Centrally acting drugs traditionally have been viewed from two different perspectives: neurologic and psychiatric. Neuropharmacology has focused on the drugs that neurologists use: those that influence movement and other aspects of brain function generally not regarded as mental or emotional. These drugs have been used to treat such disorders as Parkinson's disease, migraine headaches, and epilepsy. Psychopharmacology, on the other hand, has focused on drugs that influence the mind. These drugs comprise the armamentarium of the psychiatrist and include the antidepressants, the anxiolytic agents, and the antipsychotic drugs used to treat schizophrenia.

The neurologic/psychiatric dichotomy still exists, but it appears increasingly artificial in light of recent research. It is based in part on the assumptions that motor and mental activities arise from distinctly different systems. However, the known effects of drugs on the brain simply do not support such a dichotomy. With few exceptions, drugs used to treat movement disorders affect emotion while drug treatment of the disordered mind influences movement. Although these effects are, in part, a consequence of nonspecific drug action, some drugs can alter both motor and mental function by influencing activity within the same region of the brain. Thus, as we learn more about how these drugs act, we are beginning to realize that the way they influence motor activity is similar to the way they affect mental function. The approach in this text represents a synthesis of neuropharmacology and psychopharmacology. This seems more consistent with the emerging view that motor and mental functions are intricately interrelated.

In my own experience teaching neuropsychopharmacology, I've come to appreciate that when students learn about drugs within a neurobiological and neuropathological context, they understand more quickly and retain the knowledge longer than if they memorize drug names and side effects without reference to causation or content. For example, having a basic understanding of the symptoms of depression and of the current views of their biological basis provides a framework for understanding antidepressant drug action. Moreover, learning about drugs in this way allows students to challenge the validity of a proposed drug action and also to adapt the model as knowledge of CNS disorders evolves. This approach guided the organization of this text.

The first three chapters give an overview of brain function and present the basic principles of drug delivery and receptor function. These chapters introduce many of the terms and concepts that are used by working pharmacologists and are needed to appreciate the subtleties of drug action. These chapters also briefly review the autonomic nervous system (ANS) and the effects drugs have on it. Most centrally acting drugs alter autonomic function either directly or indirectly. The autonomic side effects that accompany treatment with centrally acting drugs are so common that it is virtually impossible to describe these drugs' actions without a solid grasp of autonomic pharmacology.

The nine chapters that follow this background section provide a comprehensive overview of the pharmacodynamics of the most commonly used centrally acting drugs. Each chapter is organized in the same way. The neurobiology underlying the disorder treated by the drug class under discussion is briefly reviewed in an introductory section. This section is followed by an in-depth discussion of the drug mechanism of action and therapeutic effects. The major side effects are then described. Again, the neurobiological mechanisms responsible for these side effects are emphasized. This section is followed by a discussion of the relevant pharmacokinetics for the drug class being considered. I believe that this sequence of presentation provides the most appropriate framework within which to learn the pharmacodynamics of centrally acting drugs.

This text is designed to ease student use, particularly review of the material for exams. In the appendix is a list of review questions that identify the main points of each chapter. In addition, a chapter-by-chapter drug list is included in the appendix. Throughout the text, figures are designed to emphasize key ideas or points that cannot be readily explained in words. The accompanying figure legends not only describe the contents of the figure but also reiterate the major idea behind the figures. Several tables are included in each chapter. They provide the *DSM-IV* criteria for the disease being considered and lists of drug effects, side effects, toxic reactions, and other salient treatment considerations.

Many people have contributed in one way or another to the completion of this book and deserve my thanks. My students have been my greatest inspiration. Their probing questions made me verify facts and examine alternative views. I want to give special thanks to my parents, Matthew and Gertrude Carvey. My mother always encouraged me in science and gave me the opportunity to enjoy it. My father, a professional golfer, taught me the most important lesson of all about teaching. I worked my way through graduate school giving golf lessons, a skill I learned from him. He always emphasized that if a student does not understand some aspect of a golf swing you are trying to teach, it is generally not the student's fault; rather, it is because "you are not conveying the idea in a way the student can understand."

I am indebted to the specialists who read the various chapters and offered constructive criticism. Many thanks to M. Victor Nora, Michael Smith, Byong Moon, Arthur V. Prancan, Robert McCarthy, Christopher Goetz, and Harold L. Klawans, my lifelong mentor to whom this book is dedicated. Judy Rosner, director of the United Parkinson Foundation, graciously consented to edit the text. I would also like to thank Michele

Einert and Joann Kern, who spend innumerable hours helping me put together the working drafts of this text, and Heather Robie, who compiled the references and index. I also wish to thank Jeff House of Oxford University Press, who kept me focused on the intent of this book. Finally, I simply could not have written this book without the continuous understanding of my wife Jane and my two sons, Chris and Pat, who underwent many sacrifices to give me the time I needed to complete it.

Contents

Drug Action in the Central Nervous System

1

Introduction

SITES OF DRUG ACTION

The fundamental unit of the central nervous system (CNS) is the neuron (Fig. 1–1), which conducts an electrical signal from its dendritic field to its terminal. This is accomplished by the activation of voltage-gated sodium channels that allow Na^+ to move down an electrochemical gradient and K^+ to exit the cell. Drugs can disrupt this process by interfering with the function of these voltage-gated channels. Local anesthetics, for instance, enter Na^+ channels from the inside of the nerve cell and block the channel while certain antiseizure drugs such as phenytoin prevent the Na^+ channel from becoming reactivated following a depolarization. In addition, the electrical activity of neurons can be disrupted by drugs that open other types of ion channels. The barbiturates, for instance, activate ligand-gated (neurotransmitter-activated) Cl^- channels. This allows Cl^- to enter nerve cells and effectively neutralizes the depolarizing effect of Na^+. Other drugs, including alcohol, the gas anesthetics, and tetrahydrocannabinol (THC—the main intoxicating component in marijuana), disrupt the fluidity of the neuronal membrane and thus disrupt the normal function of ion channels embedded within it.

The function of electrical activity within a neuron is to transfer signals to other nerve cells. Although neurons can communicate with one another through electrotonic synapses where electrical current is passed between the two, by far the most common method of neuronal communication is the release of chemical neurotransmitters.

1

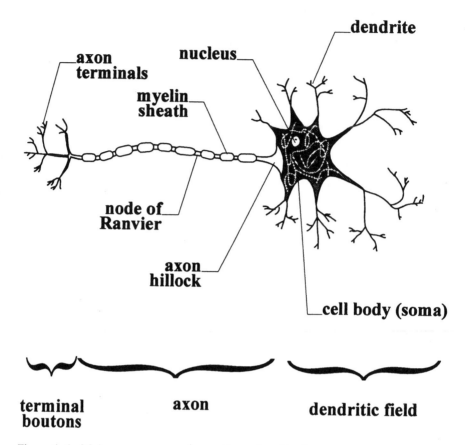

Figure 1–1. Major components of a myelinated multipolar neuron.

The action potential that propagates down the axon in an all-or-none fashion eventually reaches the neurotransmitter release site. In most neurons this occurs at a specialized region of the axon called the terminal bouton. In other neurons, neurotransmitters can be released all along the axon at specialized regions called varicosities that are functionally similar to terminal boutons. As in Na^+ channels, depolarization leads to the activation of N-type (N for neurotransmitter), voltage-gated Ca^{2+} channels, allowing Ca^{2+} to enter the nerve. The Ca^{2+} that enters the terminal then initiates the release of the neurotransmitter. The release site contains several specialized proteins that bind Ca^{2+} (Fig. 1–2), initiating a cascade of events that leads to the extrusion of the synaptic vesicle and its contents into the synapse in a process called exocytosis. Drugs that act on neurotransmitter receptors located near release sites can influence the function of the proteins involved in release and thereby decrease (most commonly) or increase (less commonly) the amount of neurotransmitter released.

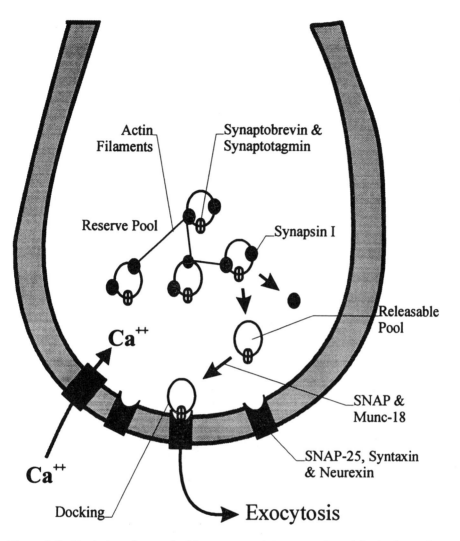

Figure 1–2. Depiction of a terminal bouton containing synaptic vesicles in the resting state and following Ca²⁺ influx. In the resting state most vesicles are bound to actin filaments, not docked at the membrane, and Ca²⁺ channels are closed. Once depolarization invades the terminal, voltage-gated Ca²⁺ channels open and Ca²⁺ triggers the docking and exocytosis of the vesicles by binding to specific proteins.

The vast majority of neurotransmitter released into the synapse is taken back into the nerve terminal in a process called reuptake. For instance, acetylcholine (ACh) is hydrolyzed to acetate and choline and the choline is taken up by the nerve terminal. In the case of norepinephrine (NE), the whole molecule is taken up. Specialized transporter proteins specific for a given neurotransmitter mediate this process. Antidepressant drugs such as desipramine bind to these transporter proteins, prevent reuptake, and extend the duration of action of the neurotransmitter. Drugs such as amphetamine bind to the transporter protein, are transported into the neuron, and promote the release of neurotransmitter.

Once the neurotransmitter binds to the transporter protein, it is "shuttled" across the membrane to the cytoplasmic side of the release site. The cytoplasm at the release site is often referred to as the mobile pool. Once in the mobile pool, the neurotransmitter that is taken back up by the transport protein or that is newly synthesized by the neuron is concentrated in synaptic vesicles (vesicular pool) by a specialized transporter protein found in the vesicular membrane. This process can be disrupted by drugs such as reserpine that deplete the vesicular pool and thereby prevent neurotransmission.

Neurotransmitter that is not taken up by transport proteins can bind to specialized receptor proteins that activate ligand-gated ion channels on other neurons (postsynaptic sites) or on specialized receptors which are located on the membrane at the release site (presynaptic sites) and are called autoreceptors. Drugs that mimic or antagonize the action of neurotransmitters bind to these receptors and alter neuronal function. Many of these receptors initiate the production of second messengers that carry the neurotransmitter signal into the cell to perform specific functions. Drugs such as caffeine influence the production of certain second messengers and thereby influence neuronal function.

Neurotransmitter receptors located at various sites on neurons influence their electrical activity in different ways. Since most drugs influence neurotransmission, the effect a drug has on a neuron will be determined, in part, by the location of the synapse where the affected neurotransmitter acts. A variety of presynaptic/postsynaptic configurations exist (Fig. 1–3). By far the most common type is the axodendritic synapse. (The prefix always refers to the presynaptic side and the main word refers to the postsynaptic side.) In an axodendritic synapse, the terminal bouton or varicosity of one neuron is the presynaptic or neurotransmitter-releasing side while the postsynaptic side is the dendritic field of another. Axosomatic synapses are those in which the terminal bouton or varicosity on the presynaptic neuron synapses on the cell body or axon hillock of the postsynaptic neuron. Since the axon hillock is the site where the action potential is initiated, these types of synapses, being closer to that site, have greater control over the firing of the postsynaptic cell. In axoaxonic synapses the terminals of the presynaptic neuron make synaptic contact with the terminals of another neuron. These synapses significantly influence the release of neurotransmitter from the postsynaptic neuron, even if the cell body is fully depolarized. A less common form of synapse is found in the dendritic fields of some neurons and is called dendrodendritic. In this synapse the dendrites of one neuron release neurotransmit-

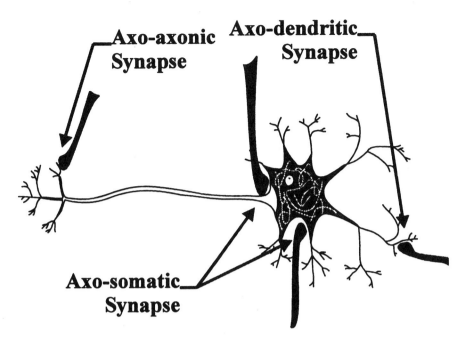

Figure 1–3. Types of synaptic configurations are shown converging on a multipolar neuron. The various types of synaptic configurations use the source of the terminal as the prefix (axonal or "axo" in all of the cases depicted) and the target of the synapse as the suffix (dendritic, somatic, or axonic in the cases depicted).

ter that interacts with postsynaptic receptors located on the dendrites of others.

Finally, neurotransmitters can be catabolized to inactive metabolites by specialized enzymes. Several drugs enhance or inhibit the function of these enzymes. The monoamine oxidase inhibitors used in the treatment of depression, for instance, inhibit the catabolism of norepinephrine (NE) and extend its duration of action.

THE NEUROTRANSMITTERS

Neurotransmitters are classified into two large groups based on their molecular weights and chemical makeup: small-molecule and large-molecule neurotransmitters. Small-molecule neurotransmitters are non-proteinaceous, have molecular weights below 1,000, and include such substances as acetylcholine, serotonin, and glutamate. In contrast, large-molecule neurotransmitters are proteins, have molecular weights greater than 1,000, and include such substances as enkephalin, substance P, and cholecystokinin. In addition to these characteristics, the two groups differ in other fundamental ways including their routes of biosynthesis and degradation, their action at synapses, and the concentrations at which they act.

Small-Molecule Neurotransmitters

The small-molecule neurotransmitters that are known to be influenced by centrally acting drugs are summarized in Table 1–1. These are the chemicals we normally think of when the term neurotransmitter is used, and they all meet the rigorous criteria for neurotransmitter status. They are all released in a Ca^{2+}-dependent fashion, act on their receptors in high-nanomolar or low-micromolar concentrations, are taken back up by transporter proteins, are reused or catabolized in the synapse, or part of the molecule is reused (e.g., acetylcholine). The small-molecule neurotransmitters are synthesized on endosomes by specific enzymes located throughout the neuron. Most of the biosynthetic pathways are subject to end-product inhibition so that high levels of mobile pool neurotransmitter can inhibit the first enzyme in the synthesizing pathway. Many pathways in the brain are characterized by the small-molecule neurotransmitter they contain: The corticostriatal glutaminergic pathway and the septohippocampal cholinergic pathway are examples.

All of the small-molecule neurotransmitters act at multiple receptor sites (Table 1–1). Acetylcholine, for instance, induces its actions through nicotinic and muscarinic receptors. Acetylcholine's activation of nicotinic and muscarinic receptors mediates different functions because the former open ion channels while the latter have this effect but also activate a second-messenger cascade. Since the distribution of these receptors is heterogenous within the neuraxis, the actions of acetylcholine in any given nuclear area will differ depending upon whether nicotinic, muscarinic, or both kinds of receptors are present. The muscarinic and nicotinic receptor families are further subdivided into receptor subtypes such as N_N and N_M. Since these receptor subtypes possess slightly different protein structures, drugs selective for a given subtype can be developed. The use of such receptor-subtype-specific drugs allows a nicotinic agonist to affect nicotinic receptors located on nerve cells without influencing nicotinic receptors on muscles.

Although more detailed descriptions of the various small-molecule neurotransmitters will be given in later chapters, it is important to point out a unique neuroanatomical characteristic of the pathways involving the neurotransmitters acetylcholine, norepinephrine, dopamine, and serotonin. Ascending neurons usually reach the cerebral cortices via the thalamus and release neurotransmitters such as gamma-aminobutyric acid or glutamate. The projection systems for acetylcholine, norepineph-

Table 1–1 Major Small-Molecule Neurotransmitters

Neurotransmitter	Receptors	Function[a]
Acetylcholine (ACh)	Muscarinic (M_1 through M_5) Nicotinic (N_N and N_M)	Memory function, sensory processing, motor coordination, neuromuscular junction neurotransmission, and ANS and PANS function
Norepinephrine (NE)	Alpha$_1$ and alpha$_2$; beta$_1$, beta$_2$, and beta$_3$.	CNS sensory processing, cerebellar function, sleep, mood, learning, memory, anxiety, and SANS
Dopamine (DA)	D_1 through D_5 in two families designated D-1 and D-2	Motor regulation, reinforcement, olfaction, mood, concentration, hormone control, and hypoxic drive
Serotonin (5HT)	Currently 18 receptors have been identified and broken into 8 families designated $5HT_1$ through $5HT_8$	Emotional processing, mood, appetite, sleep, pain processing, hallucinations, and reflex regulation
Glutamate (Glu)	NMDA, quisqualate, and kainate	Long-term potentiation, memory, major excitatory function within the CNS and PNS
Gamma-amino-butyric acid (GABA)	$GABA_A$ and $GABA_B$	Major inhibitory neurotransmitter in the CNS
Histamine (H)	H_1 and H_2	Sleep, sedation, and temperature regulation
Glycine (Gly)		Major inhibitory function within the spinal cord

[a]ANS = autonomic nervous system, PANS = parasympathetic autonomic nervous system, SANS = sympathetic autonomic nervous system

rine, dopamine, and serotonin, however, do not. Fibers containing these neurotransmitters bypass thalamic circuitry and innervate targets in the cortex directly. This innervation pattern is consistent with their role as regulators of cortical activity. They do not determine the type of activity that enters the cortex via thalamic projections but rather they modulate the activity that enters the cortex via the thalamus. Some authors have used the analogy of a radio to describe this function: Thalamic projections determine which radio station is played while extrathalamic projections determine the volume. Interestingly, most of the drugs used to treat psychiatric disorders selectively influence the function of these extrathalamic projections.

Large-Molecule Neurotransmitters

A variety of neuroactive peptides have been characterized (Table 1–2). Enkephalin, the endogenous morphine-like substance, is the best-known member of this class. This neuropeptide is released throughout the pain pathways of the neuraxis where morphine can mimic its action and reduce pain. Substance P (Sub P) is thought to be the neurotransmitter released by the primary pain fibers in the periphery and is found throughout the CNS as well. Cholecystokinin (CCK), the gut peptide known for its gall-bladder-contracting action, is also found within the CNS. Many of the neuropeptides are "colocalized" with small-molecule neurotransmitters (i.e., some dopaminergic fibers contain both dopamine and the neuropeptide neurotensin). Although none of the neuropeptides has been elevated to true neurotransmitter status, their actions in many cases are similar to those of the small-molecule neurotransmitters. Their synthesis, however, differs from that of the small-molecule neurotransmitters such as dopamine (DA). Whereas DA is synthesized from a precursor, tyrosine, the synthesis of a neuropeptide involves progressive cleavage from larger polypeptides. Neurotransmitters such as DA can also be taken back up into nerve terminals, repackaged in synaptic vesicles, and released again,

Table 1–2 Large-Molecule Neurotransmitters (Neuropeptides)[a]

Hypothalamic-releasing hormones	**Gastrointestinal peptides**
Thyrotropin-releasing hormone	Vasoactive intestinal peptide (VIP)
Gonadotropin-releasing hormone	Cholecystokinin (CCK)
Somatostatin	Substance P (Sub P)
Growth-hormone-releasing hormone	Gastrin
Corticotropin-releasing hormone	Neurotensin
	Insulin
Pituitary peptides	Glucagon
Adrenocorticotropic hormone (ACTH)	Bombesin
Thyrotropin	Met-enkephalin (met-Enk)
Luteinizing hormone	Leu-enkephalin (leu-Enk)
Prolactin	Secretin
Beta-endorphin	Motilin
Alpha-melanocyte-stimulating hormone	
Growth hormone	**Others**
	Atrial naturetic hormone
Neurohypophyseal hormones	Bradykinin
Oxytocin	Sleep peptides
Vasopressin	Calcitonin
	Calcitonin-gene-related peptide (CGRP)
	Neuropeptide Y
	Galanin
	Substance K

[a]Adapted from Kandel, Schwartz, and Jessell (1991)

but neuropeptides can only be synthesized in the cell body by ribosomes, packaged by the Golgi apparatus, and then transported to the terminal for release. Since their action is terminated exclusively by nonspecific peptidases, they cannot be reused. Colocalized neuropeptides often act at picomolar and low-nanomolar concentrations and often modulate the activity of a colocalized small-molecule neurotransmitter. There is also evidence that neuropeptides are not released in a 1 : 1 ratio with their colocalized neurotransmitters, but rather in a frequency-dependent fashion. Such frequency-dependent release may enable a neuron to alter the effect of its small-molecule neurotransmitter so that the postsynaptic effect differs depending upon the rate at which the presynaptic neuron fires.

There are no centrally acting drugs that selectively influence the action of any neuropeptide other than enkephalin or Sub P. Because the neuropeptides are proteins of large molecular weight that do not readily enter the brain, their actions in the CNS cannot be effectively studied following systemic administration. This is unfortunate since many neuropeptides are known to influence very specific regions of the brain. If they did enter the brain easily, they might provide highly selective therapeutic effects such as suppression of appetite without the wide range of side effects normally associated with the use of drugs that act on small-molecule systems. The development of small molecules that readily enter brain and regulate the effect of known large-molecule neurotransmitters is an active area of research in many pharmaceutical companies.

Centrally-Acting Gases

Within the last few years evidence has accumulated that nitric oxide (NO) and carbon monoxide (CO) are heterogenously distributed within the CNS and function as neurotransmitters although they have not yet met all the criteria needed to be classified as such. Unlike small- and large-molecule neurotransmitters, they are not synthesized for storage in synaptic vesicles. Rather, they are emitted as gases following a Ca^{2+}-calmodulin-mediated enzymatic reaction (see Chapter 3). The liberated gas then simply diffuses away from the synaptic terminal. The gas neurotransmitters bind to specific acceptor proteins inside the target cell where they activate guanine nucleotide-binding protein (G proteins), thereby elevating cyclic adenosine monophosphate (cAMP). NO and CO may also act as retrograde neurotransmitters in that they can be released by a postsynaptic neuron, diffuse to the presynaptic terminal, and facilitate future neurotransmitter release. Their action as retrograde neurotransmitters appears critical to the development of long-term potentiation which is currently thought to be responsible, at least in part, for establishing memory.

In high-enough concentrations, these gases can also induce free radical damage and thus may be involved in excitotoxicity.

Neurotrophic Factors

Although nerve growth factor (NGF) was isolated in the 1950s, its importance in neural function was not appreciated until recently. In the past few years, several peptidergic compounds called neurotrophic factors have been identified within the brain and are now known to play an important role there (Table 1–3). A neurotrophic factor (NTF), by definition, enhances the growth of neurons. The NTFs do not function as neurotransmitters but rather regulate neuronal growth within the CNS and are the molecules most likely responsible for maintaining the cytoarchitectural integrity of neuronal pathways. They are known to regulate the phenomenon of programmed cell death: In the absence of a specific NTF, neurons initiate a cascade of events leading to cell death. My laboratory and others have shown that drugs can affect NTFs, probably through their impact on neurotransmitter systems that appear to regulate NTF production and release. NTFs seem to be released at low concentrations all the time, and alterations in neurotransmission apparently increase or decrease the amount released. Thus, the administration of drugs might actually alter the physical structure of the brain by influencing the trophic environment. This raises the possibility that chronic drug treatment may permanently alter brain structure and function. Several studies involving the administration of various NTFs directly into the CNS of patients with neurodegenerative diseases are currently underway.

Table 1–3 Major Neurotrophic Factors in the CNS

Neurotrophin growth factors
Nerve growth factor (NGF)
Brain-derived neurotrophic factor (BDNF)
Neurotrophin-3 (NT-3)
Neurotrophin-4/5 (NT-4/5)
Neurotrophin-6 (NT-6)

Others
Basic fibroblast growth factor (bFGF)
Acidic fibroblast growth factor (aFGF)
Glial-derived neurotrophic factor (GDNF)
Ciliary neurotrophic factor (CNTF)
Cholinergic development factor (CDF)
Platelet-derived neurotrophic factor (PDNF)
Insulin-dependent growth factor (IDGF)
Epidermal growth factor (EGF)

CNS SYSTEMS

The complex function among the various systems of the brain makes it difficult to describe in anatomical terms. Generally, it is the complex interaction among brain regions that is responsible for the disorders that will be described in the later chapters of this book. Accordingly, six terms will be used throughout the book that reflect the joint activity of a number of interacting neural systems: motor, sensory, memory, emotional, cognitive, and autonomic.

Motor processing refers to the neuronal activity responsible for movement. The structures involved include the cerebellum, certain regions of the basal ganglia, the motor strip of the frontal cortex, and suprasegmental nuclei in the brainstem controlling posture such as the vestibular nuclei (refer to Figs. 1–4 and 1–5). Drug classes that affect motor processing include the antiparkinson agents, central stimulants, antispasmodic agents, muscle relaxers, and sedative-hypnotics.

Sensory processing refers to the neuronal activity involved in responding to and transmitting sensory information. The participating structures include those responsible for the primary senses of vision, audition, olfaction, touch, and pain as well as the thalamus, parietal cortex, occipital cortex, and parts of the temporal cortex where perceptual information, often from several different modalities, is integrated. Among the drugs that affect sensory processing are the sedative-hypnotics, local anesthetics, and hallucinogens.

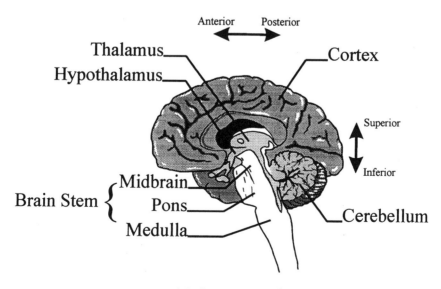

Figure 1–4. Major subdivisions of the brain in sagittal section.

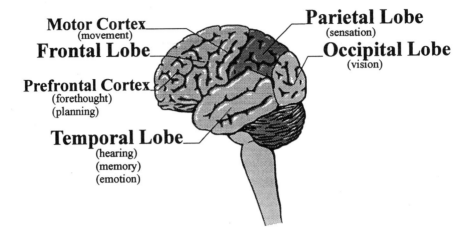

Figure 1–5. The major lobes of the cerebral cortex and their primary functions.

Memory is the ability of the brain to recall events and integrate them into ongoing activity. It is generally divided into two basic forms called procedural and declarative. Procedural memory refers to the ability to implement a set of practiced motor actions such as hitting a golf ball or driving a car. It involves a number of limbic structures as well as the cerebellum and perhaps even the caudate nucleus in the basal ganglia. Declarative memory, on the other hand, involves thoughts and associations that can be recalled and applied to influence future activity. These would include facts such as that Springfield is the capital of Illinois and knowledge of events, such as, "I was riding my bike when I heard Kennedy was assassinated." Declarative memory involves the hippocampus, amygdala, thalamus, and the cortical mantle. Memory exists in the short term (e.g., ability to redial a phone number), intermediate term (e.g., ability to recall three items from a list after ten minutes), and long term (e.g., Roger Maris hit 61 home runs in one season). Long-term memory seems to require protein synthesis and may involve alterations in the growth of dendrites or terminal boutons (neuronal plasticity). Dementia is a broad term used to describe disorders of memory such as Alzheimer's disease and multi-infarct dementia. Drugs that affect memory include most CNS depressants and cholinergic agents.

Limbic processing occurs in such regions of the brain as the hypothalamus, amygdala, septum, cingulate and entorhinal cortices of the frontal lobes, the hippocampus, and mammillary bodies. Emotion refers to the conscious perception of the neuronal activity in these structures and is best described as a state of preparedness. For instance, particular patterns of neural activity in these limbic structures are involved in preparing the brain and body for an anticipated activity and give rise to feelings that we know as fear, love, or anxiety. Drugs that affect the limbic system include the antidepressants, antipsychotics, central stimulants, anxiolytic agents, the opioids, street drugs such as phencyclidine, and all drugs possessing dependence liability.

Cognitive processing occurs in those executive regions of the brain where sensory information is interpreted and weighed before the decision to act via the motor system is made (whether consciously or unconsciously). Cognitive processing also encompasses those functions of the brain such as abstract reasoning and forethought that do not necessarily result in motor expression but may be critical to future motor acts. Cognitive processing is influenced by emotion and draws on memory. It relies heavily on associational fibers from throughout the brain that converge on prefrontal cortical structures such as the anteromedial frontal, orbitofrontal, and cingulate areas. Delirium is the broad term used to describe disorders of this function. Drugs that affect cognitive processing include the antipsychotics, the central stimulants, most street drugs, and the sedative-hypnotics.

Autonomic processing refers to the activation of the autonomic nervous system (ANS), which has three major subsystems: the sympathetic autonomic nervous system (SANS), the parasympathetic autonomic nervous system (PANS), and the enteric nervous system (Fig. 1–6). The SANS mediates the fight-or-flight reflex associated with confrontation. Thus, increased heart rate, increased flow of blood to the muscles, increased diameter of the bronchi, and dilation of the pupils (mydriasis) are part of a coordinated response involving SANS activation. In addition to these overt actions, the SANS also mediates several important metabolic processes that regulate the availability of energy needed to perform the fight-or-flight response (Table 1–4). The PANS mediates the more vegetative aspects of life such as digestion, salivation, lacrimation, and urination. The enteric system is the plexus of nerves that innervates the digestive tract. It responds to the expansion of the digestive tract resulting from the presence of food and mediates peristalsis and the propulsion of food through the gastrointestinal tract. It is under positive and negative control by the PANS and SANS, respectively. The ANS is an involuntary system over which the individual has little control.

Autonomic function is usually described according to which subsystem is predominating; e.g., increased sympathetic or parasympathetic "tone." (The term tone is often used in reference to autonomic function since it incorporates all aspects of activity including central activation by the hypothalamus, neurotransmitter release, receptor activation, second-messenger activity, and responsiveness by the effector structures.) The ac-

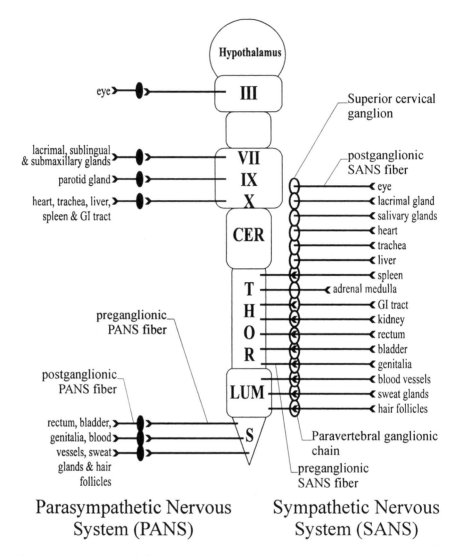

Hypothalamus

eye

III

lacrimal, sublingual
& submaxillary glands

parotid gland

VII

IX

heart, trachea, liver,
spleen & GI tract

X

CER

preganglionic
PANS fiber

T
H
O
R

postganglionic
PANS fiber

LUM

rectum, bladder,
genitalia, blood
vessels, sweat
glands & hair
follicles

S

Superior cervical
ganglion

postganglionic
SANS fiber

eye
lacrimal gland
salivary glands
heart
trachea
liver
spleen
adrenal medulla
GI tract
kidney
rectum
bladder
genitalia
blood vessels
sweat glands
hair follicles

Paravertebral ganglionic
chain

preganglionic
SANS fiber

Parasympathetic Nervous System (PANS)

Sympathetic Nervous System (SANS)

Figure 1–6. Anatomy of the autonomic nervous system (ANS). The parasympathetic autonomic nervous systems (PANS) is depicted on the left where preganglionic fibers are cranial nerves III, VII, IX, X, and the sacral (S) nerves. The sympathetic autonomic nervous system (SANS) is depicted on the right where preganglionic fibers from the thoracic (THOR) and lumbar (LUM) spinal cord synapse on the paravertebral ganglionic chain that gives off postganglionic fibers which innervate their target structures. Note that most ANS targets receive a dual innervation from both the SANS and PANS. The effects of autonomic activation are summarized in Table 1-4. Overall autonomic tone is primarily regulated by nuclear areas in the hypothalamus (CER = cervical spinal cord).

14

Table 1–4 Autonomic-mediated Effects[a]

System	Receptor	Effect
Vasculature	Alpha$_1$	**Constriction of most vascular beds**
	Beta$_2$	Relaxation of vascular smooth muscle in striated muscle and heart
	Muscarinic	Mild relaxation of vascular smooth muscle
Cardiac	Beta$_1$	Positive chronotropy and dromotropy
	Alpha$_1$	Positive inotropy
	M$_2$	**Negative ino, chrono-, and dromotropy**
Eye	Alpha$_1$	Mydriasis
	Beta$_2$	Far vision
	Muscarinic	Miosis and near vision
Stomach and intestines	Alpha$_{1 \text{ and } 2}$	Decreased smooth muscle tone and increased sphincter tone
	Beta$_2$	Decreased motility
	Muscarinic	**Increased motility and secretions with decreased sphincter tone**
Lung	Beta$_2$	Bronchodilatation and decreased secretions
	Muscarinic	**Bronchoconstriction and increased secretions**
Bladder	Alpha$_1$	Trigone and sphincter contraction
	Beta$_2$	Detrussor relaxation
	Muscarinic	**Detrussor contraction with trigone and sphincter relaxation**
Sex organs (male)	Alpha$_1$	Ejaculation
	Muscarinic	Erection
Liver	Beta$_2$	Glycogenolysis and gluconeogenesis
Salivary glands	Alpha$_1$	Minimal secretion
	Muscarinic	**Potassium and water secretion**
Lacrimal glands	Alpha	Minimal secretion
	Muscarinic	**Maximal secretion**

[a]Effects in bold depict the predominant ANS tone

tivity of an organ or organ system is generally under primary control by the SANS or PANS. Heart rate is mainly regulated by the PANS while vascular tone is mainly regulated by the SANS (Table 1–4). Moreover, the central regulation of SANS and PANS tone is not mutually exclusive; a reduction in the tone of one system usually increases activity in the other. Thus, to state that the antidepressant drug imipramine reduces sympathetic tone not only implies that it blocks activity of the SANS but also that PANS activity has increased.

The anatomy of the ANS is such that activation of the SANS produces a global response. Impulses in preganglionic fibers of the SANS increase the activity of several postganglionic fibers whose neurotransmit-

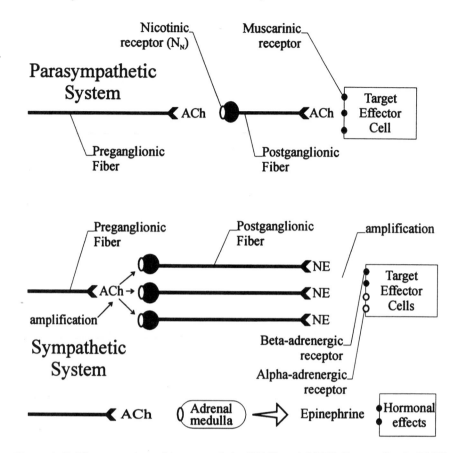

Figure 1–7. The synaptic architecture of the PANS and SANS. Preganglionic PANS fibers release ACh that acts through nicotinic type N (N_N) receptors to depolarize only a few postganglionic fibers, the action of which is mediated by ACh working through muscarinic receptors located on the target cell. The preganglionic fibers of the SANS also release ACh that acts through nicotinic type N (N_N) receptors that, in contrast to the PANS, depolarize several postganglionic fibers each of which can influence many effector cells via alpha- and beta-adrenergic receptors. The SANS system thus amplifies autonomic activity. This is especially true for SANS preganglionic activation of the adrenal medulla which, by virtue of the epinephrine released, can produce systemic alpha- and beta-adrenergic receptor effects.

ter (most often norepinephrine) diffuses across a large synaptic space to affect several effector cells (Fig. 1–7). Moreover, activity in preganglionic fibers of the SANS provokes the release of epinephrine from the adrenal gland, producing hormonal effects throughout the body. In contrast, preganglionic fibers of the PANS generally activate only a few postganglionic fibers (with the exception of the PANS regulation of the

Table 1–5 Autonomic Receptor Subtypes and Second-Messenger Systems

Receptor	Designation	Second-Messenger System
Nicotinic	N_N	Ionotropic, neuronal receptor
	N_M	Ionotropic, muscle receptor
Adrenergic	$alpha_1$	PLC alters gCa^{2+}
	$alpha_2$	G_i alters gK^+
	$beta_1$	G_s increase cAMP and alters gCa^{2+}
	$beta_2$	G_s increase cAMP and alters gCa^{2+}
	$beta_3$	G_s increase cAMP and alters gCa^{2+}
Muscarinic	M_1	PLC increases gCa^{2+} contracting smooth muscle
	M_2	G_i alters gK^+
	M_3	PLC increases gCa^{2+} contracting smooth muscle
	M_4	G_i alters gK^+
	M_5	PLC increases gCa^{2+} contracting smooth muscle

PLC = phospholipase-C, g = conductance, G_i = guanine nucleotide-binding protein (inhibitory), G_s = guanine nucleotide-binding protein (stimulatory).

enteric system); the neurotransmitter from these fibers (exclusively acetylcholine) diffuses a short distance to influence activity in only a few effector cells.

Because the ANS uses small-molecule neurotransmitters that interact with receptor families and receptor subtypes (Table 1–5), SANS tone is often described in terms of alpha- or beta-adrenergic tone while the PANS is described in terms of muscarinic tone. For instance, the autonomic effects of the antidepressant drug imipramine mentioned above reduce alpha tone. Since nicotinic (N_N) receptors mediate the effects of acetylcholine released by preganglionic fibers, drugs that act at nicotinic receptors activate or inhibit both the SANS and the PANS. Many centrally acting drugs affect the activity of the ANS by acting on either the central regulatory regions of the hypothalamus or at alpha, beta or muscarinic receptors that are responsible for carrying out ANS function. Most of the drugs discussed in this text influence autonomic function as a side effect.

The Delivery of Drugs
to the CNS

*A*lthough many drugs can alter CNS function they will only be effective if they penetrate the parenchyma of the brain and spinal cord. The controlled delivery of a drug into the CNS is therefore a major consideration of physicians and scientists. Most of the brain and all of the spinal cord are segregated from the rest of the body by the blood brain barrier (BBB). This barrier reduces the ability of many drugs to enter the brain and completely blocks the entry of others. It probably evolved to restrict access to the CNS by environmental agents that might compromise its function. Despite its presence, however, numerous environmental substances can cause infection, alter neurotransmitter levels, and even produce neuronal degeneration. Thus, the BBB is not an absolute barrier. Yet it also restricts chemicals present in the brain from entering the general circulation, where they might interfere with peripheral nervous system function. The BBB thus creates a compartment more or less separating the brain from the rest of the body. Notwithstanding the unique problems of getting drugs into this compartment, many of the basic principles of drug delivery to the body apply to the special circumstances of CNS drug delivery. A review of these principles is therefore appropriate.

LADME

Throughout my career as a pharmacologist, few mnemonic devices have helped me recall a set of principles as well as the LADME system has.

This acronym stands for *l*iberation, *a*bsorption, *d*istribution, *m*etabolism, and *e*xcretion (Fig. 2–1). When delivering a drug to any biologic system, these are the fundamental processes that influence the amount of drug that will reach the target. Although the LADME framework is most commonly used to organize thinking about drug delivery to the body, its principles apply to the movement of drugs from the body to the brain as well.

Liberation

Liberation is the release of a drug into a biologic system from its administered form. Drugs come in many forms. The same drug can be adminis-

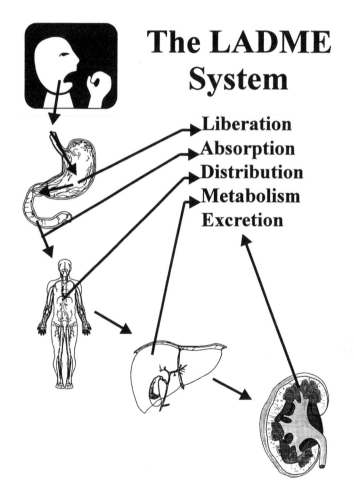

The LADME System

Liberation
Absorption
Distribution
Metabolism
Excretion

Figure 2–1. The LADME acronym stands for liberation, absorption, distribution, metabolism (biotransformation), and excretion, and it describes how most drugs are handled by the body.

tered as a pill, a liquid, a suppository, an inhaler or a sterile, buffered solution that is intravenously injected. Additional chemicals (termed excipients) are often used to facilitate the ability of the drug to exist in these various forms. The combination of a drug with its excipients is called a formulation. In many cases the excipients are simply fillers so that the pill can be made large enough to be used conveniently. In other cases, the excipients form a very complex mix of chemicals that release the drug into the system slowly. Such timed-release formulations usually are in the form of a tablet or a capsule that liberates the drug over several hours. To achieve an even longer release (up to one month), sustained-release formulations that are usually administered intramuscularly in an oil-based excipient can be used. Antipsychotic drugs can be administered in this formulation, which is also called a depot form of a drug. Even more complex methods of drug delivery have been developed such as drug pumps and other implantable devices that are especially useful in delivering proteinaceous drugs to the brain. All of these different formulations can influence the speed with which a drug is released into a biologic system.

The rate of liberation of a drug from its particular formulation can control the rate of delivery of the drug to a biologic system when the liberation rate is slower than the absorption rate of the drug. This is true of many timed-release and sustained-release formulations and can apply to some immediate-release formulations as well. For instance, the immediate-release formulation of the anticonvulsant drug phenytoin is now distributed by several companies in a generic form. Phenytoin is very insoluble in most biologic systems and generic drug producers use different excipients to enhance its solubility. When two formulations of a drug have the same degree of bioavailability (see below) and the same rate of absorption, the resulting plasma level curves will be similar and the two formulations are said to be bioequivalent. The Food and Drug Administration (FDA) sets standards for bioequivalence to reduce the incidence of problems associated with differing formulations made by generic drug producers. Although generic formulations are bioequivalent, they generally liberate phenytoin more rapidly than the phenytoin sold under the trade name of Dilantin. Thus, a patient stabilized on a particular dosage of Dilantin in New York who moves to California where a generic formulation is substituted would be expected to exhibit a different plasma level curve, which could affect the patient's seizures.

Liberation problems are especially prevalent in sustained-release formulations. For instance, children with attention deficit/hyperactivity disorder (AD/HD) may take two or three doses of immediate-release methylphenidate a day. Switching to a timed-release formulation offers greater convenience but has its own drawbacks. In the traditional immediate-release tablet formulation, methylphenidate reaches its peak plasma level in one hour. Timed-release formulations, however, can sometimes take up to four hours to release methylphenidate, thereby delaying absorption. A timed-release formulation taken at 7 A.M. therefore may not provide adequate plasma levels to help the child maintain attention during the first three or four classes that morning.

Despite their problems, timed-release and depot formulations can be very helpful. They are convenient to use and can significantly improve patient compliance. Compliance refers to whether or not patients take prescribed drugs when they are supposed to. The more times a day patients need to take drugs, the more "noncompliant" they tend to be. Psychotic patients are a notoriously noncompliant population since they often do not take their medication at all. In these patients, injecting depot formulations once a month ensures compliance.

In addition to the excipients used, several additional factors can influence the liberation of a drug. The liberation of many drugs is influenced by stomach acidity and antacids, what foods are consumed with the drug, and even which side a patient lies on after taking pills. For drugs that are released and inactivated by the low pH of the stomach, enteric-coated formulations have been developed. Drugs that increase stomach acidity and produce irritation can be formulated with buffers (as in buffered aspirin) to reduce this problem.

Absorption

Once a drug has been liberated from its administered form, it must be absorbed by the target system. Following enteral (oral) administration, the drug must move from the gastrointestinal tract into the systemic circulation that will distribute it to the body. Parenteral (other than oral) administration includes such routes as intravenous (i.v.), intramuscular (i.m.), and subcutaneous (s.c.). These routes are generally associated with faster absorption rates because of their better access to blood. Many of the same factors that determine drug liberation can also influence drug absorption. Thus, pH, the foods eaten, and the effects of other drugs can all influence absorption in much the same way that they influence liberation. But other factors such as drug concentration, the lipid solubility of the drug, the blood flow to the area, and especially the surface area over which a drug is absorbed also have an impact on the absorption rate. For instance, smoking cocaine, which involves the enormous surface area of the lungs, has dramatically changed the abuse patterns that were formerly associated with insufflation ("snorting") in which a small surface area absorbed the drug. The higher peak levels of cocaine achieved with inhalation are associated with greater euphoria and a significantly increased incidence of side effects and drug dependence.

In general, most enterally administered drugs are absorbed from the duodenum, primarily because of the enormous surface area of the villi located there. Thus, the time it takes a drug to move from the stomach to the duodenum can affect the absorption rate. A full stomach that stimulates gastric motility may speed transit time through the duodenum so that less of the drug enters the circulation and more is passed out in the feces. Opioids and antimuscarinic agents can slow gastrointestinal (GI) transit time and thereby delay absorption. In contrast, drugs that enhance transit time and increase the absorption rate are called prokinetic agents. Drugs such as metoclopramide are often used for this purpose in the management of migraine headache, which causes G.I. stasis.

The term used to describe the quantity of a drug that reaches the circulation is bioavailability, and it is defined as the percentage of the administered dose that reaches the circulation. Drugs administered intravenously are 100% bioavailable whereas the bioavailability of drugs administered by any other route is generally less than 100%. With enteral administration, the bioavailability of many drugs varies considerably between subjects and, within the same subject, can also change from day to day.

In order for a drug to be absorbed and reach the nervous system, it must cross membranes even if administered intravascularly. Drugs can cross membranes in three different ways: passive diffusion, facilitated diffusion, or active transport. Most drugs are absorbed via passive diffusion. Passive diffusion, "bulk diffusion," or simply "diffusion" refers to the movement of a drug down its concentration gradient into an area of lesser concentration. The rate of diffusion in an aqueous solution depends exclusively upon this concentration gradient. In the body, however, a drug has to move across a membrane to enter the blood or brain and the diffusion rate then depends not only on the concentration gradient but also on the drug's lipid solubility. Since membranes are primarily lipid structures, a lipid-soluble drug can move into the membrane and its achieved concentration there will be greater than in the cytoplasm of the cell. A diffusion gradient from the membrane itself into the cytoplasm is thus established and a percentage of the drug will then diffuse from the membrane into the cell. Even in the presence of a steep concentration gradient, a drug that cannot penetrate a membrane will not be absorbed. In contrast, drugs that are extremely lipid-soluble may not enter the aqueous phase of the blood or may dissolve so extensively in a membrane that they do not achieve effective concentrations at their sites of action. The lipid solubility of a drug depends on its physical characteristics and is generally determined by that proportion of the drug that dissolves in oil relative to water (this ratio is called the oil : water partition coefficient and is a physical characteristic of a drug).

Blood flow can have a strong impact on concentration gradients. Most anesthetics are moderately lipid soluble and can be absorbed more quickly from the lung compartment if the rate of pulmonary blood perfusion is increased. With increased blood flow, blood that has already absorbed the anesthetic is circulated away from the lungs, bringing in fresh blood. This newly circulated blood has no anesthetic in it so the concentration gradient for the anesthetic to diffuse across the membranes of the lung and into the blood remains steep. The absorption rate is therefore very high. As the concentration of the anesthetic in blood increases, however, blood circulated into the lungs will already have anesthetic in it, the concentration gradient will decline, and the absorption rate will decrease.

Drugs that cannot be absorbed passively need a transport protein to carry them across the membrane. This form of diffusion is called carrier-mediated transport. If carrier-mediated transport involves the direct input of energy (generally in the form of ATP adenosine triphosphate–), it is called active transport. If an energy gradient is set up by an electrical difference across a membrane and the transport protein utilizes this potential energy, (*i.e.*, the energy utilized is indirect as in Na^+ or H^+ moving down their concentration gradients), the method of transport is called facilitated diffusion. Active transport can move drugs up a concentration gradient, although no centrally acting drug I am aware of has this mode of absorption. Active transport does, however, remove certain antibiotics from the cerebrospinal fluid. Facilitated diffusion, on the other hand, involves a carrier protein but cannot move a drug against a concentration gradient. Glucose is usually transported by facilitated diffusion and thus requires an ionic gradient to facilitate its carrier-mediated transport. It is important to recognize that a facilitated diffusion pump is a "shuttle protein" since it can move a substrate into or out of a cell depending on the concentration gradient and the distribution of ions. As we will see, this ability of a shuttle protein to move a drug in both directions is responsible, at least in part, for amphetamine's release of DA and NE from nerve terminals.

Many drugs are formulated in the so-called salt form. A salt of a drug is usually made by substituting a more aqueous ion such as hydrobromide or sulfate for hydrogen ion. Formulating a drug in a salt form increases its aqueous solubility, thereby facilitating its ability to dissolve in gastrointestinal fluids or blood. Once in an aqueous medium, the salt dissociates from the drug and is replaced, generally by H^+. Depending on the salt used, errors in a delivered dose can occur. The sulfate used to facilitate the aqueous solubility of amphetamine sulfate comprises 42% of the drug's formula weight (*i.e.*, 230). Administering 10 mg of amphetamine sulfate will therefore deliver only 5.8 mg of amphetamine to the system (a 42% error) because the molecular weight of amphetamine is only 134.

Once a drug is in solution, the question is, How much of it is actually in a diffusible form? The hydrogen ion concentration (pH) of the medium carrying a drug has a significant effect on the proportion of the drug present in its lipid-soluble and therefore diffusible form. A high concentration of H^+ ions in the medium can "force" positive charges onto certain molecules. In the case of a drug that is a weak base (a proton acceptor in aqueous solutions), the addition of an H^+ ion to the molecule renders the molecule positively charged, hydrophilic, and therefore less lipid soluble. In the case of a drug that is a weak acid (a proton donator in aqueous solutions), the addition of an H^+ ion renders the molecule electrically neutral, lipophilic, and more lipid soluble. The pH of the medium carrying the drug thus will influence the percentage of the drug present in its ionized (nondiffusible) and un-ionized (diffusible) form. Consider the following formula:

$$pH - pKa = \log ([ionized]/[un\text{-}ionized])$$

This is called the Henderson-Hassalbalch equation and it describes the proportion of an acidic drug that is in its soluble form at any given pH (my graduate students remember the right side of the equation as I over U or I.O.U. which stands for *[I]/[u]*). In the case of a weak acid, once the drug has detached from its salt, the solubilized drug will separate into two forms in solution:

$$AH = A^- + H^+$$

This H^+ ion donor, or weak acid, can only pass through membranes in its non-ionized or AH form. The drug in its ionized form (A^-) is unable to cross the membrane unless it is pumped. The propensity to yield an H^+ ion in solution is a physical characteristic and therefore a constant for that particular drug. This constant is termed the pKa. Suppose a weakly acidic drug has a pKa of 4.4. Using the Henderson-Hassalbalch equation, we see the following degree of dissociation at physiologic pH (*i.e.*, 7.4):

$$pH - pKa = \log(I/u)$$
$$7.4 - 4.4 = \log(I/u)$$
$$3 = \log(I/u)$$

Since we are working in log units, the ratio of the ionized to the unionized form of the drug is the antilog of 3 or 1,000. Thus, for every molecule of the drug that is in the un-ionized and diffusible form, there are 1,000 parts of the nondiffusible drug in the ionic form ($I/u = 1,000/1 =$

1,000 which is the antilog of 3). Because of the pH, there is very little diffusible drug. This effectively decreases the concentration gradient since only the un-ionized form can diffuse, resulting in a slow rate of absorption. However, in the acidic environment of the stomach where the pH is around 1.4, the equation yields -3 (*i.e.,* 1.4 $-4.4 = -3$), the antilog of which is 1/1,000. In the stomach, therefore, for every one part ionized drug, there will be 1,000 parts unionized drug. Since most of the drug in the stomach is in a diffusible form, the concentration gradient between the stomach and the blood is very high and the absorption rate is therefore rapid. If the stomach had a large surface area, a weak acid would be readily absorbed from the stomach. Regardless of the amount of drug available for absorption, however, surface area is extremely important, and even weak acids are predominantly absorbed in the duodenum, even though the pH significantly reduces the proportion of the drug in the AH or diffusible form.

As straightforward as the Henderson-Hassalbalch equation is, students still get confused because weak bases respond oppositely. Remember that weak bases are proton acceptors, and thus:

$$BH^+ = B + H^+$$

This equation would be applicable to the use of cocaine which is often sold as "crack" on the streets in the free-base (B) form (that portion of a weak base that is not ionized). In contrast to a weak acid, which must be hydrogenated to be diffusible, it is the free-base form of a weak base that is lipid soluble and therefore diffusible. Since the dissolution is opposite, the Henderson-Hassalbalch equation must be reversed. The Henderson-Hassalbalch equation for a weak base is:

$$pH - pKa = \log([un\text{-}ionized]/[ionized])$$

If the acid is I.O.U. (*I/u*), then the weak base is U.O.I., or un-ionized/ionized. Using the weak base phencyclidine (pKa = 9.4) in blood (pH 7.4) as an example, the result is $7.4 - 9.4 = -2$ or 1/100. In the stomach, where the pH is 1.4, the equation is $1.4 - 9.4 = -8$, which equals 1/100,000,000. Now apply these results to U.O.I. and you should be able to see that in blood, 1% of phencyclidine is in the free-base, diffusible form while in the stomach the vast majority is in the ionized, nondiffusible form.

The impact that pH has on diffusion is especially relevant to understanding the actions of some drugs, especially when there are highly disparate hydrogen ion concentrations on either side of a membrane. Using the example of the blood and the stomach again, certain situations arise in which a drug can diffuse into the stomach and, because of its low pH, become trapped there since the drug is converted predominantly into a nondiffusible, ionized form. When a substance that can become ionized gets trapped because of pH differences, the process is called ion trapping. The cyclic coma associated with phencyclidine (PCP) overdose illustrates this principle (see Fig. 2–2).

PCP is a widely abused street drug that is a weak base (pKa = 9.4). It is readily absorbed following enteral administration although it can also be burned in a pipe and inhaled into the lungs (pyrolysis). Once absorbed into the circulation, it can produce a coma as part of its toxic profile. In many cases the coma is not continuous, but rather cyclical. As a weak base, PCP is mostly in the ionized form (u/I = 1/100,000,000) in the stomach and is absorbed mainly in the duodenum. Once in the blood, where a much higher percentage of the drug exists in the free-base form (u/I = 1/100), the free base can diffuse across lipid barriers. When it circulates past the

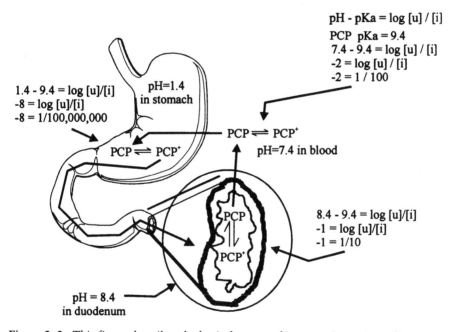

Figure 2–2. This figure describes the basic features of ion trapping as it applies to enterogastric recirculation of phencyclidine (PCP). Since PCP is a weak base with a pKa of 9.4, it exists in a 1/100 ratio of un-ionized (*u*) to ionized (*i*) in the blood. Once the un-ionized portion enters the extremely acidic environment of the stomach, the Henderson-Hassalbach equation results in a *[u]/[i]* ratio of 1 : 100,000,000 effectively trapping the ionized drug in the stomach—thus, ion trapping. When the drug eventually reaches the duodenum, a much larger percentage of the drug is in the un-ionized and therefore diffusible form, and it can then enter the portal circulation readily. This pattern of ion trapping in the stomach and diffusion back into the circulation is called enterogastric recirculation.

stomach, some PCP will diffuse out of the blood and into the acidic environment of the stomach. When it does, the acidic environment of the stomach converts most of the free base into the ionized form. Since the ionized form cannot cross membranes, ionized PCP becomes trapped in the stomach. In fact, the stomach becomes a "sink" for circulating PCP through ion trapping. In a sense the stomach draws PCP from the circulation, thereby reducing the plasma concentration. As the plasma concentration decreases, PCP is drawn out of the brain and the patient comes out of the coma. When the PCP eventually reenters the duodenum, much of the ionized PCP is converted to the free-base form and is again absorbed, raising plasma concentration. Drug levels in the brain rise and the patient again becomes comatose. This cycle continues to repeat itself until the overall body burden of PCP is reduced by biotransformation or excretion. This pattern of absorption and distribution into the stomach followed by reabsorption is referred to as enterogastric recirculation. In later chapters you will see that ion trapping is also pivotal to the actions of amphetamine and local anesthetics.

Distribution

The term distribution refers to the circulation of a drug to its target sites within a biological system. As one would assume, distribution is greatly influenced by blood flow and by diffusion of the drug out of the blood into its target system. The term generally used to describe the distribution of a drug is the apparent volume of distribution (Vd). The volume of distribution is the amount of drug that leaves the circulation and enters the organs. Its units are liters. A drug that has a Vd of three liters has been distributed to three liters of body fluid. Since three liters is approximately the volume of plasma in the circulation and we know that the drug first enters blood because Vd is usually determined following intravenous administration, we assume that a Vd of three describes a drug that does not leave the blood very readily. Drugs that distribute in total body water have a Vd of about 42 liters. An example is lithium, which is used in the treatment of manic-depression. Drugs that are more lipid soluble, such as diazepam, can have Vds in the thousands. Obviously, we do not have 1,000 liters of body fluid. A Vd in the thousands means that the drug concentration in blood, on which Vd is based, is very low because most of it has left the blood and entered other compartments of the body such as fat or brain.

The distribution of drugs, especially when they are reasonably lipid soluble, occurs in phases. Diazepam (Valium), for instance, first enters brain because of preferential blood flow to the brain (see below). The plasma concentration drops rapidly as the drug enters the brain. This is the first phase. Because diazepam is also soluble in muscle, circulation to muscle eventually delivers diazepam to this tissue, reducing the concentration in the blood. This reduced blood concentration effectively reverses the gradient from blood to brain so that diazepam leaves the brain, representing a second phase of distribution. A third phase takes place when diazepam leaves blood to enter fat. Since diazepam is a moderately lipid-soluble drug, most of the drug will eventually end up in fat. Acting as a long-term reservoir for moderately lipophilic drugs, fat allows the slow leaching out of drugs into the general circulation, where they can continue to influence brain function much longer than one might anticipate. This phenomenon contributes to the so-called drug hangover, in which low levels of sedative-hypnotic drugs remain in the circulation the next day, leaving the patient lethargic. The fact that diazepam entered the brain in its first phase and then left the brain during the second phase is responsible for its short duration of effect in the brain. This process of leaving one target site and entering another based on preferential blood flow and lipid solubility is referred to as redistribution. As we will see, the duration of action of many drugs that affect the CNS is reduced by redistribution. In general, it can be assumed that the more lipid soluble a drug is, the more likely it is to be redistributed because the potential reservoir for a drug in the body's fat store increases as lipid solubility increases.

Metabolism (Biotransformation)

The *M* in LADME stands for metabolism. Drug metabolism is usually regarded as the breakdown of drugs. Yet the term metabolism commonly refers to both the breakdown (catabolism) and the synthesis (anabolism) of chemicals. In addition, it is often used to describe the production of energy by the body. Because of this potential for confusion, biotransformation is a more appropriate term used to describe the breakdown of drugs. Even this term can be somewhat confusing since it is also appropriately used to describe the conversion of a prodrug to its active form. A prodrug is a substance that is administered in an inactive form requiring biotransformation by the body to produce the active form.

Most drugs are biotransformed and thus rendered less active by specialized enzymes associated with the endoplasmic reticulum of the liver. Because these enzymes can be isolated using differential centrifugation and are found in the microsomal fraction (that portion of a tissue pellet resulting from centrifugation of a homogenate of the liver that contains formed vesicles termed microsomes), the biotransformation system of the liver is often referred to as the microsomal system (it can also be called the mixed-function enzymatic oxidative system (MEOS) or the P-450 system because of its requirement for cytochrome P-450). Although the liver is primarily responsible for biotransformation, enzyme systems found in blood, kidneys, and lungs as well as other tissues also contribute to this process.

It is generally assumed that the microsomal system evolved to biotransform environmental substances that could be potentially harmful to the body. Animals with this capability would be less likely to fall prey to environmental toxins. Several isoforms of the biotransforming enzymes exist. (The term isoform is used here to describe enzymes that are structurally similar but functionally different.) The various oxidative enzymes are part of a large gene family that evolved through mutations from a single original protein (Nebert and Gonzalez, 1987). Isoforms of the oxidative enzymes may have varying capacities to biotransform certain drugs and, since they are genetically inherited, genetic differences in biotransformation exist. This genetic polymorphism of biotransforming enzymes enables some individuals, for instance, to consume more alcohol than can others without getting drunk. Pharmacogenetics is the study of the genetic variability in the way the body interacts with drugs and genetic variation in biotransforming enzymes is an important part of this variability.

Like distribution, biotransformation also can occur in phases. Phase I reactions involve oxidation, hydrolysis, and reduction of the parent structure. The resulting polar metabolite can then be eliminated from the body in urine or conjugated with glucuronide, sulfate, acetate, or an amino acid. These conjugation reactions are referred to as phase II reactions. Converting the parent drugs to polar metabolites or conjugating them generally, but not always, inactivates the drugs and makes them more water soluble and therefore easier to excrete.

Usually, there are many more molecules of converting enzymes than there are molecules of drug to biotransform. In this situation, the biotransformation rate depends on the quantity of the drug in the plasma and is said to be first order. As is true of any enzyme system, however, the number of drug molecules can greatly exceed the number of enzymes, and saturation of the converting enzymes will then occur. Under saturation, or zero-order conditions, the biotransformation rate is fixed and dependent upon the concentration of enzymes. The biotransformation rate of a drug is often first order at one concentration and zero order at a higher concentration. A classic example is alcohol. Normally, alcohol is biotransformed by the enzyme alcohol dehydrogenase. If one drink is consumed, there are more molecules of alcohol dehydrogenase than of alcohol and the biotransformation rate is first order. The alcohol concentration in the blood will drop very rapidly because the enzyme is not saturated. However, if two or three or more drinks are consumed in a short period of time so that the number of molecules of alcohol in the blood exceeds the number of molecules of alcohol dehydrogenase, the biotransformation rate will shift to zero order. Under zero-order kinetics, the next drink consumed will enter the blood and, because of saturation of alcohol dehydrogenase, it will raise the blood alcohol level dramatically, leading to intoxication. Thus, getting drunk depends not so much on how much alcohol is consumed as on the rate at which it is consumed.

The bioavailability of many drugs is reduced by biotransformation that occurs in transit from the gastrointestinal tract to the general circulation. Once a drug is liberated, it can be catabolized by enzymes in the gastrointestinal tract as well as by biotransformation in the liver after it is absorbed into the portal circulation. Enzymes in the gastric mucosa and especially in the liver can dramatically reduce the amount of drug made available to the rest of the body. The reduction in bioavailability that occurs as a result of biotransformation in the G.I. tract and liver is called the first-pass effect or first-pass metabolism. A significant reduction in the bioavailability of a drug can therefore take place during the drug's initial ("first") passage into the system. Some degree of first-pass metabolism is unavoidable following enteral administration. However, other routes of administration can be chosen to circumvent the first-pass effect by delivering the drug to a location from which it is not immediately absorbed into the portal circulation. These sites would include intravenous (i.v.), intramuscular (i.m.), and subcutaneous (s.c.) routes as well as rectal and sublingual administration. Using these alternative routes of administration does not prevent biotransformation since all blood eventually reaches the liver, but avoiding the first-pass effect does allow a higher plasma level to be achieved. Since the peak plasma levels that are achieved by an administered dose can have a profound effect on the efficacy of a drug, avoiding first-pass metabolism can be important in delivering a higher dose of drug to the brain.

The capacity of the biotransformation system can be changed. The most common change observed is induction (an increase in the number of enzymes available for biotransformation). Chronic treatment with drugs such as phenobarbital or phenytoin and long-term exposure to environmental toxins and the tars found in cigarettes can increase, or induce, the synthesis of the biotransformation enzymes. An induction can be so profound that the overall size and weight of the liver can increase. In general, it is assumed that the biotransformation rate of the average healthy human can increase approximately two- to threefold. In contrast, certain drugs can inhibit the biotransformation rate. The classic examples are cimetidine or alcohol. Liver disease can also reduce the biotransformation rate and thereby increase the plasma concentrations of some drugs.

Drugs that are biotransformed and subsequently conjugated (especially glucuronides) can be secreted by the liver into bile. When bile enters the digestive environment of the gastrointestinal tract, conjugated drugs can be catabolized back to the parent compound, which can be re-absorbed by the intestines. Once reabsorbed, the drug is again free to produce its desired effects, thus extending its duration of action. This phenomenon is termed enterohepatic recirculation. Diazepam is one ex-ample of a drug that undergoes enterohepatic recirculation.

Excretion

Excretion refers to the elimination of a drug from the body. The major organ of excretion is the kidney but the bowel, sweat glands, saliva, skin, and lungs can also participate. With the exception of the lung, excretion involves an aqueous medium and the associated requirement for aqueous solubility. Although excretion of the unchanged parent drugs does occur, especially when they are water soluble, more efficient excretion is gener-ally achieved by enhancing their aqueous solubility through biotransfor-mation. The excretion of drugs and their metabolites involves both pas-sive and active processes. Drugs conjugated with glucuronide are actively excreted in the kidneys by the pumps that normally excrete uric acid. Other drugs are simply excreted passively in the urine since the majority of the biotransformed drugs are in a polar form and cannot be reab-sorbed by the distal tubules of the kidneys. The fact that a drug is usually metabolized to a more polar form does not, however, mean that it will not have a less polar and therefore diffusible form. Based on the Hender-son-Hassalbalch equation, a lipid-soluble and therefore diffusible per-centage of a drug will always exist unless it is an ion such as lithium. The excretion rates of a drug can therefore be influenced by the pH of the urine. Acidifying the urine by administering ammonium chloride intra-venously reduces urinary pH and allows a considerably higher percentage of a weak-base drug to exist in the ionized and therefore excretable form. Acidifying the urine can increase the excretion rate of amphetamine for instance and, in some cases, shorten the duration of a toxic overdose episode. Treating an overdose victim with sodium bicarbonate to alkalin-ize the urine enhances the excretion rate of weak acids such as aspirin.

Drug Half-life

The half-life of a drug $(t_{1/2})$ is the amount of time it takes for the plasma level to decrease by 50%. A drug's half-life is influenced by several fac-tors, the most important of which are biotransformation and excretion. Under first-order kinetics the plasma half-life will be independent of plasma concentration. Thus, if there are 1,000 ng/ml of a drug with a half-life of four hours in the plasma, after four hours the plasma concentrations will be 500 ng/ml. In contrast, if this drug is saturating the bio-transformation system, it may take 12 hours to reduce a plasma level of 1,000 ng/ml to 500 ng/ml. The saturation of the biotransformation enzymes (zero-order kinetics) therefore changes the half-life. Once the plasma level falls below saturation and first-order kinetics are reinstated, it will only take four hours to halve the plasma level. As would be expected, the conversion from first-order to zero-order kinetics can have a significant impact on the efficacy and toxicity of a drug.

Plasma Binding

Drug being distributed to the body often binds to plasma proteins such as albumin. The consequence is a reduced quantity of drug available for diffusion across a membrane. Obviously, drug bound to large plasma proteins is not available to enter the brain. Only unbound, un-ionized drug will cross into the brain. Plasma protein binding, by reducing the percentage of drug in its soluble, diffusible form, influences concentration gradients and hence the diffusion of a drug into brain. A plasma blood level can be measured at 100 ng/ml, but only 10% of that drug is available for diffusion if 90% of the drug is bound to plasma albumin. Moreover, depending upon the pKa of the drug, only a certain portion of the 10% of the unbound drug is in a diffusible form. Plasma binding thus can significantly influence the efficacy of an administered drug. On the other hand, drug that is bound to plasma proteins cannot be biotransformed or excreted, which tends to increase its duration of action.

Drug that is bound to plasma proteins is in equilibrium with the unbound, soluble pool in blood (Fig. 2–3). Since the ratio of bound to unbound drug is fixed by the physical properties of the drug (its affinity for plasma protein), drug bound to plasma proteins can act as a reservoir of drug available for diffusion. As diffusible drug leaves the circulation and enters the brain, the unbound concentration will be reduced and then replaced by drug from the bound pool.

Drugs that readily bind to plasma proteins can present problems when several drugs are being taken by a patient. The anticonvulsant agent phenytoin is highly protein bound (more than 90%). Aspirin can displace a portion of the phenytoin from its plasma binding sites because aspirin has a higher affinity for these binding sites. Phenytoin is displaced from its binding sites by aspirin and its unbound concentration increases rapidly. In most cases, this will result in increased biotransformation and excretion that will rapidly attenuate the increased concentration of unbound phenytoin. If the patient is bordering on toxicity, however, the increase in unbound plasma concentration of phenytoin brought about by aspirin co-administration, even if it is transient, can have deleterious ef-

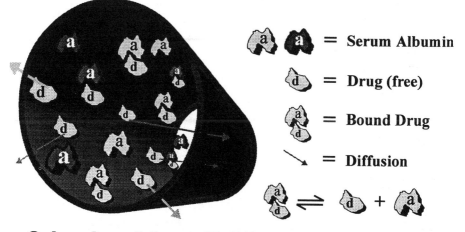

Only unbound drug will diffuse from blood vessels.

Figure 2–3. Plasma contains several types of proteins that can bind drugs (d). In this figure, serum albumin (a) is used as an example. Drug molecules bound to plasma proteins are not free to diffuse from the vascular compartment and are thus sequestered from their sites of actions. This bound pool of drug can, however, act as a reservoir for drug molecules, effectively preventing their biotransformation and excretion, which thereby extends the half-life of the drug in the body.

fects. Moreover, since the biotransformation of phenytoin is generally zero order at therapeutic dosages, the increase in unbound drug will have an even more profound effect since the biotransforming enzymes are already saturated, leaving only excretion to reduce the displaced quantity of unbound drug.

SYSTEMIC DELIVERY WITH CENTRAL ACTION

The underlying assumption in most of the preceding discussion has been that this is a one-compartment model: A drug enters the circulation (or compartment) and moves unimpeded to a target site. In such a model, the rate constants for absorption, distribution, metabolism, and excretion that describe the movement of drug into the target structure from the blood are basically similar to the rate constants that characterize the drug in blood. However, the factors that influence the diffusion of drug out of the circulation and into an organ such as the heart can be very different from those that affect diffusion into the brain because of the presence of the BBB. The way a drug is handled in the "brain compartment" can be dramatically different from that observed in the peripheral circulation. Thus, a two-compartment model is needed to explain the kinetics of a drug working on the brain: one set of rate constants for the blood and another for the brain. This is not to say that the two separate compartments are not in equilibrium with one another, because they are. Rather, the kinetics differ because, compared to blood, the brain is characterized by reduced extracellular space, increased numbers of uptake sites, and in some cases different biotransforming enzymes. Therefore, although many of the factors discussed above apply to the delivery of drugs to the brain, several additional factors are unique to the environment of the brain, the most important being the BBB.

The Blood Brain Barrier

The vascular epithelial cells that form the capillary walls in the brain are connected by tight junctions. These cells also secrete an additional layer of lipid called a basement membrane (Fig. 2–4). This architecture is strikingly different from that of most other perivascular tissues in the body where the cells are connected by gap junctions. As the name implies, gap junctions allow large bulky molecules to pass through the gaps between the cells. In contrast, tight junctions and the basement membrane "force" molecules to diffuse through the membrane matrix. This cytoarchitecture is not the only factor that contributes to the BBB. Glial cells form astrocytic feet on the vasculature that further restrict the passage of materials into the brain. Tight junctions, a basement membrane, and astrocytic feet ensheathe the vasculature and force drugs to diffuse across membranes, thereby presenting a barrier to the diffusion of polar compounds. The BBB should not be viewed as an absolute barrier, however, since extremely high doses of water-soluble drugs can cross into the brain compartment. Rather, it should be considered a significant impediment to the entry of water-soluble drugs. Because of the BBB, the diffusion of a drug into the brain is, in general, inversely proportional to its water solubility. In addition, certain enzymes are found in the perivascular tissues of the brain. Drugs such as levodopa that enter the brain are immediately biotransformed by these enzymes, thereby reducing the amount of drug entering. Such enzymatic barriers should also be considered a part of the BBB.

The BBB can be opened by administering the osmotic diuretic mannitol. The osmotic pressure induced by mannitol is thought to dehydrate the perivascular tissues comprising the BBB, causing tight junctions to separate and leak. Mannitol might be delivered before a chemotherapeutic agent to facilitate the entry of an anticancer agent that would not otherwise penetrate the barrier. Alterations in the integrity of the BBB can accompany high doses of ethanol and can also occur in certain forms of meningitis. A lack of tight-junction patency due to incomplete develop-

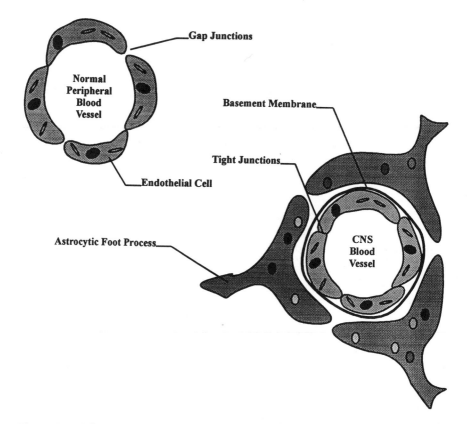

Figure 2–4. The various components of the blood brain barrier (BBB) are depicted. Note that brain blood vessels have endothelial cells with tight junctions, are surrounded by a basement membrane, and are apposed by foot processes from astrocytes. Together, these components severely restrict the diffusion of drug into the brain compartment.

ment contributes to the increased potency and toxicity of certain drugs in neonates while in some elderly patients tight junction patency is reduced by the aging process.

Like glucose, many drugs gain entry into the CNS via carrier-mediated transport (facilitated diffusion). Unlike the facilitated diffusion of glucose in the periphery, however, the transport of glucose across the BBB does not require the presence of insulin. The brain, like muscle and the liver, is insulin-independent. (The facilitated diffusion pump protein does not require activation by insulin.) Since nerves have a very limited capacity to store glucose as glycogen, the brain uses glucose as its primary energy source, and metabolic need draws glucose from the blood into the CNS on an "on-demand" basis. Thus, hypoglycemia reduces available glucose, leading to unconsciousness. Insulin-induced hypoglycemia can also occur when an overdose of insulin leads to reduced vascular glucose and subsequent unconsciousness. (This procedure was used in the past by psychiatrists in a misguided attempt to treat schizophrenia and depression.) Drugs that utilize facilitated diffusion to cross the BBB will have to compete with other chemicals that normally use the same transport protein. Drugs such as levodopa, which are transported by the large neutral amino acid pump, will have to compete with other large neutral amino acids such as tryptophan. Indeed, high protein meals rich in large neutral amino acids will reduce the amount of levodopa that enters the brain.

Although the BBB prevents the access of many drugs to the CNS, it can also be used to advantage in certain therapeutic maneuvers because of its very ability to restrict entry. The treatment of diarrhea with diphenoxylate is based on such a strategy. Diphenoxylate is a morphine-like compound that does not readily enter the CNS because its low lipid solubility reduces its diffusion across the BBB. It therefore induces an antidiarrheal effect in the periphery without the CNS effects, notably respiratory depression and dependency, that would attend the use of this drug if it penetrated the BBB readily.

Other Barriers to Drug Diffusion

Once a drug gets past the BBB, it meets additional barriers to effective diffusion. These further impediments to drug action include myelin sheaths, densely packed glial cells, reuptake sites, catabolic enzymes, and little extracellular space. Indeed, the brain has the least extracellular space of any organ in the body. This small extracellular volume does not readily lend itself to diffusion. In addition, since many agents that influence neurotransmitter systems exert their effects on catabolic, anabolic, or termination mechanisms in these systems, diffusion distances become limited by the incorporation of drugs into these processes. For example, levodopa is converted to DA to produce its antiparkinson effect. Once levodopa enters the brain, it is converted to DA which in turn is catabolized by monoamine oxidase B (MAO-B) or catechol-O-methyltransferase (COMT) or it can be taken up by DA reuptake pumps. These processes remove DA from the extracellular space, thereby reducing its diffusion. As a result, the diffusion distance of levodopa converted to DA is extremely limited (about 1.5 mm, Kroin et al., 1991). The net effect of these combined actions is reduced diffusion and a need to increase the delivered dose to attain a concentration gradient that is sufficient to reach all brain target tissues.

The BBB can also influence the elimination of a drug from the brain. Once a drug finally reaches its site of action in the CNS, it can be catabolized (generally to a more water-soluble form). Such catabolic products will not cross the BBB and therefore must exit the brain at a different site—the cerebrospinal fluid (CSF). The extracellular space of the brain is separated from the CSF by the so-called brain CSF barrier. This barrier is composed of a layer of ependymal cells connected by gap junctions. It is a leaky barrier and polar substances readily pass through it. Since CSF is being continuously made (total volume of 150 ml every three to four hours), there is generally a net diffusion gradient across this barrier and a net flux out of brain and into CSF. CSF eventually diffuses across the arachnoid granulations in the superior sagittal sinus (and other locations), carrying drugs with it into the general circulation. On the other hand, drugs that are not metabolized can also leave the brain by the same route as they entered: diffusion back across the BBB.

The Choroid Plexus and its Effects on Drug Kinetics

The choroid plexus of the brain is responsible for making CSF and can also act as a portal of entry into the CNS for some drugs. It produces an ultrafiltrate of the blood in much the same way as the kidney produces urine. Choroid epithelial cells form tight junctions with one another, impeding the passage of most substances into the CSF. The basolateral surface of the choroid plexus is in contact with the vasculature and is leaky (gap junctions are present; Fig. 2–5). The apical surface, adjacent to the ventricles of the brain, forms villi that actively transport Na^+ into the ventricle. Chloride and obligatory water (water that moves to maintain osmotic pressure) follow the Na^+ into the CSF. The apical surface also has facilitated diffusion pumps that carry certain trace nutrients into the brain such as vitamin C, folate, B_6, deoxyribonucleosides, and small amounts of glucose and thiamine. The choroid plexus thus seems responsible for supplying certain trace nutrients to the brain.

The choroid plexus is not only the site of entry of vitamins and other trace nutrients: It is also a housekeeper that can remove certain substances from the brain. Systemically administered antibiotics such as penicillin and cephalosporin enter the brain but are actively and rapidly pumped out of the CSF by the choroid plexus. (Apparently the structures of some antibiotics are such that they bind to a transport protein whose normal function is currently unknown.) This has significant implications for treating CNS infections. For example, the inflammation caused by bacterial meningitis produces a leaky BBB and choroid plexus. As a result, when penicillin is given for these infections it enters the CNS readily and levels decrease dramatically (2,000%). However, as the inflammation is reduced by penicillin's antibacterial action, the BBB returns to normal, penicillin enters the CNS less readily, and it is pumped out by the choroid plexus. The result is reduced penicillin levels in the CNS leading to enhanced bacterial growth and a potential recurrence of symptoms.

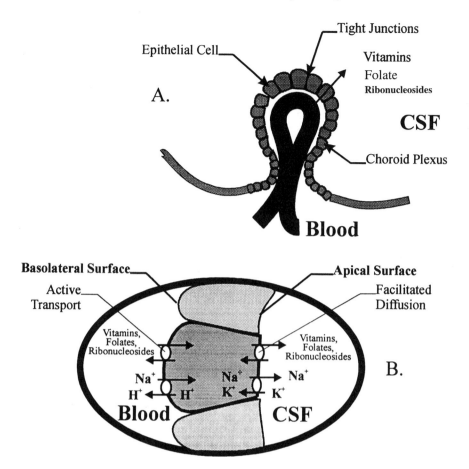

Figure 2–5. The choroid plexus is the site in the brain where cerebrospinal fluid (CSF) is produced. In A the configuration of the plexus relative to the vasculature is depicted where tight junctions restrict the bulk flow of fluids between the blood and the ventricular system. In B one of the cells is depicted where active transport moves Na^+ from the blood into the CSF in exchange for K^+ and H^+ with water following the Na^+ to maintain osmotic pressure. In this way, fluid moves from the blood and into the brain. Certain vitamins, folic acids, and ribonucleosides have affinity for transport proteins and can gain access to the brain compartment at this site.

This cycle of enhanced entry and removal is avoided by administering antibiotics such as ceftriaxone that are not substrates for the pumps in the choroid plexus (Spector and Johanson, 1989).

Brain Regions Not Protected by the BBB

Not all regions of the brain are guarded by the BBB. Apparently, some brain structures require unhindered access to blood to fulfill their functional requirements. One of the more notable unprotected areas is the chemoreceptor trigger zone (CTZ), or area postrema, which acts as the vomiting center of the brain. The CTZ lies in the floor of the fourth ventricle and is considered part of the periventricular organ (a group of brain nuclei lining the ventricles of the brain, many of which are not protected by the BBB). Exposed to vasculature unguarded by the BBB, the CTZ can react quickly to agents that have just entered the blood from the gut so that the stomach contents can be expelled before more absorption takes place. The CTZ is known to possess dopaminergic and serotonergic receptors. The dopaminergic drug apomorphine can be used effectively to induce emesis. Syrup of ipecac has the same property. Its active ingredient (emetine) is an alkaloid obtained from ipecac (Brazil roots), and many alkaloid compounds have dopaminergic properties. On the other hand, metoclopramide, a DA antagonist and ondansetron, a serotonin (5HT) antagonist, block receptors on the CTZ and are often effective in reducing vomiting caused by cancer chemotherapeutic agents. Among other regions of the CNS not protected by the BBB is the hypothalamus, which must sense alterations in peripheral proteins in its role of regulating the pituitary/body feedback axis.

How can the chemical integrity of the brain be maintained if several of its regions are not protected by the BBB? Recall that even after molecules cross the BBB, diffusion distances are severely limited. Thus, although molecules in the blood can gain easy access to these unprotected areas of the brain, they will not readily diffuse into adjacent brain regions because of the severe limitations to diffusion.

We tend to think that centrally acting drugs produce their effects exclusively because of their entry into the CNS. However, systemically administered agents produce peripheral actions carried into the CNS by afferent pathways. By acting on afferent sensory systems, drugs that do not readily cross the BBB can still produce CNS effects. A good example involves the neuropeptide cholecystokinin (CCK). This "gut" peptide reduces feeding behavior when administered peripherally. It was originally thought that CCK inhibited the feeding center in the hypothalamus by direct entry into brain areas not protected by the BBB. Later studies showed, however, that if the vagus nerve were cut and CCK was administered, feeding behavior would not be suppressed. It has now been shown that terminal sensory fibers of the X cranial nerve (the vagus) possess CCK receptors. Once the receptors are activated by CCK released by the gut, the sensory signal is conveyed back to the hypothalamus where it stimulates the nuclear areas mediating satiety, thereby suppressing feeding (Smith et al., 1981). Thus, this gut peptide, which is normally released with a large meal to facilitate digestion through gallbladder contraction, also represents a peripheral stimulus to inhibit further feeding behavior.

The converse action occurs as well. Suppose we administer an agent known to act within the CNS that also influences peripheral vascular tone. One might think that the SANS activation by such a drug is the result of its direct action on alpha receptors in the peripheral vascular beds. However, the drug may have no peripheral action, but rather may influence peripheral vascular tone by activating CNS vasomotor centers, or alternatively by changing the sensitivity of the CNS response to alterations in, for example, baroreceptor afferent activity. Thus, one must be cautious when ascribing an effect of a centrally acting drug to either a central or peripheral action.

Brain Perfusion Rate and CNS Drug Action

Many lipophilic drugs, such as the barbiturates, benzodiazepines, and anesthetic gases, are very effective in the CNS although they ultimately end up in body fat. Since the brain is the most perfused organ of the body (approximately 2% of body weight while receiving 20% of cardiac output), drugs will be circulated more to brain than other organs. This is especially true since body fat normally receives a disproportionately low percentage of cardiac output compared with other tissues. Therefore, although a benzodiazepine such as diazepam would prefer a nice warm fat globule in which to spend its half-life, it will distribute to the brain first. Despite the fact that its half-life is 96 hours, however, the sedative-hypnotic effect of diazepam will only last for six to eight hours due to phase II redistribution as described above.

Blood flow to the brain is tightly regulated so that the overall percentage of cardiac output it receives remains quite constant. Despite this regulation, the regional distribution of blood flow within the brain is highly variable because of several factors, most notably CO_2. Indeed, CO_2 is the most important regulator of regional blood flow in the brain. CO_2 induces vasodilation, probably by reducing perivascular pH. Regional metabolism is thought to increase as a result of neuronal activity; the associated increase in CO_2 production leads to a decrease in perivascular pH that, in some unknown way, induces vasodilation. This vasodilation leads to enhanced perfusion of the brain region in question. The effects of metabolism—increased CO_2 production and subsequent vasodilation—are so pronounced that regional blood flow techniques are used to identify areas of the brain that are metabolically active (e.g., a person using vision while evaluating an object would exhibit increased blood flow to the visual cortex in the occipital lobe because of the increased neuronal metabolism associated with visual processing there). The CO_2-induced vasodilation associated with regional increases in neuronal activity can lead to local increases in the availability of a drug as well. For example, the increased metabolic activity associated with a seizure focus results in dramatically increased CO_2 production and compensatory vasodilation in that focus. This enhances the delivery of the anticonvulsant phenytoin to the region of the brain in greatest need of phenytoin—the seizure focus. As a result, the level of this drug in brain regions affected by seizures can be much higher than the plasma level.

Other factors also influence regional blood flow within the brain. Adenosine (released by nerves and resulting from metabolism), as well as local increases in extracellular K^+ resulting from excessive depolarization, induces local vasodilation. The smooth muscle of the cerebral vasculature also seems able to respond to alterations in pulse pressure independent of chemically mediated actions. A variety of factors can therefore influence the delivery of drugs to the brain by altering its vascular flow.

Lipophilicity and CNS Drug Action

The brain is a moderately fatty structure protected by many fatty membranes. Drugs that are fat soluble enter the brain faster than do drugs that are not. Pharmaceutical efforts to enhance the lipid solubility of drugs at physiologic pH will generally increase central action. The classic example used to illustrate this point is heroin. Heroin (diacetylmorphine) is metabolized to morphine in the brain. Although it is a prodrug of morphine, heroin is more potent than morphine. The presence of the acetyl groups on the morphine molecule makes heroin more lipid soluble than morphine. At equally administered dosages, more heroin than morphine enters the brain. Heroin is therefore more potent than morphine even though the actions of both drugs are mediated by the same morphine molecule. Moreover, the increased lipid solubility of heroin affects not only the resulting concentration of morphine achieved in brain, but because it enters so much more easily, also the rate at which a peak drug level is obtained. For the heroin user, the faster the drug can enter the brain, the more pronounced the "rush." The euphorogenic properties of opioid drugs are thus enhanced by increasing the rates of drug entry into the CNS.

TOLERANCE

The chronic administration of many drugs can change their potencies. Potency is defined as the quantity of drug needed to produce a specified effect. A decrease in the potency of a drug resulting from chronic exposure to that drug is termed tolerance. Tolerance implies a reduction in the response of a biologic system to a drug. There are seven categories of tolerance: pharmacodynamic, pharmacokinetic, physiologic, behavioral, rapid tolerance, cross tolerance, and reverse tolerance.

Pharmacodynamic tolerance is said to occur when potency has been lowered by a reduction in the efficiency through which a drug carries out its mechanism of action. The prototypical mechanism is a decrease in the number of receptors to which the drug binds (see Chapter 3). If a drug is binding to a neurotransmitter receptor to produce its effect and the system compensates for this increased activity by decreasing the number of those receptors, more drug will be needed to achieve the same effect. Another type of pharmacodynamic tolerance is desensitization, which results from phosphorylation of the receptor, reducing its ability to produce second messengers. In both examples, the mechanism by which the drug exerts its effects is altered by chronic drug exposure and the result is pharmacodynamic tolerance.

Pharmacokinetic tolerance (also called biodispositional tolerance) occurs when a biologic system reduces the concentration of a drug delivered to its effector site as a result of an alteration in a pharmacokinetic parameter. The barbiturates induce the microsomal enzyme biotransformation system. The resulting increase in number of enzymes will biotransform an administered dose of phenobarbital faster. As a result, a higher dose of the drug will be required to deliver the same amount of drug to the brain. Since the action of the drug in the brain has not changed but the drug's availability at its site of action has, this is accurately described as pharmacokinetic tolerance.

Biological systems compensate for a chronic change in neurotransmission in several ways. Pharmacodynamic tolerance is one example. Neuropharmacologic agents tend to affect a single neurotransmitter system that represents but one set of synapses in a series of neuronal connections. Alterations at one set of synapses often change neurotransmitter activity at other synapses. An example serves to illustrate this point. The antipsychotic drug haloperidol blocks the action of DA in the striatum. As a result of chronic treatment, DA receptor number increases. More haloperidol is subsequently needed to achieve the same level of DA-receptor blockade (pharmacodynamic tolerance). However, DA inhibits striatal neurons that release the neurotransmitter ACh. Blocking DA reduces the normal inhibitory action of DA on these striatal cholinergic neurons, resulting in increased ACh release that can activate muscarinic receptors on the next neuron. This increased ACh release decreases the number of muscarinic ACh-receptor sites, resulting in reduced potency of ACh at this synapse. Since the effect of ACh has been decreased because of decreased numbers of muscarinic receptors, a higher dose of haloperidol would have to be administered to achieve the same level of ACh activity; again tolerance has developed. In this case, however, the mechanism responsible for the decrease in muscarinic receptors and the associated tolerance is not directly related to the mechanism of action of haloperidol, but is rather a secondary consequence of the action of the drug. This describes a physiologic tolerance that is defined as a reduction in the potency of an administered drug following chronic administration because of compensatory changes in the biologic system not directly related to the mechanism of action of the drug. Since chronic haloperidol treatment results in DA-receptor and muscarinic-receptor alterations, pharmacodynamic as well as physiologic tolerance has occurred in this case.

Understanding the difference between pharmacodynamic and physiologic tolerance is extremely important since it enables you to appreciate some of the more subtle aspects of drug action. The development of pharmacodynamic or physiologic tolerance indicates that the brain is adjusting to the continued presence of a drug. These adjustments occur through a variety of compensatory mechanisms that are designed to reestablish the predrug state. When the drug is removed, the pharmacodynamic and physiologic tolerance that have developed subside slowly. Neurotransmitters that are now acting in the absence of the drug will then produce hypersensitive or hyposensitive rebound effects because of the tolerance. These rebound effects produce the signs and symptoms of the withdrawal syndromes that accompany the rapid discontinuation of most centrally acting drugs. The pharmacodynamic changes that occur are reasonably easy to understand since they are directly related to the mechanisms of action of the drug. However, physiologic tolerance also contributes to withdrawal symptoms. By not appreciating that physiologic tolerance has developed, you might inappropriately assume that a component of the withdrawal syndrome is a direct consequence of the drug's action even though it was not. This applies to side effects as well. Levodopa therapy can produce a movement disorder called myoclonus (uncontrollable muscle jerks). Since this side effect is associated with levodopa therapy it could readily be assumed that it results from the pharmacodynamic action of levodopa (increased DA): More likely, it is a consequence of physiologic neuroadaptation in the serotonin system. If we do not appreciate physiologic tolerance, we may be perplexed to find that antiserotonergic agents are effective in reducing this side effect.

Behavioral tolerance is defined as a reduction in the potency of a drug secondary to an intentional change in the behavior of the consumer based on cognitive anticipation of the possibility of adverse effects. This type of tolerance is unique to the centrally acting drugs. Heavy alcohol consumption produces predictable motor dysfunction that the alcoholic anticipates. The gait becomes wobbly (ataxia) and, as a result, intoxicated individuals walk with their feet wider apart (a broad-based gait). Coordination and reflex time also suffer: Intoxicated individuals tend to stumble and fall a lot. Alcoholics learn that if they stand up quickly and make rapid movements, they are more likely to fall, or at least draw attention to themselves because of uncoordinated movements. They therefore adapt their behaviors so that the effects of the drug are less pronounced. They often walk next to solid objects so quick adjustments of vertical posture can be made with the hands. Marijuana users tend not to bend over so as not to induce orthostatic hypotension. Heroin users tend to inject their drugs in a comfortable location so that they can sit or lie down during the initial "rush" when they would be most likely to fall. Of course, the reverse is also true. As will be discussed, hallucinogenic drug users will often adapt their behaviors to intensify the effects of the drug.

A special case of tolerance can occur very rapidly (two to 24 hours) during exposure to certain drugs. The effects of drugs such as tyramine and lysergic acid diethylamide (LSD) can produce such a rapid reduction in potency that the dosage needed to induce an equivalent effect on the second day of administration can be three to five times higher. In the case of tyramine, the dramatic reduction in potency is the result of depletion of NE and is therefore pharmacodynamic in nature. In the case of LSD the mechanism is not completely known. Such rapid changes in potency following acute exposure to a drug are called rapid tolerance or, more commonly, tachyphylaxis.

Another special case of tolerance is cross tolerance, which is defined as a reduction in the potency of one drug because of exposure (usually chronic) to another drug, that is generally, although not always, in the same drug class. Following chronic use of diazepam to facilitate sleep, tolerance to its sedative effects often develops. Switching to another member of the benzodiazepine class to induce sedation is pointless since the patient will be equally tolerant to that drug (cross tolerance). Even attempts at substituting a drug from a completely different chemical class, such as a barbiturate or alcohol, will often yield similar reductions in potency. The ability of drugs of different classes to induce cross tolerance suggests that they act via similar mechanisms (pharmacodynamic tolerance). One alternative explanation is that cross tolerance is the result of similar forms of physiologic tolerance that have occurred in response to the actions of the drugs regardless of their mechanisms of action.

All the forms of tolerance described thus far involve reductions in potency. Reverse tolerance (also called sensitization) is defined as an increase in potency following continued exposure to a drug. The classic teaching example is cocaine. The administration of cocaine to an animal increases motor activity. After several exposures to the drug, administering the original dose of cocaine produces a greater motor response. Performing dose-response studies following chronic exposure to cocaine reveals that the ability to induce the same degree of locomotion observed acutely can be elicited by a lower administered dose of cocaine. The animal has been "sensitized" to the drug. The term priming has also been used to describe this phenomenon. Priming, however, should be used in a more restrictive sense and refers to the need to expose a biologic system to a drug at least once before the desired effect is obtained (comparable to priming a hand-pump with water to get it to pump water). Reverse tolerance is thought to underlie the increased ability of levodopa to induce dyskinetic movements in the symptomatic treatment of Parkinson's disease and cocaine's ability to produce drug dependence. Reverse tolerance may explain, at least in part, the inability of the marijuana users to get "high" the first couple of times they use the drug although this may be an example of priming. The mechanism(s) responsible for reverse tolerance does not appear to involve an alteration in the bioavailability of the drug to the brain, so it may not be a special case of biodispositional tolerance. Nor does a behavioral adaptation seem responsible for this phenomenon. The mechanism(s) involved in reverse tolerance is a very active area of research and probably involves both pharmacodynamic and physiologic changes.

3

Drugs and Receptors

The receptor is the key to understanding the functions of neuro-transmitters and the drugs that mimic their actions. It is the neu-rotransmitter receptor that will determine if a hormone is se-creted, a muscle contracted, or a nerve depolarized or inhibited. The receptor and the proteins it acts through also determine whether the re-sponse will last only for a few milliseconds or for 50 years. Since most centrally acting drugs mimic the action of neurotransmitters, the interac-tion between a drug and its receptor will similarly determine the biologi-cal response produced.

Broadly, the term receptor means a biological site to which a chemical binds and thus produces a biological action. Most neurotransmitter re-ceptors are formed by the extracellular domains of proteins that span the membrane. However, receptors may also be soluble proteins, nucleic acids, or glycolipids found within the cytoplasm or nucleus of a cell. Thus, if a drug inhibits an intracellular enzyme and produces a biological response, that site can be considered a receptor. Likewise, a drug that blocks a reuptake pump may do so by binding to a transporter protein. Referring to these sites as receptors is technically correct although often confusing. Consequently, the use of the term receptor in this book will be reserved for sites where a neurotransmitter acts to induce a specific bio-logic response. The terms binding site and acceptor will be used to iden-tify all other sites of drug action associated with a biologic response in-cluding enzymes, allosteric regulatory sites, and transporter proteins.

The term nonspecific binding site adds to the semantic confusion sur-rounding receptors. These are defined as biological sites where drugs bind but do not perform biological actions. Nonspecific binding sites include serum albumin, proteins, and other molecules found throughout the brain and periphery that generally, although not always, have lower affinities for a drug than receptors or acceptor sites. These nonspecific sites often segregate a drug from its unbound pool and thereby prevent it from binding to a specific site where a biological action might otherwise occur.

Most of the drugs discussed in this text work by interacting with receptors or acceptors. Knowing what receptors a drug interacts with and where those receptors are located helps predict its actions and side effects. We usually think that a centrally acting drug is aimed at a specific receptor in a specific region of the brain to produce its target-specific effects (Fig. 3–1). Unfortunately, few currently available drugs possess such specificity. Dopamine (DA) antagonists, for instance, block several DA-receptor subtypes throughout the brain and thus also produce target-nonspecific effects. Moreover, many DA antagonists also block muscarinic, serotonergic, and noradrenergic receptors and thereby produce receptor-nonspecific effects. The pharmacodynamic actions of a drug involve the target-specific effects that represent its desired action as well as target- and receptor-nonspecific effects that represent side effects. "Clean" receptor- and target-specific drugs are now a major focus of drug development.

NEUROTRANSMITTER–RECEPTOR INTERACTIONS

The traditional view of synaptic transmission was that the released neurotransmitter interacted with its specific receptor in a "lock-and-key" fashion and opened an ion channel that changed membrane potential. The receptor and ionophore were thus viewed as separate parts of the same protein. When the neurotransmitter bound to its receptor, the conformation of the receptor protein was altered and this, in turn, altered the conformation of the ionophore, allowing ions to pass through. Since such channels are activated by a neurotransmitter or drug rather than by a change in voltage, they are called ligand-gated channels to distinguish them from voltage-gated channels. (The term ligand is used to refer to any chemical entity that can bind specifically to a receptor.)

It is now known that the lock-and-key model describes only a small proportion of neurotransmitter–receptor interactions. Most receptors are comprised of an acceptor site that binds the neurotransmitter and sets off a cascade of tertiary structural changes in other subunits of the same protein, inducing conformational changes in other proteins associated with the receptor complex. The result of these conformational changes is the

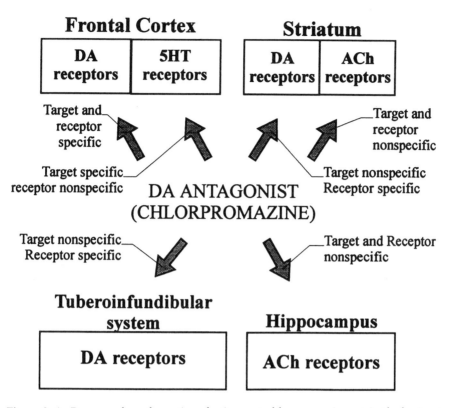

Figure 3–1. Drugs such as the antipsychotic agent chlorpromazine act in the brain at their intended site of action (target specific), at unintended sites (target nonspecific), at intended receptors (receptor specific), and at unintended receptor sites (receptor nonspecific). In the case depicted, chlorpromazine (DA antagonist) is blocking DA receptors in the frontal cortex (target- and receptor-specific action) to produce its desired effect. Chlorpromazine can also bind to DA receptors at other locations (target-nonspecific effects) where DA antagonism can lead to side effects. Chlorpromazine's structure also has affinity for other receptors such as acetylcholine (ACh) and serotonin (5HT), the blockade of which can also result in side effects within the target structure (target specific but receptor nonspecific) as well as in nontarget structures (target- and receptor-nonspecific effects).

synthesis or release of second messengers that include such important regulators of cell function as cyclic adenosine monophosphate (cAMP), diacylglycerol (DAG), and Ca^{2+}. The effects of some of these second messengers can even regulate gene transcription. Thus, besides their traditional roles as ion conductance regulators, receptors also influence intracellular metabolism, translation, and transcription. These responses can produce profound and long-lasting effects on neuronal function.

Since neurotransmitter–receptor interactions result in either ligand-gated alterations in ion conductance or conductance changes accompanied by second-messenger production, neurotransmitter receptors fall into two broad categories. Those that only change the conductance of an ion are called ionotropic receptors. They include the nicotinic, $5HT_3$, $GABA_A$, and glutamate receptors. Ionotropic receptors are generally formed by one protein that has several different subunits. The various subunits not only bind to the neurotransmitter but also form the ionophore (the ion channel) and anchor the receptor in the lipid bilayer (membrane-spanning domains). Alternatively, neurotransmitter–receptor interactions may alter the structure of a coupling protein called a guanine nucleotide-binding protein (G protein). As discussed below, activation of the G protein alters the structure of another protein that initiates the production of a second messenger initiating other intracellular actions that regulate neural function. Receptors that directly alter the production of second messengers are called metabotropic receptors since the receptor–neurotransmitter interaction initiates a metabolic (enzyme mediated) activity. A metabotropic receptor can bind a single, released neurotransmitter molecule and transform that signal into the production of numerous second-messenger molecules that can produce an even greater increase in the number of third and fourth messengers. Unlike ionotropic receptors, therefore, metabotropic receptors can dramatically amplify the initial signal carried by the neurotransmitter.

The interaction between a ligand (drug or neurotransmitter) and its binding site generally involves noncovalent bonding and is reversible. Thus, once the ligand dissociates from its binding site, it can collide with the receptor again, and if the receptor has not been altered by the prior ligand–receptor interaction, a response will again occur. Therefore, whether it is an ionotropic, metabotropic, or other type of drug–acceptor interaction, the magnitude of the response will depend on the number of collisions per unit of time. The residence time of neurotransmitters in the synapse is such that multiple collisions generally occur, and this determines the duration of ionic conductance or amount of second messenger produced. Drugs that remain in the synapse or increase the duration of time a neurotransmitter spends in the synapse consequently increase the receptor's effect. However, many receptors shift from a high-affinity to a low-affinity state following ligand interaction. When a ligand binds to the receptor in its low-affinity state, the response that occurs is markedly attenuated. Since shifting back to the high-affinity state requires time, additional collisions that might occur during this time are less effective at producing a response. Rarely, a drug may bind to its receptor irreversibly through covalent bonds so that the ligand and the receptor are irrevocably transformed. These agents are referred to as irreversible inhibitors. An example is mustard gas, which covalently binds to ACh receptors. In such cases, new receptors must be synthesized in order for an effect to occur again. Other drugs are transformed into highly reactive intermediates by the acceptor interaction (generally an enzyme) and these intermediates bind irreversibly to the acceptor site, thereby inactivating it. These agents are called suicide inhibitors because the drug, in a sense, "commits suicide" to carry out its biologic effect. The monoamine oxidase inhibitors used to treat depression are classic examples.

Ionotropic Receptors

The interaction of a drug or a neurotransmitter with an ionotropic receptor can increase the conductance of several different ions. Whether or not the neuron is depolarized or inhibited by the action of the receptor will depend on the ion involved. The ionotropic receptors found at the neuromuscular junction are the traditional excitatory neurotransmitter receptors one first learns about in introductory biology classes. At these receptors, the interaction with a neurotransmitter or drug causes an immediate conformational change in the structure of the protein that forms the ligand-gated ion channel. This conformational change directly causes the channel to open, permitting ionic conductance. At the neuromuscular junction Na^+ passes into the muscle cell, bringing with it a positive charge that results in depolarization and muscle contraction. Other ligand-gated channels produce depolarization by opening Ca^{2+} channels. In contrast, ionotropic receptor–ligand interactions can open K^+ channels, allowing positive charge to leave the nerve cell. This loss of positive charge renders the neuron more electrically negative relative to its environment (hyperpolarized) and therefore more difficult to depolarize (i.e., inhibited). Ionotropic receptors that open Cl^- channels usually do not change the resting membrane potential of a neuron, although they produce an inhibitory effect. Opening a Cl^- channel makes the membrane "leaky" to negative current. Because the normal resting potential of a neuron is close to the equilibrium potential for Cl^-, chloride neither enters nor leaves the cell once its conductance channels are open. However, if Cl^- channels were open when another neurotransmitter opened a Na^+ channel on the same neuron, Cl^- ions would move into the cell, neutralizing the depolarizing effect of the Na^+ ions that entered.

Since the ionotropic receptor is intimately associated with the ion channel protein (they are subunits of the same protein), the consequence of neurotransmitter–receptor interaction is immediate. The resulting change in the polarity of the neuron happens quickly and the neuron then repolarizes quickly. Thus, ionotropic receptors are fast-acting receptors that perturb the target neuron for only a few milliseconds. These perturbations may or may not be of sufficient magnitude to produce an action potential in the neuron.

Metabotropic Receptors

In contrast to the speed with which ionotropic neurotransmitter–receptor interactions induce a change in the resting potential of a neuron, metabotropic receptors are slow. Because the interaction between the neurotransmitter and the binding site initiates a cascade of structural changes in coupling proteins and enzymes that make second messengers, hundreds of milliseconds are generally needed to observe a change in a neuron activated by these receptors. Although metabotropic receptors are called by that name because they induce the metabolism of another chemical to produce a second messenger, they all appear to influence the conductance of ions across the membrane as well, albeit with a time delay. In addition, since the activation of these receptors sometimes alters the transcription of DNA in the nucleus of the target neuron via second-messenger systems, the actions of metabotropic receptors can induce permanent changes in the target neuron. Metabotropic receptors thus can induce short-latency changes (hundreds of milliseconds) mediated by ion conductance changes as well as long-lasting changes mediated by second messengers. Several second-messenger systems are currently known, including the cAMP system, the phospholipase A-2 system, Ca^{2+}-calmodulin, and the phosphoinositide cascade. Besides these established second-messenger systems, other intracellular messengers including serine/ threonine kinases and tyrosine kinases are also involved with intracellular signal transduction. More second-messenger systems probably are awaiting discovery.

Despite the variety of second messengers in the brain, the neurotransmitter metabotropic receptors thus far characterized all use the same type of coupling protein to initiate the sequence of events that leads to second-messenger production. These coupling proteins are called G proteins because they bind to guanine-nucleotide proteins. The G proteins have been well characterized. They are found on the cytoplasmic side of the membrane and are activated by the intracellular domain of the receptor protein. They are composed of three functional subunits called alpha, beta, and gamma (Fig. 3–2). Several different types of G proteins exist including G_i and G_s. The subscripts *i* and *s* stand for inhibitory and stimulatory. Thus, activation of a G_i protein inhibits while activation of a G_s protein stimulates the production of the second-messenger cAMP. In addition to these G proteins, several others are currently known. G_o (for "other") will be used to designate the numerous isoforms of this G_o protein. Whether or not a G protein is G_o, G_i, or G_s depends primarily on the structure of the alpha subunit; the same beta and gamma subunits are shared by all the G proteins.

G proteins have a quaternary structure formed by three functional subunits. In its resting state the alpha subunit is bound to guanine-

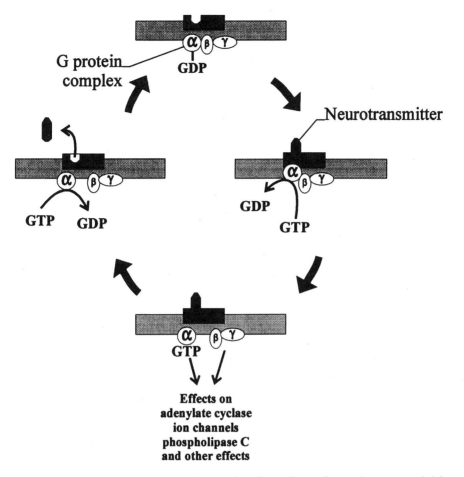

G protein complex

GDP

Neurotransmitter

GDP

GTP

GTP   GDP

GTP

**Effects on
adenylate cyclase
ion channels
phospholipase C
and other effects**

Figure 3–2. Drugs or neurotransmitters acting through metabotropic receptors initiate their intracellular events by activating various G proteins. In its resting state the three subunits of the G protein have potential GTPase activity that is initiated by a drug or neurotransmitter binding to its receptor. GTP then becomes bound to the alpha subunit and the beta and gamma subunits dissociate from the alpha-GTP complex. The alpha subunit can then transfer the energy from the GTP to activate adenylate cyclase, ion channels, and other second-messenger cascades. After the energy transfer, GDP remains bound to the alpha subunit, causing a tertiary structural alteration in the neurotransmitter receptor, displacing the drug or neurotransmitter from the binding site. After displacement, the alpha-GDP complex again binds to the beta and gamma subunits in preparation for the next binding event.

diphosphate (GDP). Activation of the receptor protein by a neurotransmitter or drug causes a conformational change in the protein that binds to and in turn causes a conformational change in the alpha subunit of the G protein. This change in the alpha subunit has three consequences: (1) guanine triphosphate (GTP) is exchanged for guanine diphosphate

(GDP); (2) the beta and gamma subunits dissociate together as a single unit from the alpha subunit; and (3) the G protein dissociates from the neurotransmitter receptor. The alpha subunit, which is now bound to a high-energy substrate, GTP, is free to activate another protein to produce a second messenger. Whether or not the beta-gamma subunit has this capability is still in question. The dissociated alpha subunit possesses enzymatic activity and can therefore cleave a phosphate group from the GTP. The energy released can then be used by the alpha subunit to activate another protein that, in turn, produces the second messenger (Fig. 3–2). Following this energy transfer, the alpha-GDP subunit is again free to bind with the beta and gamma subunits and form the original quaternary structure of the G protein. The activation of this receptor–G-protein cascade generates a second messenger. Typically, the activation of the G-protein is also associated with an opening of an ion channel. The mechanism responsible for this ionotropic action of the G protein is currently unknown. (For an extensive review of second-messenger systems and their molecular biology see Hyman and Nestler, 1996.)

Cyclic nucleotide second-messenger systems
Once the alpha subunit has exchanged the GDP for guanosine triphosphate (GTP), it has GTPase (enzymatic) activity (Fig. 3–2). The G_s protein cleaves a high-energy phosphate group off GTP and transfers the resulting energy to adenylate cyclase. Thus, the alpha-GTP complex becomes coupled to a third protein that possesses enzymatic activity, adenylate cyclase, to which the energy from the cleavage of GTP to GDP is transferred. This energy is subsequently used to cleave adenosine triphosphate (ATP) into cAMP and adenosine diphosphate (ADP). The cAMP formed is water soluble and can diffuse away from the membrane to induce a structural change in still another protein (see below). G_s proteins therefore stimulate adenylate cyclase. Alternatively, the activation of G_i proteins inhibits the activity of adenylate cyclase, thereby reducing the production of cAMP that may be occurring in the cell as a result of G_s activation. D_1 and D_2 receptor families exhibit this antagonistic action on cAMP production. D_1 receptors are coupled to G_s receptors while D_2 receptors are coupled to G_i receptors. DA released in nanomolar quantities stimulates D_2 receptors, inhibiting cAMP production, while D_1 receptors activated at micromolar quantities stimulate cAMP production. Thus, depending on the amount of DA released, cAMP synthesis can be increased or decreased. Other receptors such as the beta-adrenergic and vasoactive intestinal peptide (VIP) receptors are coupled to the G_s protein while opiate and alpha$_2$ receptors are coupled with the G_i protein.

Several drugs can raise or lower levels of cAMP by altering the synthesis or catabolism of the second messengers independent of the receptor protein. Phosphodiesterase inhibitors such as theophylline and caffeine are the best-known class. Since the enzyme phosphodiesterase catabolizes cAMP, drugs that inhibit phosphodiesterase enhance the effects of neurotransmitters or drugs that act by increasing cAMP levels. By binding to the alpha subunit of the G protein, cholera toxins can permanently activate the G_s protein initiating the pathologic cascade responsible for cholera. Pertussis toxin, which is responsible for whooping cough, can permanently deactivate G_i and G_o.

Phospholipase A$_2$ (PLA$_2$) and the arachidonic acid pathway
Histamine (and probably other neurotransmitters) binds to its receptor and activates a G_o protein, which activates the enzyme PLA$_2$ (Fig. 3–3). PLA$_2$ hydrolyzes phosphoinositol in the membrane, releasing arachidonic acid from the cell membrane. Arachidonic acid is then rapidly converted to a family of active metabolites called the eicosanoids. The enzyme cyclooxygenase convert's arachidonic acid to a group of compounds called the prostaglandins and thromboxanes. These metabolites are involved in peripheral inflammatory processes. Their actions in the brain are not well characterized although they are known to play a role in the production of fever. Arachidonic acid can also be metabolized by lipoxygenases to yield hydroperoxyeicosatrienoic acid (HPETE). The production of this second messenger has been shown to influence the phosphorylation status of ion channels (see below).

As with the cAMP system, several drugs can influence the activity of the arachidonic acid pathway. Corticosteroids prevent the mobilization of arachidonic acid from the membrane. Among several other actions, these drugs can reduce the production of a variety of second messengers emanating from the release of arachidonic acid. Aspirin, indomethacin, and the nonsteroidal antiinflammatory drugs (NSAIDs) such as ibuprofen inhibit the enzyme cyclooxygenase. Because the prostaglandins can influence pain thresholds, they also possess analgesic actions. The release of prostaglandins into a wound area reduces the threshold for pain, probably by altering the phosphorylation status of the pain fiber. The NSAIDs prevent this sensitization and are therefore useful in pain management.

The DAG-IP$_3$ cascade
The activation of G_o proteins by muscarinic receptors is responsible for the production of two second messengers via the enzyme phospholipase C (Fig. 3–4). Phosphatidylinositol (PI) is a phospholipid found on the cytoplasmic side of the membrane. Activation of phospholipase C cleaves PI into two primary components called inositol triphosphate (IP$_3$) and diacylglycerol (DAG). IP$_3$ is water soluble and therefore diffuses into the cytosol where it interacts with mitochondria and especially with the en-

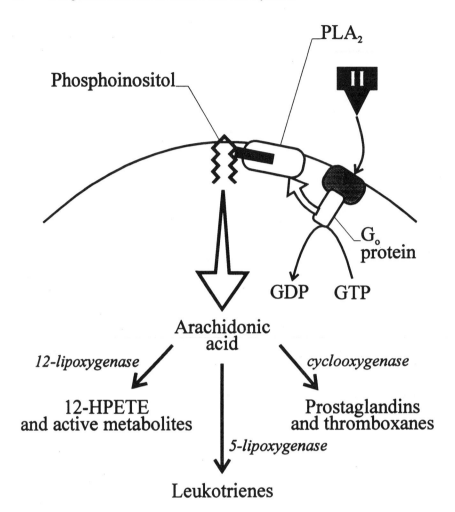

Figure 3–3. Some drugs and neurotransmitters (such as histamine [H]) acting through G_o proteins activate the enzyme phospholipase A_2 (PLA_2) drawing energy from GTP. PLA_2 hydrolyzes phosphoinositol embedded on the cytosolic side of the membrane to yield the important intermediate arachidonic acid. Arachidonic acid can be converted into the prostaglandins and thromboxanes by the enzyme cyclooxygenase (italics). Arachidonic acid can also be converted to the leukotrienes and hydroperoxyeicosatrienoic acids (HPETE) by the two forms of lipoxygenase enzymes shown in italics.

doplasmic reticulum to release intracellular stores of Ca^{2+}. The increase in intracellular Ca^{2+} concentration resulting from IP_3 may have several functions in the cell, including (1) depolarization by the addition of intracellular unbound positive charge, (2) activation of several intracellular proteins, (3) activation of Ca^{2+}-sensitive K^+ channels, and (4) binding to another protein called calmodulin. The Ca^{2+}-calmodulin complex can ac-

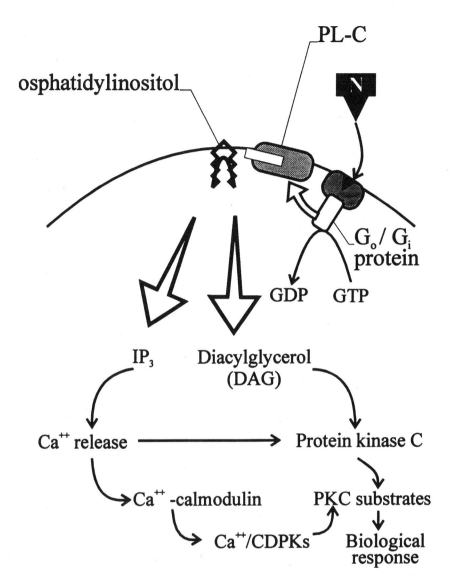

Figure 3–4. The phospholipase C (phosphoinositide cascade) is initiated when a neurotransmitter (N) binds to a receptor coupled with various G_o proteins. Phospholipase C (PL-C) converts phosphatidylinositol into the second messengers inositol triphosphate (IP_3) and diacylglycerol (DAG). IP_3 induces the release of intracellular stores of Ca^{2+} that can directly activate protein kinase C or its substrates (PKC substrates) through calmodulin and its calmodulin-dependent protein kinases (CDPKs). DAG can also directly activate PKC and through its substrates produces several biological responses.

tivate another family of protein kinases called Ca^{2+}-calmodulin-dependent protein kinases that have several intracellular functions (see below).

The phosphoinositides are recycled back into the membrane by a series of enzymes that are not yet completely characterized. One of these enzymes, inositol 1-phosphatase, is blocked by the drug lithium. Lithium's ability to reduce the activation of phosphatidylinositol is probably responsible for its action in combating manic-depressive disorder.

DAG, the other product of phospholipase C activation, is a water-insoluble compound that remains bound to the cytoplasmic side of the membrane. From its membrane-bound position DAG activates an important cytosolic enzyme called protein kinase C (PKC). When activated by DAG in the presence of Ca^{2+}, PKC either remains bound to the membrane or diffuses into the cytoplasm, activating or deactivating other proteins.

Consequences of Metabotropic Receptor Activation

We have seen how G proteins, via their various isoforms, can activate several different second-messenger systems. These second messengers are usually specific for given neurotransmitters. Thus, DA generally produces its postsynaptic action by altering cAMP while ACh, acting on muscarinic receptors, initiates the phosphoinositide cascade to carry the signal into the cell. Several different second-messenger systems can exist within the same neuron and the products of different metabotropic receptor interactions can therefore interact in complex ways. Since neurons often make synaptic contact with several other neurons, a single cell may have several different metabotropic receptors simultaneously activated by their respective neurotransmitters. These various second-messenger systems can act additively or synergistically or counteract one another, as well. Through these interactions, second messengers can regulate important functions of the cell including neurotransmitter–receptor transduction, cytoskeletal assembly, and ion channel conductance. Second-messenger systems can also regulate translation rates and even initiate gene transcription. Most often, these neuronal activities are not directly regulated by the second messengers themselves but rather by third and fourth messengers activated by the second messengers. Thus, the generation of a second messenger by a neurotransmitter–receptor interaction is only the first step in a cascade of events that subsequently alters the function of molecules within the target neuron. Functional alterations in intracellular molecules mediated by second messengers are regulated by adding or removing phosphates.

The activity of a protein can be dramatically increased or decreased by phosphorylation. Proteins that add phosphate groups to other proteins are called protein kinases while those that take phosphate groups off other proteins are called phosphatases. Protein kinases and phosphatases together regulate the phosphorylation status of a molecule or cell. Phosphorylation status refers to the overall level of phosphorylation present in a cell. The factors that are responsible for regulating phosphatase activity are not well known, whereas numerous protein kinase systems have been well characterized. Some receptors can activate protein kinases directly by binding to tyrosine residues in the enzymes. These tyrosine kinases can regulate cell growth and differentiation when activated by neurotrophic factors such as nerve growth factor (NGF). Other protein kinases, such as those activated by PKC and PLA_2, phosphorylate the amino acids serine and threonine (serine/threonine kinases). The regulation of protein activity by phosphorylation is so common that it is probably fair to say that almost every chemical activity in a cell is influenced to a certain extent by phosphorylation. Moreover, since a given target protein usually has several potential phosphorylation sites and several different protein kinases can independently phosphorylate these sites, a given target protein can be activated or inhibited by several kinases and phosphatases, yielding an extremely complex pattern of regulation. This ability of several second-messenger systems to interact within a cell is called cross talk.

A phosphate group $(PO_4{}^{-3})$ has a strong net negative charge and a bulky molecular configuration. Because of its molecular size and charge distribution, phosphorylation or dephosphorylation can dramatically alter the tertiary and quaternary structures of target proteins. The resulting conformational changes brought about by a change in the phosphorylation status of a protein can therefore dramatically alter protein activity. Altering the phosphorylation status of certain intracellular elements can even turn on and turn off cell functions. It is difficult to understate the importance of this activity.

Phosphorylation and dephosphorylation are able to influence neuronal events for seconds or hours and their effects are readily reversible. However, the activation of second-messenger systems can also influence neuronal function for days, weeks, and maybe even permanently by modifying genetic activity within the cell. Many second-messenger systems activate cAMP-dependent protein kinases that enter the nucleus of a cell (Fig. 3–5). Inside the nucleus, genetic transcription (DNA to messenger RNA [mRNA]) is controlled by RNA polymerase. The polymerase binds to an area of DNA called the promoter that is just upstream to the DNA to be transcribed. RNA polymerase does not bind directly to the DNA in the promoter region. Rather, a set of proteins called transcription factors bind to the promoter region and the polymerase to guide transcription. The transcriptional process can also be regulated by a stretch of DNA

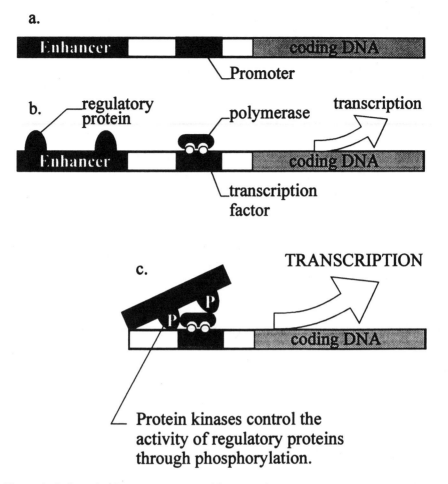

Figure 3–5. Protein kinases are activated by several messenger systems such as cyclic adenosine monophosphate (cAMP). These kinases can, in turn, activate regulatory proteins to enhance the transcription rate as depicted in this figure. Messenger RNAs resulting from polymerase-mediated transcription of a coding DNA sequence (a) are regulated by several upstream regions of the DNA (promoter and enhancer). In order for the polymerase to initiate transcription it must first bind to the promoter via proteinaceous transcription factors (b). Transcription rates can be increased significantly as a result of protein kinase-mediated phosphorylation (P) of regulatory proteins on enhancer regions several thousand base pairs upstream from the coding region. Drugs, by influencing the production of transcription factors or by increasing the production of protein kinases, can significantly alter the production of new messenger RNAs which, in turn, can influence protein synthesis and cell function.

60

called the enhancer region that is generally found some distance from the promoter region. In the presence of regulatory proteins that bind to the enhancer region, transcription is greatly facilitated. By phosphorylating the regulatory proteins in the enhancer region, protein kinases facilitate the enhancer's ability to increase the activity of the polymerase thereby speeding the synthesis of mRNA. Consequently, the synthesis of tyrosine hydroxylase, for example, a key enzyme in the synthesis of DA and NE, would be increased.

The capacity of a neuron to alter the rate of production of an enzyme such as tyrosine hydroxylase or turn on the synthesis of a new enzyme would undoubtedly influence its function. If, as a result of metabotropic receptor activation, a protein-kinase-mediated event turns on a series of genes that regulates a neuron's growth, or determines the type of neuron a progenitor cell develops into, the effects of a metabotropic receptor can be permanent. Phosphorylation status is influenced by neurotransmitters that act on metabotropic receptors; several drugs discussed in the following chapters mimic, block, or enhance the actions of those neurotransmitters; drug-induced alterations in phosphorylation status thus are pivotal in this text to an understanding of the pharmacodynamics of centrally acting drugs.

Multiple Receptors

All small-molecule neurotransmitters and many neuropeptides produce their effects through multiple-receptor subtypes. Some neurotransmitters such as GABA act through only two receptor subtypes while others, such as 5HT, have as many as 18. Receptor subtypes have different amino acid sequences in their extracellular domains that can all bind the same neurotransmitter, although with different affinities. Neurotransmitter receptors are often categorized into families as well. Each family uses different intracellular domains to generate second messengers. Thus, DA is currently known to act through five receptors that are divided into two families designated D-1 and D-2. The two D-1 receptors activate G_s while the three D-2 receptors activate G_i. Some D-2 receptors become activated in the presence of nanomolar concentrations of DA while the D-1 receptors are activated by micromolar concentrations. Since D-1 receptors increase cAMP production while D-2 receptors inhibit adenylate cyclase, the generation of cAMP depends not only on the receptor family activated, but also on the frequency of DA neuron stimulation, which determines the synaptic concentration of DA. Multiple receptors therefore offer greater versatility in synaptic signaling. Receptor subtypes can even determine the type of the response that will occur in response to neurotransmitter release, as well. Thus, at lower levels of SANS activation, alpha receptors are predominantly activated. At higher levels of SANS activation where epinephrine is released, beta-adrenergic receptors are activated and will convert a pure vasoconstrictive response to one where vasoconstriction and vasodilation occur. From an evolutionary perspective, multiple-receptor subtypes diversify the response characteristics of a neurotransmitter without the need to evolve a completely different neurotransmitter system. From a pharmacologist's viewpoint, the existence of multiple-receptor subtypes helps us develop receptor-subtype-selective drugs that can enhance target specificity and thereby reduce the number of side effects.

MODE OF DRUG ACTION

Drugs that work via receptor systems can be divided into four categories based on their mechanisms of action: (1) direct-acting agonists, (2) indirect-acting agonists, (3) direct-acting antagonists, and (4) indirect-acting antagonists. These categories can be very helpful in understanding the pharmacodynamics of most drugs.

Direct-Acting Agonist

A direct-acting agonist has both affinity and efficacy (produces a response) at a receptor. It binds to a receptor and mimics the normal action of the neurotransmitter. Such drugs can be receptor-subtype selective (e.g., bromocriptine, a D_2 agonist) or receptor-subtype nonselective (e.g., apomorphine, a D_1 and D_2 agonist), in which case they are called mixed agonists.

Indirect-Acting Agonist

An indirect-acting agonist enhances the action of a neurotransmitter in an indirect fashion. Usually, these drugs act by increasing the levels of a neurotransmitter or by extending the time a neurotransmitter resides in the synapse. Their mechanisms include (1) blocking catabolic enzymes (e.g., acetylcholinesterase inhibitors that increase ACh levels or monoamine-oxidase inhibitors that increase the biogenic amines DA, NE, and 5HT, (2) stimulating the release of a neurotransmitter (e.g., amphetamine for DA and NE), and (3) inhibiting reuptake of a neurotransmitter (e.g., amphetamine, the tricyclic antidepressants, and cocaine, all of which can inhibit the reuptake of biogenic amines).

Direct-Acting Antagonist

A direct-acting antagonist has affinity for a receptor but does not have efficacy for a receptor. These drugs bind to a receptor but do not induce a biological action. When direct-acting antagonists bind to a receptor, they interfere with the neurotransmitter's ability to gain access to the binding site and thereby reduce neurotransmitter actions (e.g., antipsychotic agents that are DA antagonists, or propranolol, which blocks beta receptors). Like direct-acting agonists, antagonists can be receptor-subtype selective or mixed. Most antagonists bind in a noncovalent fashion at the same site where the neurotransmitter binds and are called competitive antagonists. Rarely, antagonists can bind to the receptor covalently and are called irreversible antagonists. Still, other drugs can inhibit access to the receptor by binding to a regulatory site on the receptor protein. Drugs that act in this manner are called noncompetitive antagonists.

Indirect-Acting Antagonist

Indirect-acting antagonists reduce the action of a neurotransmitter, usually by depleting its presynaptic stores (e.g., reserpine for DA, NE, and 5HT or marijuana for ACh). Drugs that are autoreceptor-selective agonists (see below), such as clonidine, can also act as indirect-acting antagonists by reducing neurotransmitter release.

Characterizing the mode of action of a drug as either direct or indirect will provide an immediate indication of the specificity and probable range of side effects that are likely to occur following its administration. Whereas direct-acting agents can be receptor-subtype specific, indirect-acting agents are not and will therefore have mixed actions. This lack of receptor specificity is more likely to produce several actions and a broader range of side effects than a receptor-subtype-selective agent. This characteristic of centrally acting drug action should always be considered when choosing a drug in a clinical or experimental situation.

RECEPTOR REGULATION

We have already seen how the sensitivity of receptors can be altered by the directed phosphorylation that second messengers and protein kinases initiate. The actual number of receptors on a neuron can also change. Indeed, before the role of phosphorylation in receptor sensitivity was appreciated, the major mechanism by which receptors were thought to affect neurotransmitter efficacy was alteration of receptor number. The number of receptors a neurotransmitter can bind to within a given terminal field is not static, but rather a dynamic aspect of neurotransmission. Such changes can dramatically alter the effectiveness of released neurotransmitter or administered drug.

The change in receptor number that accompanies chronic drug administration is well known and is commonly referred to as receptor up-

or down-regulation. Although exceptions exist, the brain usually responds to prolonged increases in neurotransmission by reducing the number of receptors (i.e., down-regulation). Conversely, prolonged decreases in neurotransmission are associated with compensatory increases in receptor numbers (up-regulation). These changes may be regarded as the brain's attempt to maintain a normal level of neurotransmission at a synapse when the effectiveness of transynaptic signaling has been altered. The changes that occur are almost invariably in number while the affinity a receptor has for its ligand generally remains unchanged. (This general rule disregards the rapid transitions between the high- and low-affinity states that receptors undergo in response to ligand interactions, as described above.) They do not appear to involve a change in mRNA production, suggesting that the mechanism responsible for these changes involves alterations in the receptor protein translation rate. Significant changes in receptor number generally require seven to 14 days of continuously altered neurotransmission. Thus, receptor-site up- and down-regulation represents a more chronic form of homeostatic regulation.

Receptor number changes have been well documented under both experimental and clinical conditions. For example, toxin-induced ablation of DA neurons in rats or that which occurs naturally in patients with Parkinson's disease increases DA receptor number in target structures of DA neurons. Since drugs generally alter neurotransmitter action, they can similarly influence receptor number. The chronic administration of a DA agonist, for instance, leads to compensatory DA receptor down-regulation which reduces the drug's potency and leads to pharmacodynamic tolerance. Such down-regulation, of course, also reduces the efficacy of any released DA. Conversely, chronic administration of a DA antagonist leads to a compensatory up-regulation of DA receptors. This is often called "receptor hypersensitivity"—a misnomer because it suggests alterations in affinity or second-messenger coupling rather than a change in receptor number. Such up-regulation also leads to pharmacodynamic tolerance since a larger dose of an antagonist would need to be administered to block the increased number of receptors. Just as up- and down-regulation require a period to develop, they also take weeks, and in some cases, months to revert to normal. Discontinuation of chronic DA antagonist treatment and clearance of the drug from the body "unmasks" an up-regulated field of receptors. As a result, normal levels of released DA will be interacting with an increased density of DA receptors, producing increased DA activity across the synapse. If this occurs in the striatum, dyskinetic movements will result. Such a mechanism is thought to contribute to the development of the movement disorder called tardive dyskinesia: a frequent complication of withdrawal from antipsychotic therapy. Since receptor alterations can dramatically influence drug effectiveness, various strategies have been developed to minimize their impact on drug effectiveness. These strategies will be described in later chapters.

RECEPTOR LOCATION AND ACTION

Where a receptor is located on a neuron influences its function. Receptor locations fall into two general categories: postsynaptic and presynaptic. Postsynaptic receptors are found on the membrane of a target neuron at a synapse. In axodendritic and axosomatic synapses, the postsynaptic receptor is on the dendrites and cell body, respectively, of the target neuron. Postsynaptic receptors situated on the cell body, especially if they are near the axon hillock, will have a more profound effect on the postsynaptic neuron's ability to generate an action potential than those located on the dendrites. Since an axon hillock integrates the effects of all the alterations in polarity that have occurred in its dendritic field and cell body, the closer a synapse is to this area of integration, the more influential the graded potential generated by that synapse is likely to be. Within the dendritic field, receptors that mediate depolarization are often located more distally while receptors that mediate inhibition, especially those employing Cl^-, are more proximal.

Presynaptic receptors are located on the membrane of the neuron that is releasing the neurotransmitter. They fall into two broad categories: autoreceptors and heteroreceptors.

An autoreceptor is a presynaptic receptor located on the cell body, terminal bouton, or varicosity that binds the neurotransmitter released by that neuron. Thus, when a presynaptic terminal releases a neurotransmitter, it can bind to postsynaptic receptors located on another neuron or to autoreceptors on the presynaptic terminal. Agonist action at the autoreceptor by the released neurotransmitter reduces future release of that same neurotransmitter. Release of NE, for example, activates the NE autoreceptor on the noradrenergic terminal (designated alpha$_2$), reducing the amount of NE the next depolarization will release. All small-molecule neurotransmitters have this form of autoreceptor-mediated regulation. Since the autoreceptor is found on the presynaptic terminal beside the actual release site, autoreceptor activation occurs only when there is enough neurotransmitter at the release site to diffuse away from postsynaptic receptors or catabolic enzymes. This negative feedback thus conserves neurotransmitter. Autoreceptors are generally metabotropic and their activation reduces future neurotransmitter release by altering the phosphorylation status of proteins at the release site (Fig. 3–6). Such alterations can decrease neurotransmitter synthesis (e.g., reduce affinity of synthesizing enzymes for cofactors), reduce activity of the voltage-gated

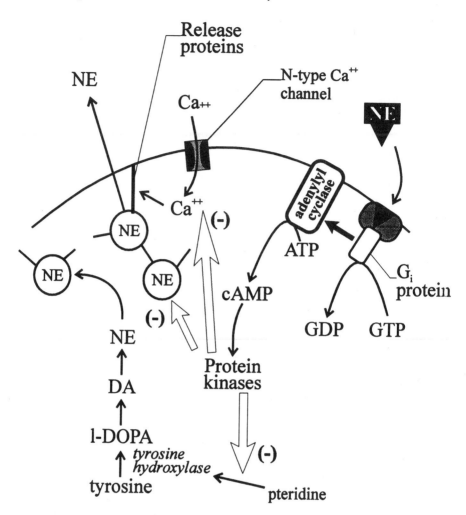

Figure 3–6. Activation of the alpha$_2$ autoreceptor has a net inhibitory effect on future neurotransmitter release through a variety of potential mechanisms. By inhibiting the activation of protein kinases which in turn influence the affinity of the cofactor pteridine for the enzyme tyrosine hydroxylase, the activity of proteins involved in vesicular exocytosis, or the activity of the voltage-gated Ca^{2+} channel, subsequent depolarizations will release less norepinephrine (NE).

Ca^{2+} channel, and reduce function of proteins responsible for neurotransmitter mobilization.

Heteroreceptors are also located presynaptically but they bind neurotransmitters other than those released by the terminal bouton on which they reside. Like autoreceptors, heteroreceptors regulate how much neurotransmitter is released. However, this regulation occurs as a result of the release of a neurotransmitter from another neuron. A heteroreceptor is therefore the postsynaptic receptor of an axoaxonic synapse. Unlike autoreceptors, heteroreceptors can be ionotropic or metabotropic. Since the amount of neurotransmitter released depends on the magnitude and duration of terminal depolarization, ionotropic heteroreceptors that depolarize the neuron potentiate neurotransmitter release. Ionotropic heteroreceptors that enhance K^+ or Cl^- conductance would neutralize the degree of depolarization and reduce neurotransmitter release. Metabotropic heteroreceptors can alter phosphorylation status and this could also influence voltage-gated channels or any of the other processes regulating Ca^{2+} conductance and neurotransmitter release. A heteroreceptor action that increases neurotransmitter release produces presynaptic facilitation, while a heteroreceptor action that reduces transmitter release would produce presynaptic inhibition. Enkephalin, released by a local interneuron in the substantia gelatinosa of the spinal cord, reduces the release of Sub P via a heteroreceptor and provides an excellent example of presynaptic inhibition (see Chapter 4). It is important to appreciate that presynaptic facilitation and inhibition do not influence the ability of the neuron to fire an action potential; they only affect its ability to release neurotransmitter. Only axodendritic, axosomatic, and dendrodendritic synapses regulate the generation of an action potential.

DOSE-RESPONSE RELATIONSHIPS

The action of a neurotransmitter or drug at its receptor is often described in terms of its dose dependency. Whether an ionotropic or metabotropic receptor is involved, the greater the number of receptors occupied, the greater the response. These dose-response relationships are most appropriately described as the log of the concentration of the ligand (generally plotted on the x-axis) vs. the percentage of maximum response (plotted on the y-axis). When plotted in these units, the resulting curve exhibits a typical sigmoidal or S shape (Fig. 3–7). Three basic assumptions underlie this relationship: (1) Only one molecule can occupy the receptor at any one time, (2) the ligand–receptor interaction is reversible and is governed by the rules of mass action, and (3) the action at the receptor is responsible for the response measured—i.e., the number of receptors occupied is proportional to the observed effect. Although these assumptions apply to any ligand–substrate interaction, we will be concerned only with the drug–receptor interaction.

"Mass action" means that a drug interacts with its receptor in the totally random fashion of Brownian motion that is not directed in any way. A direct collision results in the drug molecule binding to its receptor reversibly. Based on this assumption, the probability of collision is small if

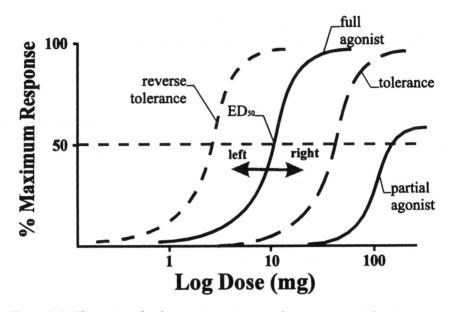

Figure 3–7. The action of a drug at its receptor produces a response that is proportional to the log of the dose administered. Log-dose response curves are generally plotted against the percent maximal response as shown in this figure. Dose-response curves can shift left or right as a result of reverse tolerance or normal tolerance, respectively. This would also alter the effective dose 50% (ED_{50}) for that drug. If a drug cannot induce a full response it is a partial agonist.

the drug is present at a low concentration while the collision rate is high at saturating concentrations of the drug. It is further assumed that the response observed is proportional to the number of receptors occupied. Thus, when low concentrations of a drug are present, the response is small, while at saturating concentrations, the response is maximal. In the middle or linear region of the S-shaped response curve, the response observed is directly proportional to the concentration. Within this range, it can be shown mathematically that the slope of the concentration–effect curve is measuring the rate of channel activation. As drug concentrations increase, however, the rate of channel activation reaches a maximal response and further increases have no effect.

Dose-response relationships can be very informative about the efficacy of a drug under study. Efficacy is defined in terms of a drug's ability to produce a maximal response. In the brain, drugs often mimic the actions of neurotransmitters, so they have full efficacy if they induce a response equivalent to that of the endogenous neurotransmitter under study (full agonists). Note that the use of the term efficacy does not require a unit of concentration. All it suggests is that at some administered dose, a maximal response can be achieved. Drugs that do not have full efficacy are called partial agonists. The administration of a partial agonist produces a sigmoidal dose-response curve but one that does not achieve a maximal effect (Fig. 3-7). A partial agonist has affinity for the receptor but not full efficacy, presumably because the molecule does not fit into the binding site of the receptor protein well enough to induce the complete conformational change needed to produce the response.

The term potency refers to the amount of drug required to achieve a specified response. Its units are generally stated in mg/kg. In medicine potency is best determined by examining the effects of a drug on a population of study subjects (although it can also be derived from a log–dose-response curve). If the desired drug effect is vasoconstriction that produces a 10-mmHg rise in blood pressure, various doses will be administered to a group of animals and their blood pressures will be measured. As dosage is increased, a greater percentage of the population will achieve the 10-mmHg rise in blood pressure. If a drug is working through a single receptor subtype (alpha$_1$ in this case) to produce its effect, there will be an administered dose that does not produce the criterion in any animal and one that produces the effect in all of the animals. The x-axis is mg/kg drug and the y-axis is the percentage of subjects achieving a criterion response. Like the dose-response curve, the effective dose-response curve is sigmoidal. The points on the curve determine the percentage of the population in which the drug is effective, i.e., the effective dose. Thus, the ED$_{50}$ is the *effective dose* at which 50% of the population would respond appropriately to the drug. The relative potencies of different drugs are generally determined by comparing their ED$_{50}$ values.

Potency is often confused with efficacy. This confusion over terms is commonly exploited in the promotion of over-the-counter medications to the public. Thus, "our headache medicine is three times more potent than aspirin" is often taken to mean that the drug possesses three times the headache relief capability. This is not true. It just means that the consumer has to take only one-third the amount of drug to obtain the same effect.

Therapeutic Index

The discussion thus far has focused on the efficacy and potency of a drug in exerting its desired actions. However, a drug may not be useful if it produces intolerable side effects at the same dose at which it produces efficacy. Just as the efficacy and potency of a drug in producing a desired effect are determined by performing dose-response studies, the same strategy can be used to examine toxic effects. For toxicity studies, however, the effect being measured is a side effect (toxic effect). Like the potency dose-response curve, toxicity is best measured in a study population.

When a drug is being developed, one aspect of its action that is assessed is its ability to kill a test animal. The dose at which half of the animals die is referred to as the LD_{50} or lethal dose 50%. This value is then used to establish a meaningful potency measure called the therapeutic index. Therapeutic index (TI) is defined as LD_{50}/ED_{50}. A drug with a high therapeutic index such as diazepam (TI > 1,000) can be used safely under most circumstances because, barring an idiosyncratic response, the dose needed to induce a useful clinical effect is more than 1,000 times lower than the dose that kills. In contrast, the general anesthetics have very low TIs because the dose needed to induce full anesthesia is usually only two to four times lower than that which will cause death.

As defined above, TI cannot be measured in humans. One cannot increase the dose until it kills a human subject. The underlying premise associated with the TI, however, is still useful in comparing the relative safety of drugs. A second convention has therefore been adopted that defines TI as TD_{50}/ED_{50}, where TD_{50} stands for toxic-dose 50%. To determine the therapeutic index in this way, a specified toxic response is monitored in patients. Drugs that induce vasoconstriction, for instance, often produce headaches. In dose-response studies on the vasoconstricting action of an $alpha_1$ agonist, the number of patients complaining of headaches would be monitored. During such studies, enough data are usually collected to establish the dose that produces headaches. Although the higher ends of these types of curves must often be extrapolated for ethical reasons, a toxic profile of the drug can be obtained.

To be completely accurate, a drug's TI should always be stated in terms of a specific side effect. Suppose the TI is 4.3 for headaches and 10.4 for heart palpitations. This means that if a drug is effective in half the population at 10 mg/kg, 50% of the population would be expected to experience a headache at 43 mg/kg while the dose needed to produce heart palpitations in 50% would be 104 mg/kg. This is not to say that the drug would not produce headaches or heart palpitations in a small percentage of patients at 10 mg/kg. The slopes of the dose-response curves for desired efficacy, headaches, and heart palpitations can be dramatically different from one another. Therefore, the TI can only be used as a relative reference point for drug comparisons and not as an absolute index of safety. In addition, one must always remember that when a drug is administered to large populations, the probability of an idiosyncratic response increases. Just because a drug has a high TI does not mean it is safe for use in all patients.

Therapeutic Range

To produce a desired effect, some minimum or threshold concentration of a drug must be present in the plasma. If plasma levels are above a certain range however, toxic effects are often observed. The minimum plasma concentration at which patients receive therapeutic benefit from a drug defines the low end while the plasma level at which intolerable side effects occur defines the high end of a therapeutic range. The therapeutic range thus establishes an acceptable working range of plasma concentrations in which least efficacy is obtained and unwanted side effects are not observed. (A variation of this notion is the therapeutic window where the high end of the plasma concentration is not associated with side effects but rather with loss of therapeutic efficacy.) Plasma levels of a drug are often measured to determine if an administered dose is yielding blood levels that fall within the therapeutic range. Perhaps a patient or animal is not exhibiting the desired effect because biotransformation rates are idiosyncratically high in the test subject. Perhaps the prescription is appropriate but the patient is not taking the drug (noncompliance). Without measuring plasma levels of a drug to determine whether they are within the therapeutic range, one cannot tell whether the individual is not responding to the drug or simply not taking enough of the drug.

Therapeutic ranges have been established for many peripherally acting drugs and can be narrow or wide depending on the side effect being evaluated and the tolerableness needed. (Drugs that induced emesis in 35% of the general population would not be tolerated in over-the-counter medications but are quite common in chemotherapy.) Unfortunately, plasma levels are not always useful for many centrally acting drugs because of the BBB. Brain levels of a drug are generally lower than plasma levels but can sometimes be higher. Generally, CSF drug levels are more reliable predictors of efficacy when they can be obtained. However, even if plasma levels do reflect the level of a drug in the brain, other factors, such as the stage of disease and drug tolerance, can influence the relationship between plasma drug level and therapeutic efficacy. Presuming that a drug can enter the CNS, other measures have been used to establish a therapeutic range and will be discussed with the appropriate drug classes in the chapters that follow.

As anyone with children knows, the dose administered to a child is generally lower than that given to an adult. Since the child's body is smaller, less volume is available for drug distribution. Therefore, given the same administered dose of a drug to a child and an adult, the child will have a higher plasma concentration than the adult. The actual dose of the drug administered to a patient is called the absolute dose. When a dose is based on some unit of body weight (i.e., mg/kg), it is termed a relative dose. Normally the relative dose of a drug is determined by the kg weight of the body. It is important to note, however, that brain weight and body weight do not necessarily increase at the same rate and can be an important consideration when administering drugs to neonates.

One final point should be made concerning dose-response curves. I call it "wiggle room." Drugs that are very potent often have steep linear phases in their dose-response curves. With these drugs, a slight increase in an administered dose can produce a dramatic increase in effect because the slope of the dose-response curve is so steep. The slight increase can readily produce toxic effects, especially if the drug has a low TI. In contrast, with drugs that have a broad dose-response curve, slight increases in an administered dose do not increase the desired effect or induce toxicity as readily. The plasma levels of drugs with broad dose-response curves can therefore be adjusted more smoothly to generate better control over the desired effect while minimizing the risk of side effects. You have more "wiggle room" in the dosing schedule. Highly potent street drugs often produce overdoses because their dose-response curves have too little wiggle room.

Shifts in the Dose-Response Curve

A number of factors can alter the dose-response curve, especially in a lateral direction. The classic example is tolerance. If an agonist is administered and pharmacokinetic, physiologic, or behavioral tolerance develops, the curve shifts to the right (Fig. 3–7). The drug, by definition, becomes less potent. In the case of reverse tolerance, the dose-response curve would shift to the left (increase in potency). Pharmacodynamic tolerance also results in a shift to the right. However, if receptor down-regulation or desensitization occurs, it is easy to envision that 100% receptor occupancy might not yield a 100% maximal response relative to the pretreatment dose-response curve. The curve would then take on the shape of that produced by a partial agonist (sigmoidal but not able to achieve a 100% response). Since the measured response depends on receptor occupancy at a given dose and, in the case of metabotropic receptors, involves a cascade of protein structural alterations, a drug may have the same affinity for its acceptor site but reduced ability to induce a response. Thus, the drug still binds to the receptor with the same avidity but the receptor may have become uncoupled from the G protein. Dose-response curves, although they are very useful for comparing drugs, do not necessarily reveal the subtle alterations in the receptor–response alterations that can sometimes occur. More sophisticated analyses are often required to determine the mechanisms responsible for alterations in the shapes of dose-response curves.

A shift to the right of a dose-response curve would also be seen when an agonist is administered in the presence of an antagonist. This shift would be parallel, indicating a reduction in potency if the agonist and antagonist were competing for the same binding site. If a percentage of the receptor population were occupied by the antagonist, fewer receptors would be available for activation by the agonist drug and its potency would consequently decline. Because the agonist and antagonist were both competing for the same site, an administered dose of an agonist sufficient to "out-compete" the antagonist could eventually be administered. If, for example, 500 molecules of agonist and 500 of an antagonist were administered, the probability of receptor occupancy by the agonist or antagonist would be 50%. However, if 5,000,000 molecules of agonist and 500 of an antagonist were administered, according to the law of mass action, the probability of an agonist occupying the receptor would be 99.99%. The action of an antagonist that competes for the same binding site as does the agonist is thus said to be surmountable. If the effect of an antagonist is surmountable by its respective agonist, the antagonist is called a competitive antagonist (the same applies for agonists; i.e., the effect of a competitive agonist is surmountable by excess neurotransmitter). In contrast, the administration of an antagonist that does not compete for the same site as does the agonist is generally not surmountable and produces not only a shift to the right in the dose-response curve, but a change in the shape of the curve itself. (The shift is not parallel but the slope of the linear phase changes.) This type of noncompetitive inhibition would occur if the antagonist's binding site alters the affinity of the drug acceptor for the agonist. The shape of dose-response curves can therefore be very informative about the action of an unknown drug and is commonly used in research.

Opioid Analgesics and Pain

Prototypic agent: *Morphine*

*E*veryone reading this book has experienced pain. It varies in intensity and quality and has been defined as an "unpleasant sensory and emotional experience associated with actual or potential tissue damage" (Mersky, 1986). Pain serves a critical protective function by alerting the organism to the existence of tissue damage. Without it, an organism would continue an activity that could potentially worsen the damage. Pain fibers initiate withdrawal reflexes within the spinal cord to provide protection prior to the conscious perception of pain. Pain fibers entering the brain permit a conscious perception of pain that helps identify the location and extent of tissue damage. Collateral pathways of this system may also disrupt ongoing neuronal activity and alter behavior such that it interferes with the healing process. Thus, just as pain serves a protective purpose, the act of alleviating it with analgesic agents can also serve a purpose beyond simple relief.

Three types of pain exist: somatic, visceral, and deafferentation. Somatic pain is the traditional form of pain associated with tissue injury. It results from the stimulation of nociceptive pain fibers, is well localized, and can be readily described by the patient as an aching or sharp sensation. After the initial sharp, pain sensation (fast pain), a dull, aching pain (slow pain) often follows. Visceral pain is qualitatively similar to somatic pain and has the same kind of source but is experienced in the thoracic or abdominal cavity and is often poorly localized or perceived in a location other than the actual site of tissue damage (referred pain). Deafferentation pain is often an extremely intense pain that is unfamiliar to the patient. Described as "vise-like," "shooting," or "electric-like," it is thought to result from neural damage (thus deafferentation) not associated with the nociceptive system. Peripheral neuropathies, postherpetic neuralgia, trigeminal neuralgia (tic douloureux), and thalamic pain secondary to stroke are examples. The anticonvulsants carbamazepine, phenytoin, and valproic acid (Swerdlow, 1984) or corticosteroids (Foley, 1985) are useful in managing deafferentation pain.

Just as the sensation of pain varies in its intensity and quality, so, too, does the emotional response to that sensation. Pain should thus be characterized on both a physical and an emotional plane—the nature of pain is dual. The highly complex interaction between these two planes influences not only the patient's ability to cope with the pain but also the physician's ability to control that pain with drugs. The complex nature of the pain experience is reflected in the anatomy of the pain pathway.

PAIN AND THE PAIN PATHWAY

The sensation of pain originates at specific nociceptive transducers that, in contrast to other sensory modalities, do not possess specialized nerve endings. Nociceptive transducers are simply free nerve endings (Fig. 4–1) that respond to a variety of noxious stimuli including heat, pressure, pH changes, caustic chemicals, and transection. Pain terminals possess specific receptors for bradykinin, histamine, acetylcholine (ACh), and serotonin (5HT), all of which induce depolarization in the sensory afferent nerves that we eventually come to recognize as pain.

Pain is transmitted to the CNS by thinly myelinated or unmyelinated peripheral nerves. Fast pain is thought to result from activation of thinly myelinated, small-diameter fibers (A-delta fibers) that conduct impulses rapidly into the CNS, inducing an immediate response. These A-delta fibers participate in withdrawal reflexes and are thought to be primarily responsible for pain localization. Their activation produces an intense, sharp, or stinging type of pain. Slow pain is transmitted along unmyelinated C fibers. It is the slow, burning, or aching pain that produces most of the perceptual discomfort and is also the pain most readily relieved by the opioid analgesics (Torebjork and Hallin, 1979). These fibers use substance P (Sub P) or glutamate (Glu) as neurotransmitter (Evans, Hammond, and Frederickson, 1988).

As with most sensations, the intensity of pain is coded by frequency. Stimulation of the nociceptive free nerve endings induces a graded or local depolarization that activates a special segment (initial segment) near the terminal. Like the axon hillock of most neurons, the initial segment has a high density of voltage-gated Na^+ channels so it is likely to activate an action potential following an influx of positive current. The degree of

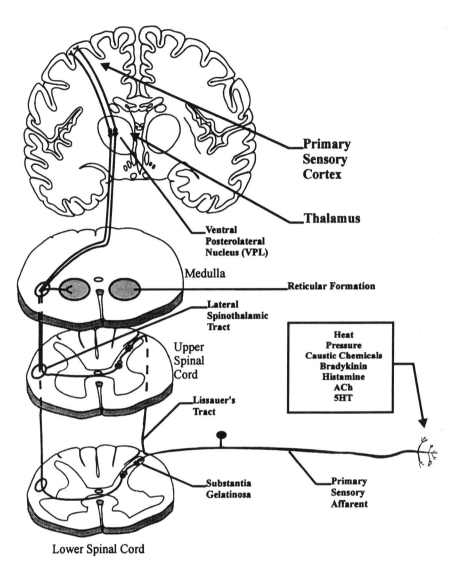

Figure 4–1. The neospinothalamic tract is excited by a variety of conditions (box) that induce depolarization in the primary sensory afferent which projects to the spinal cord. Branches of this nerve ascend or descend a few segments in Lissauer's tract and synapse on interneurons in the substantia gelatinosa. Most fibers cross at the segmental level and ascend, giving off collaterals in the medulla to excite the reticular formation. The fibers continue up to the ventral posterolateral nucleus of the thalamus where they synapse on fibers that project to the primary sensory cortex for pain localization.

terminal stimulation does not adapt and continues to initiate generator potentials, the frequency of which determines the intensity of the pain sensation.

The vast majority of pain fibers enter the spinal cord through the dorsal root and synapse predominantly in the substantia gelatinosa (see Payne and Pasternak, 1992). A-delta fibers synapse in the substantia gelatinosa; then they give rise to fibers that mostly cross the spinal cord and ascend in the neospinothalamic tract carrying nociceptive information to the ventroposterolateral (VPL) nucleus of the thalamus where they synapse on fibers that project to the ipsilateral primary sensory cortex in the parietal lobe. This pathway gives off collaterals to the reticular formation, as well. The neospinothalamic tract thus primarily carries A-delta, fast-pain activity and is thought to be largely responsible for pain localization.

C fibers primarily synapse in the substantia gelatinosa (lamina II) and make multiple synaptic connections with fibers that then enter laminae I and V. Fibers from these nerves again mostly cross to the contralateral side and ascend in the spinothalamic tract via the paleospinothalamic tract. Unlike fibers of the neospinothalamic tract, paleospinothalamic fibers make multiple connections in the brain as they ascend to the thalamus. Collaterals of these fibers invade the reticular formation and the periaqueductal gray (PAG) before entering the medial and posterior thalamic nuclei and intralaminar nuclei of the thalamus (Fig. 4–2). Neurons in the thalamus innervated by the ascending fibers of the paleospinothalamic tract project heavily to a variety of cortical and subcortical limbic regions while only a few fibers project to the primary sensory cortex. Projections to the hypothalamus likely mediate the autonomic response to pain while projections to the amygdala likely play a central role in pain memory. Unlike the neospinothalamic pathway, the paleospinothalamic pathway is not topographically organized and, as a result, the slow-pain component carried by this pathway is not as readily localized. Thus, the ascending nociceptive pathway localizes pain through the topographically organized neospinothalamic tract while the paleospinothalamic tract activates limbic regions of the brain that are most likely involved in pain discomfort—the dual nature of pain is therefore reflected in its afferent pathways.

The notion of a "pain gate" suggests that the intensity of pain can be controlled. Just as a gate in a fence swings open and then closed, the intensity of pain can wax and wane. The observation that rubbing a painful area can reduce the intensity of the pain led to the hypothesis that stimulation of non-nociceptive afferent fibers entering the spinal cord from the area of the painful stimulus somehow reduced activity in the nociceptive system (Melzack and Wall, 1984). The gate metaphor expressed the view

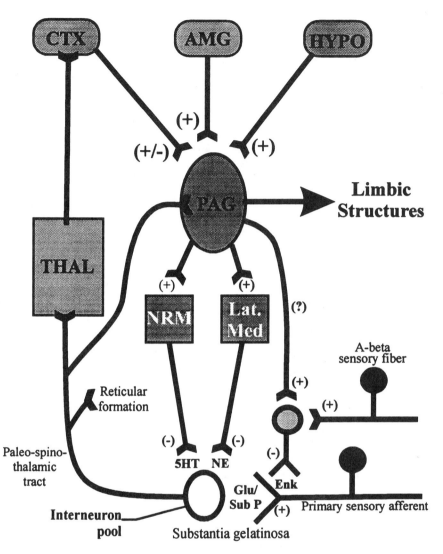

Figure 4–2. The various connections of the periaqueductal gray (PAG) system are depicted in this schematic. The PAG is rich in enkephalin (Enk) receptors that regulate several target structures. Efferent fibers from the PAG are known to enhance activity in the nucleus raphe magnus (NRM) and the lateral medulla (Lat Med), both of which descend into the spinal cord to influence activity in the interneuron pool in the dorsal horn using serotonin (5HT) and norepinephrine (NE) as neurotransmitters, respectively. Efferent fibers from the PAG may also descend to activate Enk interneurons in the substantia gelatinosa region of the dorsal horn. Activity in the PAG is regulated by the cerebral cortex (CTX), the amygdala (AMG), and the hypothalamus (HYPO). Ascending collaterals from the lateral paleospinothalamic tract that invade the PAG make connections that eventually invade several forebrain limbic regions. These connections are thought to be responsible for the dull-pain-and-suffering component of pain.

that activity in the primary pain afferent was not affected and indicated that the pain "gate" could be closed, open, or partially open depending on the intensity of the activity in other sensory fibers. The exact mechanism which gate theory presupposes remains unknown but is thought to involve vibration-sensitive fiber activation of the polysynaptic pathways in the dorsal horn that reduce the release of Sub P from the primary nociceptive afferent (Fig. 4–2). Mechanical devices are still used today in some patients to "vibrate" tissue in painful areas, thereby reducing the intensity of intractable pain. It was also recognized early on that the emotional state of an individual or the ability to consciously suppress the perception of pain might also be involved with this hypothesized gate system. This suggested that the pain gate was also regulated by suprasegmental systems that descended into the spinal cord to regulate the degree to which primary nociceptive activity could enter the spinal cord. Thus, soldiers returning home from World War II with severe injuries reported significantly less pain than did individuals with similar injuries here in the United States, presumably because the relief of surviving the war resulted in suprasegmental activity patterns that suppressed afferent pain perception (Beecher, 1946). The principles involved in the gate theory were the impetus for a long series of studies that eventually led to the discovery of the endogenous substances responsible for regulating the gate: the opioid peptides.

THE OPIOID PEPTIDES

It was known for centuries that extracts of the poppy seed (opium) could reduce pain and induce a "dream-like" euphoric state. From extractions of opium, morphine (named after the Greek god of dreams, Morpheus) was identified as the most active component. Codeine and papaverine are also active components in opium. The later discovery of the enkephalin system resulted from a search for the endogenous site where morphine is bound (Lasagna and Beecher, 1954; Pert and Snyder, 1973). After the receptor was identified, three major families of endogenous opium-like substances referred to today as the opioid peptides were discovered. (In today's nomenclature, the term opioid includes all endogenous and synthetic agents with opium-like properties.)

The three major endogenous opioid families are the enkephalins, the dynorphins, and the endorphins, all of which are peptides of varying length that produce analgesic effects and other CNS actions. Like all neuropeptides, these opioids are derived from larger precursor proteins that undergo progressive cleavage to yield smaller polypeptides with differing properties. The best-known opioid precursor peptide is pro-opiomelanocortin (POMC) (Fig. 4–3). As a result of the action of various peptidases, POMC can yield adrenocorticotrophin (ACTH), alpha-melanocyte-stimulating hormone (alpha-MSH), beta-lipotropin (B-LPH), beta-endorphin, and beta-MSH. Although POMC contains the sequence for the primary morphine-like neurotransmitter met-enkephalin, this is not a normal product of POMC. Rather, nerves that release enkephalin (enkephalinergic neurons) contain proenkephalin precursor molecules that yield many copies of the pentapeptides met- and leu-enkephalin (Enk) (Fig. 4–3). Met- and leu-Enk share the same four-amino-acid sequence (Tyr-Gly-Gly-Phe-*) but differ in one amino acid. (* = leucine or methionine for Leu- and Met-Enk, respectively). The precursor molecule for the dynorphins is prodynorphin. Prodynorphin is biotransformed to dynorphins A and B. Neurons containing these substances are found throughout the CNS and spinal cord. With the probable exception of met- and leu-Enk, the products of these precursor polypeptides may also have paracrine- or even hormone-like effects. Thus, they may be released from a neuron or other cell and diffuse locally through the extracellular space (paracrine) or through the blood (hormone) to influence target systems some distance away.

Enkephalin (Enk) as a Neurotransmitter

Although not yet elevated to true neurotransmitter status, the pentapeptides leu- and met-Enk released from enkephalinergic neurons are found throughout the pain axis and also in other areas of the brain. As large-molecule neurotransmitters, the enkephalins are synthesized in the neuronal cell body by the Golgi apparatus, transported to the terminal by axoplasmic transport, and stored in large vesicles. In addition, once they are released, they are not taken back up into the nerve terminal but rather are biotransformed by nonspecific peptidases.

Where studied, enkephalin acts through G proteins to inhibit cAMP formation (see Herz, 1993, for review). As a result, enkephalin increases outward K^+ conductance, leading to reduced excitability or hyperpolarization. Enkephalin also inhibits N-type Ca^{2+} channels thereby reducing neurotransmitter release. The enkephalins are often colocalized with small-molecule neurotransmitters such as GABA but the implications of this colocalization are unknown.

At several locations along the pain pathway, activation of enkephalin receptors can reduce pain at both the spinal and the suprasegmental level. (In discussions of pain pathways, "supraspinal" is the convention used to refer to "suprasegmental," a convention that will be used in the remainder of this chapter for consistency.) In the substantia gelatinosa, Enk reduces the release of Sub P from C fiber terminals (Basbaum, 1984). As a

Pro-opiomelanocortin

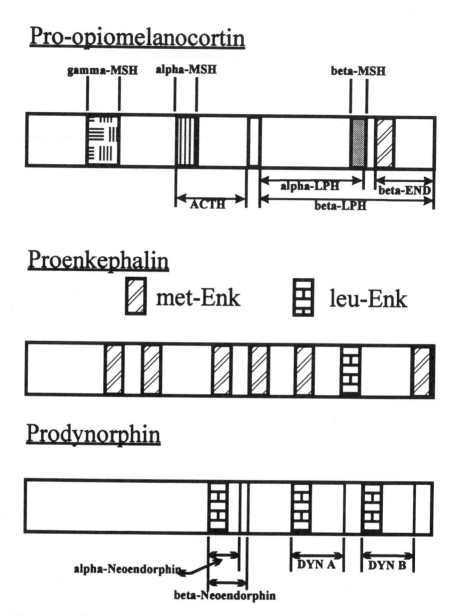

Figure 4–3. The three currently known opioid precursor proteins are shown. Each peptide is successively cleaved into smaller peptides. Pro-opiomelanocortin yields several active peptides including gamma-, alpha-, and beta-melanocyte-stimulating hormone (MSH), adrenocorticotropic hormone (ACTH), alpha- and beta-lipotropin (LPH), and beta-endorphin (END). Proenkephalin is degraded to yield six copies of methionine enkephalin (met-Enk) and one copy of leucine enkephalin (leu-Enk). The third opiate precursor protein is prodynorphin. Embedded within its structure are the endorphins alpha and beta neoendorphin as well as dynorphin (DYN) A and B. (Adapted from Cooper, Bloom, and Roth, 1996, with permission.)

result, nociceptive activity is reduced at its site of entry into the CNS (the dorsal horn), consistent with gate theory. Enkephalins are also found in the periaqueductal gray where they produce profound analgesia following the infusion of opiates or electrical stimulation (Bodnar et al., 1988). The action of opioids in the periaqueductal gray likely reduces ascending paleospinothalamic activity while enhancing the activity of antinociceptive fibers descending into the dorsal horn. As seen in Figure 4–2, activation of the periaqueductal gray increases activity in the nucleus raphe magnus that, via descending serotonergic projections into the spinal cord, inhibits the activity of the spinothalamic tract. The periaqueductal gray also activates lateral medullary groups whose descending noradrenergic projections similarly reduce pain transmission. Drugs such as amitriptyline and amphetamine that increase the activity of 5HT and NE, respectively, enhance the analgesic efficacy of opioid drugs. In addition, drugs that influence limbic, cortical areas, the amygdala, and the hypothalamus can also alter pain thresholds, by virtue of their efferent projections to the periaqueductal gray. The periaqueductal gray system is therefore consistent with gate theory and explains the analgesic-potentiating effects of several drugs outside the opioid class. This system is also consistent with the putative involvement of the enkephalins with other phenomena including the runner's high (Heitkamp, Huber, and Schieb, 1996), "placebo effects" (Levine, Gordon, and Fields, 1979), and acupuncture (Mayer, Price, and Rafii, 1977).

The Opioid Receptor System

Three opioid receptor families exist: mu, kappa, and delta (Table 4–1). An epsilon receptor has also been proposed and may selectively mediate the analgesic actions of beta-endorphin (Schultz, Wuster, and Herz, 1981). As in all the receptor families thus far studied, subtypes also exist.

Mu receptors

The original analgesic binding site was designated mu because of its association with morphine binding. It eventually became apparent, however, that there were two distinct binding sites that are now designated mu_1 and mu_2 (Pasternak, Childers, and Snyder, 1980). Mu_1 binding sites are predominantly located at supraspinal levels and are most concentrated in the periaqueductal gray, the raphe, the locus ceruleus, and the gigantocellular region of the brainstem. They are thought to mediate supraspinal analgesia and participate in the euphoric and sedative effects of the opioid agents. In addition, mu_1 receptors modulate the actions of other neurotransmitters within the CNS such as GABA and DA which are likely involved with the rigidity, dependence liability,

Table 4–1 Opioid Receptor Subtypes and Functions[a]

Receptor Subtype	Analgesia Location	Other Actions
Mu		Miosis
Mu$_1$	Supraspinal (PAG, NRM, and LC)	Euphoria, sedation, dependence, increases prolactin release and DA turnover; decreases GABA release
Mu$_2$	Spinal, lower brainstem, and myenteric plexus	Spinal analgesia, respiratory depression; decreases GH release and gastrointestinal transit; antitussive actions, and emetic effects
Kappa		Miosis, reduced DA activity
Kappa$_1$	Spinal and cerebellum	ADH inhibition, constipation, and sedation
Kappa$_2$	Unknown	Unknown
Kappa$_3$	Supraspinal (similar to mu$_1$)	Analgesia
Delta		Increased GH release (?) Increased DA turnover
Delta$_1$	Supraspinal	Analgesia
Delta$_2$	Spinal	
Epsilon	(?)	Beta-endorphin mediation

[a]PAG = periaqueductal gray, NRM = n. raphe magnus, LC = locus ceruleus, GH = growth hormone, ADH = antidiuretic hormone

and effects on prolactin release associated with morphine use. Mu$_2$ receptors are found predominantly in the lower brainstem, the spinal cord, and the myenteric plexus. Mu$_2$ receptors mediate spinal analgesia, constipation, and respiratory depression and may participate in the antitussive and emetic actions of opioid agents as well. While morphine binds to both sites with approximately equal affinity, the endogenous enkephalins prefer the mu$_2$ site. Mu receptors, by activating PANS innervation of the pupil, produce miosis that characteristically accompanies opioid use, although the receptor subtype responsible has not been determined.

Kappa receptors

Three subtypes have currently been characterized in receptor binding studies (Payne and Pasternak, 1992). Kappa$_1$ receptors contribute to the sedative actions of the opioids and participate in their constipating effects, as well. Kappa$_3$ receptors clearly participate in supraspinal analgesia. Their supraspinal distribution is similar to that of the mu$_1$ receptor although they are less concentrated in the periaqueductal gray. Little is known about the actions of the kappa$_2$ receptor.

Delta receptors

Two delta-receptor subtypes are currently known (Pasternak, 1993). Delta$_1$ receptors are thought to participate in supraspinal analgesia although controversy still surrounds their analgesic mechanism. Delta$_1$ receptors are found throughout the limbic system. Delta$_2$ sites are distributed predominantly in the spinal cord where they mediate spinal analgesia. Delta receptors have very high affinity for Enk and may be responsible for many enkephalin-mediated effects.

It is assumed that the actions and side effects that accompany opioid use are mediated through these receptor subtypes. Unfortunately, numerous questions involving receptor-subtype distribution, actions, and relationships with the varied effects of the opioid drug class remain. Although our understanding is incomplete, several of the effects of opioid drugs have been well characterized, revealing the rich pharmacodynamic diversity of this important and widely prescribed drug class.

PHARMACODYNAMICS OF THE OPIOID DRUG CLASS

As a drug class, the opioids can reduce pain without significant sedation or interference with other sensory modalities. Other drugs with analgesic properties, including the nonbenzodiazepine sedative-hypnotics, the anesthetics, phencyclidine (PCP), and even alcohol, alleviate pain only at doses associated with significant sedation. Thus, their analgesic actions differ from those of the opioids and the aspirin-like drugs. This is not to say that the opioids do not induce sedation. Rather, it is their ability to reduce pain at doses that do not cause sedation that is their distinguishing characteristic and that which defines a pure analgesic drug.

The opioid drugs can be classified into three groups: full agonists, partial agonists/antagonists, and full antagonists. The drugs in these classes possess varied affinities for the different receptor subtypes, and although they are all direct-acting agonists and antagonists, none of the currently available drugs is receptor-subtype specific. All members of the receptor drug class are therefore mixed agonists or antagonists. As we will see, however, some drugs prefer one receptor subtype over another and consequently possess different analgesic qualities.

Opioid Receptor Agonists

Morphine

The pharmaceutic industrial standard to which all other opioid analgesics are compared is morphine. Since it is the prototypic opioid agent, the following discussion of morphine will serve as an introduction to all of the major pharmacologic actions of the full agonists (Table 4–2).

Analgesia. Invariably, morphine is prescribed for its analgesic effects. As a highly potent agonist at mu and kappa receptors with moderate affinity for delta receptors, morphine acts at several locations throughout the neuraxis including the sinal cord. However, the analgesic action of morphine is thought to occur predominantly at the supraspinal level through mu_1- and $kappa_3$-receptor activation (Bodnar et al., 1988). Local infusion of morphine into the periaqueductal gray induces the greatest analgesic effects of all the areas studied. But many supraspinal regions where morphine binds send direct or indirect projections to the dorsal horn of the spinal cord. Thus, activation of opioid receptors in the raphe and locus ceruleus increase 5HT and NE, respectively, both of which potentiate analgesic action. Destruction of these pathways reduces morphine's analgesic potency following systemic administration (Basbaum, 1984). The involvement of 5HT and NE in pain modulation explains the increased efficacy of morphine in the presence of 5HT reuptake inhibitors such as amitriptyline and indirect-acting NE agonists such as amphetamine.

Morphine does not affect signal transduction in the terminal fields of the primary nociceptive afferent nor does it alter conduction down the primary sensory afferent. Acting through a mu_2 heteroreceptor, however, it does reduce Sub P release by C-fiber terminal boutons in the substantia gelatinosa. Delta and $kappa_1$ receptors may also participate in this action (Ling and Pasternak, 1983). Although morphine is known to act in the spinal cord, its ability to achieve adequate analgesic concentrations there is limited. Spinal-mediated analgesia following systemic morphine administration is therefore minimal. Following other routes of administration (intrathecal), however, the mu_2-, delta-, and $kappa_3$-mediated effects can become very important.

Reduction of Sub P release attenuates the ability of the primary nociceptive afferent C fiber to activate fibers that eventually form the paleospinothalamic tract. Thus, at the spinal level, morphine predominantly affects slow pain but does not significantly attenuate sharp, shooting fast pain. From a clinical perspective this is important. The thinly myelinated A-delta fibers that give rise to the neospinothalamic tract are primarily responsible for pain localization and mediate the reflex responses to pain at the spinal cord level. Remaining painfully aware of the location in which tissue damage has occurred is important for patients as they then reduce activities that would cause further damage to this area. If morphine completely suppressed fast pain activity, a patient recovering from surgery might be more likely to roll over in bed and place stress on a surgical site. However, the low potency of morphine for

Table 4–2 Morphine's Actions and Mechanisms

Action	Mechanism(s)[a]
Analgesia	Mu_1 and $kappa_3$ action at supraspinal level, especially at the periaqueductal gray; Mu_2, delta, and kappa actions in the substantia gelatinosa mediate spinal analgesia
Dependence liability	Increased DA in the n. accumbens resulting from mu_2 as well as other direct actions likely involving delta and kappa receptors
Euphoria	Mu_1 (predominantly) and delta effects as well as increased DA, decreased NE, and altered 5HT in the forebrain
Respiratory depression	Mu_2-, delta-, and kappa-mediated reduction in sensitivity to CO_2 in the medulla; depression of rhythmicity in the dorsal respiratory group of the n. tractus solitarius
Sedation	Kappa-mediated reduction in NMDA activity and other direct effects in the cortex
Cough suppression	Mu_2-, delta-, and kappa-mediated actions (?) as well as direct antagonism of Glu activity
Nausea/vomiting	Direct stimulation of the CTZ; depression of vestibular system; increased DA and 5HT mediated through supraspinal actions
Rigidity	Decreased DA activity in the nigrostriatal pathway; Enk-mediated inhibition of the globus pallidus via striatal GABAergic outflow pathways
Hormonal effects & oliguria	Mu-mediated increase in ADH; mu_1-mediated increase in prolactin; minor reductions in LH, FSH, and ACTH
Miosis	Mu_2-mediated activation of Edinger-Westphal nucleus
Hypotension	Direct histamine displacement from mast cells; delta-mediated medullary depression and smooth muscle relaxation; CO_2-mediated vasodilation in brain and heart
Constipation	Mu_2-mediated inhibition of the enteric system; supraspinal depression of descending autonomic reflexes; anorexic effects; reduced defecation reflex
Hypothermia	Hypothalamic depression
Right upper quadrant pain	Sphincter of Oddi spasm
Inhibition of labor	Smooth muscle relaxation
Urticaria	Histamine release
Morphine flush	Histamine release and reduced vasomotor tone
Anorexia	Depression of hypothalamic feeding center

[a]NMDA = N-methyl-D-aspartate (glutamate receptor), ADH = antidiuretic hormone, LH = luteinizing hormone, FSH = follicle-stimulating hormone

reducing neospinothalamic activity preserves the patient's ability to identify and react to localizing fast pain.

Morphine also affects the emotional response to pain. Recall that the paleospinothalamic tract gives rise to several collaterals as it ascends to the thalamus and that its connections in the thalamus influence the activity of a variety of cortical and subcortical limbic structures where opioid receptors are found. Under the influence of morphine, pain is still recognized as such but patients will often state that they "simply do not care about it." It is as though the suffering caused by pain has been dissociated from the sensation. This reflects morphine's ability to change the affective response to pain. It may represent the action of morphine on delta receptors that are particularly dense in limbic structures. This activity would also be expected to reduce the intensity of the perception of fast pain. Thus, even though morphine does not attenuate fast pain in the spinal cord, its actions at the supraspinal level will "take the edge off" fast pain.

Analgesia and Dependence Liability. Most studies demonstrate that morphine (1) reduces pain and suffering, (2) does not significantly interfere with diagnostically relevant pain localization, (3) alters the quality of both slow and fast pain, (4) does not completely compromise protective pain reflexes, (5) improves the patient's psychological state, which may help the healing process, and (6) rarely leads to dependence in the clinical setting. With such an impressive list of positive attributes, why is it that many physicians are reluctant to aggressively manage short-term or long-term pain with drugs such as morphine? Jaffe and Martin state in *The Pharmacological Basis of Therapeutics* that

> Some clinicians, out of an exaggerated concern for the possibility of inducing addiction, tend to prescribe initial doses of opioids that are too low or too infrequent to alleviate pain, and then respond to the patient's continued complaints with an even more exaggerated concern about drug dependence, despite the probability that the request for more drug is only the expected consequence of the inadequate dosage initially prescribed. (8th edition, page 502)

This exaggerated concern is simply not supported by the scientific literature since morphine dependence rarely occurs within the time frame of the typical postprocedural recovery period (see Newman, 1983). Thus, it is fair to say that the opioid analgesics are underprescribed and that unnecessary suffering commonly occurs. This is especially true of very young and very old patients who may not be able to convey adequately the suffering they are experiencing.

Euphorogenic Actions. The euphoric, mood-altering, and reinforcing actions of morphine probably result from opioid-receptor stimulation at several sites throughout the neuraxis. The euphoria starts as a "rush" that is highly sought after by i.v. drug abusers. In the clinical setting, where routes other than i.v. are generally used, few patients experience a rush and many find the drug's initial effect unpleasant, especially if nausea and vomiting are involved. Following the initial effect, high doses can induce a pleasant, dream-like state in which hallucinations, delusions, and significant disruptions of cognitive functioning are rarely experienced. Mu and delta receptors likely mediate this effect and morphine's ability to increase DA through its actions at mu_1 receptors in the ventral tegmental area may also be involved with this effect.

Respiratory Depression. Morphine acts in a dose-dependent fashion to depress respiration. Indeed, most deaths secondary to overdose are a direct consequence of respiratory depression. All aspects of respiration are affected (rate, tidal exchange, and minute volume). This effect is primarily mediated by mu_2 receptors located in the respiratory centers of the lower brainstem (Fig. 4–4).

Respiratory depression is a consequence of reduced responsiveness to increasing levels of CO_2 in the chemosensitive areas of the brainstem. Morphine also depresses the inherent rhythmicity of the dorsal respiratory group in the nucleus tractus solitarius, further attenuating the respiratory cycle. As the administered dose of morphine increases, these combined effects can reduce ventilation to the point at which significant hypoxia occurs. However, this depressant effect is partially countered by the eventual reduction in arterial O_2 saturation that stimulates the respiratory centers. Thus, reduced O_2 increases DA release by the glomus cells of the carotid body, and this in turn increases the firing rate of the glossopharyngeal afferents projecting to the dorsal respiratory group (Graves et al., 1983). The component of respiratory activity mediated by hypoxic drive therefore remains intact—a point that is particularly relevant to the overdose victim for two reasons. First, the depressant effect of morphine on the medullary centers is, in part, offset by the increase in hypoxic drive that will develop. Thus, hypoxia will maintain respiration in a patient who would otherwise have succumbed to medullary depression. Second, the natural tendency to administer O_2 to a patient in respiratory depression can be fatal if that depression is a result of a morphine overdose. Administering O_2 will raise arterial O_2 saturation, reduce hypoxic drive, and "uncover" an otherwise fatal respiratory depression. Oxygen should therefore be used very cautiously in opioid overdose patients and 100% oxygen is contraindicated.

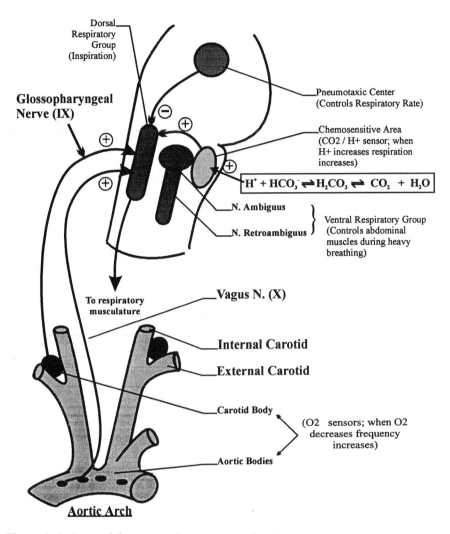

Figure 4–4. Some of the neuronal circuitry involved in respiration is depicted in this schematic. Peripheral chemoreceptors located in the carotid bodies and aortic bodies detect reductions in blood O_2 tension, which increases DA in the glomus cells and excites ascending fibers. Ascending fibers in the glossopharyngeal and vagus nerve invade the dorsal respiratory group to increase respiration. This portion of the circuit is called hypoxic drive and is not influenced by the opioids. The chemosensitive area in the brainstem responds to alterations in pH. When CO_2 plasma concentrations increase, H^+ ion concentrations increase in the cerebrospinal fluid. This increase stimulates the dorsal respiratory group to enhance respiration and reduce CO_2 concentration. This so-called chemotactic drive is blunted by the opioids.

Sedative Effects. Although significant analgesia can occur without sedation, as the administered dose of morphine increases, sedation, obtundation, and eventually coma will likely occur in all patients. Sedation is primarily the result of reduced excitatory neurotransmitter release (Glu) at several locations in the neuroaxis including the thalamus and reticular formation secondary to Enk action at kappa$_1$ heteroreceptors.

Cough Reflex. Morphine suppresses the cough reflex in a dose-dependent fashion. Although opioid receptors are undoubtedly involved in the cough reflex, opioid antagonists will not eliminate the antitussive action of morphine, suggesting that other receptors are involved as well. Glutamate has been strongly implicated in this reflex. Although the opioid receptors responsible for the antitussive effect are not known, they are apparently different from those mediating analgesic and respiratory depressant effects since drugs that effectively dissociate these effects from cough suppression have been developed (e.g., dextromethorphan).

Nausea and Vomiting. Nausea and vomiting are not uncommon at the beginning of morphine treatment. Recumbent patients are at reduced risk, suggesting the involvement of vestibular function. Morphine can directly stimulate the chemoreceptor trigger zone (CTZ) and induce nausea and vomiting. (The acid hydrolysate of morphine, apomorphine, is a potent DA agonist and a well-known emetic agent.) This effect occurs independently of motion and is only partially blocked by mu antagonists. Since DA antagonists and the 5HT antagonist ondansetron effectively block nausea and are frequently used as adjuncts to morphine treatment, the involvement of nonopioid systems is implied. However, the actions of morphine eventually depress the CTZ during prolonged therapy, obviating the need for coadministered antiemetics.

Rigidity. Morphine reduces DA activity in the substantia nigra and can produce rigidity. Enk, colocalized with GABA in the so-called indirect outflow pathway of the striatum, inhibits the external segment of the globus pallidus and probably also contributes to muscle rigidity (see Chapter 9). Whatever its mechanism, the chest-wall rigidity seen at high plasma levels can exacerbate respiratory depression and is a major consideration when high-potency opioids are used to induce neurolept-analgesia during surgery (see Chapter 7).

Hypothalamic Effects. Morphine influences several hormones. It reduces the release of gonadotrophic-releasing hormone (GnRH) and corticotropin-releasing factor (CRF), diminishing circulating levels of luteinizing hormone (LH), follicle-stimulating hormone (FSH), ACTH, and beta-endorphin. It increases prolactin release perhaps because of a mu_1-mediated reduction in hypothalamic DA that acts as prolactin-inhibitory factor. These hormonal effects are minor, however. By contrast, morphine increases the release of antidiuretic hormone (ADH) in a dose-dependent fashion and at doses that are clinically relevant. This mu-receptor-mediated effect leads to reduced urine formation as a result of increased Na^+ reabsorption in the collecting duct resulting in oliguria (scanty urine). The reduced urine output is complicated by a blunting of the sensations associated with the need to urinate that often leads to catheterization.

On the other hand, morphine can act on kappa receptors to reduce ADH release, increase urine formation, and produce polyuria. Following systemic administration, however, the predominant effect of morphine is on mu receptors and oliguria is most commonly observed. Other hypothalamic effects include depression of the "feeding center" and centrally induced hypothermia. Under conditions of severe muscular rigidity, however, excessive muscular tone induced by rigidity can produce hyperthermia.

Pupils. Morphine activates the Edinger-Westphal nucleus of the oculomotor nerve through mu_2 receptors, leading to miosis. In fact, pinpoint pupils are one sign in the pathognomonic triad for morphine overdose. But, in overdose situations associated with respiratory depression, the consequent hypoxia can lead to hypometabolism and decreased neuronal activity in the oculomotor system, producing mydriasis. Thus, when using eye signs in the diagnosis of a morphine-overdose patient, one must take into account arterial O_2 saturation and the time elapsed from drug administration.

Cardiovascular Effects. Morphine's effects include vasodilation, reduced peripheral resistance, and inhibition of the baroreceptor reflex. These arise from morphine's delta actions in the CNS that depress the medullary vasomotor system (a direct, delta-mediated smooth muscle relaxation). More importantly, morphine directly increases vascular histamine release. Morphine-induced histamine release does not involve degranulation of mast cells but rather simple displacement of histamine from the heparin–protein complex. This "histamine effect" is shared by several opioids with structures similar to morphine and is a consequence of their high affinity for the histamine-binding protein in mast cells. At higher doses, released histamine can induce bronchial constriction and increase secretions in the respiratory tree. Consequently, the opioids should not be used in asthmatics or in a patient with an otherwise obstructed airway. The release of histamine also contributes to peripheral vasodilation, producing the "morphine flush"—most notably observed in the face. histamine release is also thought to produce urticaria (itchiness), a common annoyance attending chronic morphine use. Although the increased release of ADH and its vasoconstrictive actions normally counteract the delta-receptor-induced and histamine-mediated vasodilation somewhat, the net effect of morphine on the cardiovascular system is vasodilation. These effects are not clinically relevant in a supine patient but can contribute to orthostatic hypotension when one is standing up. This state is exacerbated by CO_2 accumulation secondary to respiratory depression leading to CNS vasodilation.

The respiratory depression associated with opioid use enhances the body's total load of CO_2. This increase leads to vasodilation in the cerebral vasculature and the coronary vasculature. (Recall from Chapter 1 that CO_2 is the most important vasoregulator in the CNS.) The accumulation of CO_2 resulting from reduced respiration and the vasodilation in the cerebral vasculature that CO_2 can produce indicate that opioids such as morphine should be used cautiously in the treatment of pain resulting from head trauma. If morphine were used in a patient with intracranial bleeding, the cerebral vasodilation that would occur secondary to CO_2 accumulation would enhance bleeding, CSF production, and edema, all of which would be expected to contribute to increased intracranial pressure.

Gastrointestinal Tract. Morphine has a pronounced effect on the gastrointestinal tract, reducing secretions and decreasing propulsive activity. Indeed, the constipating effects of the opioid class are legendary and have led to the development of several drugs for treating diarrhea. These effects are mediated primarily by morphine's direct action on mu_2 receptors located in the myenteric plexus, although the CNS depression that can accompany high-dose therapy will suppress descending autonomic activity and contribute, as well. In the stomach, morphine reduces acid secretion and motility. These effects decrease emptying time, which can reduce the bioavailability of coadministered drugs. The effects on stomach motility can also contribute to esophageal reflux that is especially bothersome because of morphine's emetic effect. Paradoxically, morphine can increase antral tone so much that intubation becomes difficult—a problem in treating overdose victims. At first this seems contradictory since the overall G.I. action of morphine reduces gut motility. However, morphine enhances tone while reducing propulsive (peristaltic) activity. This might suggest that opioid receptors reduce the integration of activity in the myenteric plexus responsible for propulsive activity while having an overall excitatory effect on the plexus. The increased transit time of fecal material allows more time for water reabsorption by the large intestine, which enhances the constipating effect of this drug. Regardless of the mechanism, the net effect is to increase tone while reducing peristalsis. Coupled with its ability to reduce secretions, morphine can produce pronounced constipation that may lead to impaction. In addition, morphine's activity in the spinal cord and brain can reduce the defecation reflex and also the appreciation for the need to defecate. Together with morphine's ability to depress the feeding center in the hypothalamus, these effects combined can produce serious nutritional problems in patients on chronic therapy.

Other Effects. Morphine has effects on other smooth muscles besides those in the gastrointestinal tract and the vasculature. Morphine enhances detrusor and external sphincter tone in the urinary system. Together with the ADH increase produced by morphine and the reduction in sensations of urinary urgency stemming from mu_2 effects in the spinal cord, urination may become a problem that necessitates catheterization. Morphine increases the pressure in the intrabiliary tract by enhancing tone in the sphincter of Oddi (i.e., biliary colic). This can lead to right upper quadrant pain in the medicated patient and can be confused with the patient's primary symptoms. Morphine prolongs labor. This can cause problems since the fetus is more susceptible than the mother to the respiratory depressant effects of morphine. Thus, morphine use should be avoided during labor. An opioid that is less potent in this regard, such as meperidine, can be used instead.

Absorption, Metabolism, and Elimination. Morphine sulphate, the normally administered formulation of morphine, is absorbed well following oral, rectal, intravenous, and intramuscular administration. But it undergoes significant first-pass metabolism, so oral doses must be adjusted accordingly. Morphine's half-life is two to four hours.

Morphine's metabolism involves glucuronide conjugation of the parent compound that can occur both hepatically and extrahepatically. Recently, it has been shown that one of morphine's conjugation products (morphine-6-glucuronide) retains potent analgesic activity (Paul et al., 1989). Because of its longer half-life, morphine-6-glucuronide can accumulate during chronic therapy, enhancing the apparent potency of an administered dose of morphine. In addition, as a glucuronide, morphine-6-glucuronide is excreted mostly by the kidney (some biliary excretion can occur) and therefore accumulates in dialysis patients and in patients with renal failure, which explains the prolonged analgesic effects of morphine observed in this patient group.

Morphine Toxicity. Based on the actions described above, the acute toxic effects of a morphine overdose are easy to predict (Table 4–3). First

Table 4–3 Morphine Toxicity and Withdrawal Syndrome

Morphine toxicity	Coma
	Respiratory depression
	Pinpoint pupils
	Hypotension
	Hypothermia
	Urinary retention
Withdrawal syndrome	
Early phase	Lacrimation, yawning, sweating, rhinorrhea, drug craving, irritability, dysphoria, tremor, agitation, restlessness, anorexia, and gooseflesh
Later phase	Intensified early phase effects
	In addition, diarrhea, nausea/vomiting, G.I. spasm, increased heart rate and blood pressure, alternating chills and sweating, depression, generalized muscle spasms, dehydration, acid–base imbalances, and a reduced seizure threshold

and foremost is the pathognomonic triad of coma, respiratory depression, and pinpoint pupils. In an emergency room, these signs signify opioid overdose. Remember, however, that whether or not miotic pupils are observed will depend on the duration of respiratory depression. Prolonged respiratory depression will lead to hypoxia with pupils that can be fixed and dilated. The morphine overdose victim is hypotensive and cool (unless significant muscle rigidity preceded loss of consciousness) and will exhibit urinary retention. A patent airway must be established and an opioid antagonist administered. Opioid antagonists can induce seizures but are lifesaving.

Withdrawal Syndrome. The signs and symptoms of morphine withdrawal arise from neuroadaptation (see Chapter 12) and depend on several variables such as dosage and duration of treatment, the individual's personality, and the environment of the patient. The intensity of the syndrome can thus vary from mild to severe although it is rarely fatal. The signs and symptoms are generally observed in two phases (Table 4–3). Some of the signs have become incorporated into colloquial descriptions of drug withdrawal in general, such as "going cold turkey," which describes the gooseflesh that so characteristically accompanies intense morphine withdrawal, and "kicking the habit"—a vivid phrase related to muscle spasms observed in the arms and legs. The syndrome generally runs its course in ten days although the drug craving may require years to subside. The withdrawal syndromes associated with other opioids are qualitatively similar but can be more protracted with longer-acting drugs such as methadone. Usually, the shorter the action of the drug abused, the

Table 4–4 Full Opioid Agonists[a]

Drug Generic (Tradename)	Analgesic Dosage Required Relative to 10 mg Morphine	Unique Actions
Codeine	60 mg	High oral bioavailability Potent antitussive agent Profound constipation
Heroin	5.0 mg	Biotransformed to active morphine
Hydromorphone (Dilaudid)	1.5 mg	Shorter acting than morphine
Oxymorphone (Numorphan)	1.0 mg	
Hydrocodone (Hycodan)		Used in combination formulations
Levorphanol (Levo-dromoran)	2.0 mg	Long half-life (12 hours) Excellent oral bioavailability Less nausea and vomiting Can induce delirium and hallucinations
Methadone (Dolophine)	10 mg	Excellent oral availability Long half-life (24 hours) "Methadone program" for treatment of opioid abuse
Meperidine (Demerol)	75 mg	Metabolite normeperidine can cause CNS excitation Less biliary colic Fewer uterine effects Less constipation
Fentanyl (Sublimaze)	0.12 mg	Similar to meperidine Formulated with droperidol as Innovar
Propoxyphene (Darvon)	65 mg	Used in combination formulations Long half-life (12 hours) Toxic metabolites may produce convulsions
Other morphine-like drugs that are not analgesic		
Dextromethorphan	Not analgesic	Orally available antitussive OTC agent
Diphenoxylate	Not analgesic	Antidiarrheal agent Formulated with atropine as Lomotil
loperamide (Imodium)	Not analgesic	Antidiarrheal agent Does not cross the BBB

[a]OTC = over the counter

shorter and more intense the withdrawal syndrome is. Clonidine and other alpha$_2$ agonists can attenuate many autonomic withdrawal symptoms through their inhibition of NE release and other CNS actions (see Charney, Heninger, and Kleber, 1986). These withdrawal signs are presumably due to rebound increases in NE following a chronic course of morphine.

Drug Interactions. Several drug classes appear to have synergistic CNS-depressant effects when administered with morphine and other opioid drugs. The phenothiazine DA antagonists, the first-generation tricyclic antidepressants, and the monoamine oxidase inhibitors all produce this synergy. This must be kept in mind when the phenothiazines are used as adjuvant antiemetics or when tricyclic compounds such as amitriptyline are used in the management of chronic pain. The use of monoamine oxidase inhibitors with opioids is an absolute contraindication because of the high incidence of hyperpyrexic coma.

Other direct-acting agonists
Overall, the other direct-acting agonists share similar pharmacodynamics with morphine. Variations in potency, bioavailability after oral administration, lipid solubility (allowing transdermal administration with some), and increased penetration into the brain dominate the differences among these other drugs (Table 4–4). Chemically, they fall into several categories with structures resembling those of morphine (Fig. 4–5).

Codeine is found in the poppy and is the other major component responsible for the analgesic and euphoric effects of opium. The analgesic effects of codeine are largely the result of its biotransformation (demethylation) to morphine. Approximately 10% of an administered dose of codeine is biotransformed to morphine. The major advantage of codeine is its excellent efficacy following oral administration due to a reduced first-pass effect. Although it has a much lower affinity for mu receptors (ten- to 20-fold) than does morphine, its increased lipid solubility compared with morphine allows greater penetration into the brain and spinal cord. It is a common constituent in analgesic formulations (e.g., acetaminophen, Tylenol #3). Codeine is more potent as an antitussive agent than are other opioid compounds. This is thought to result from codeine's ability to bind to nonopioid receptors in the medullary centers that regulate the cough reflex. Codeine's ability to induce constipation is profound, perhaps because its higher lipid solubility leads to increased availability to the myenteric plexus.

Heroin, chemically, is diacetylmorphine and is rapidly converted to monoacetylmorphine (MAM) and then to morphine in the brain. Acetylation of the morphine structure results in higher lipid solubility and increased availability to the brain. Heroin therefore possesses enhanced

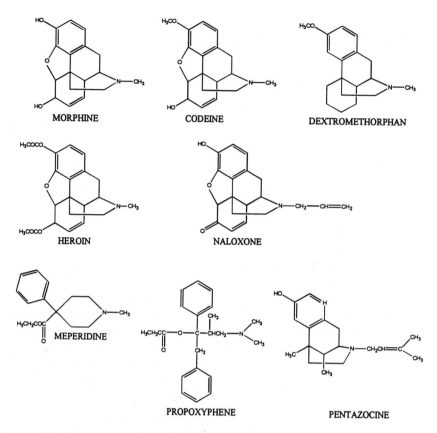

Figure 4–5. Structures of the various chemical classes that comprise the opioid drug family.

euphorogenic potency relative to morphine. Usually self-administered intravenously by addicts, it can induce death through respiratory depression due to dramatic variations in purity. Purchased on the street, heroin is often adulterated ("cut") several times with other chemicals so its street potency can consequently be much less than that of pure heroin.

Meperidine and structurally related analgesics in the phenylpiperidine family such as fentanyl (Sublimaze) are potent mu agonists. A synthetic agent with actions very similar to those of morphine, meperidine is absorbed well from all sites. Unfortunately, oral, high-dose administration can be associated with excitation due to metabolic conversion to normeperidine. This metabolite may have sigma-receptor actions that can induce psychotomimetic effects similar to those associated with phencyclidine (PCP; see Chapter 12). However, selective kappa opioid agonists can also produce paradoxic excitement and psychotomimetic effects and meperidine's kappa actions may contribute to these side effects as well.

Meperidine and the extremely potent fentanyl appear to have reduced effects on smooth muscle at doses that are equianalgesic with those of morphine. The use of these drugs is therefore associated with less constipation, fewer complications during labor, and fewer spasms of the sphincter of Oddi.

Diphenoxylate, a congener of meperidine, is combined with atropine to formulate the antidiarrheal agent Lomotil. Diphenoxylate does not readily cross the BBB and therefore does not have the CNS effects normally attending opioid use. Its extremely poor aqueous solubility makes it virtually impossible to solubilize for parenteral use, further reducing its abuse potential. However, it must always be assumed that some individuals will abuse anything; the consumption of large doses of diphenoxylate can produce euphoria and even induce dependence. To reduce this abuse potential, the pharmaceutical industry formulated diphenoxylate with atropine. Although the antimuscarinic effects of atropine would be expected to contribute to diphenoxylate's antidiarrheal effects, the low doses added are not normally effective in this regard. If an individual consumes enough Lomotil to induce diphenoxylate-mediated euphoria, however, that person will also consume enough atropine to produce a very unpleasant antimuscarinic toxicity. Loperamide, on the other hand, is a meperidine congener that does not penetrate the BBB at all. Like diphenoxylate it, too, is an effective antidiarrheal agent and, because of its veritable exclusion from the CNS, it is sold over the counter as Imodium.

Methadone is a long-acting, orally active, morphine-like substance with less emetic potency. It is used primarily in treatment programs for dependent patients since it produces effects similar to morphine or heroin. Since it is given free of charge, methadone programs reduce crime. Its high oral bioavailability reduces the infectious disease problems associated with needle use and its long duration of effect produces a less intense withdrawal syndrome if the addict tries to stop. The effectiveness of this program has been modest and remains controversial (see Stimson and Oppenheimer, 1982).

Dextromethorphan is an over-the-counter (OTC) drug most commonly used for suppression of cough. It is the d-isomer of levorphanol, has little affinity for mu receptors, and does not produce analgesia, respiratory depression, or dependence. Its ability to suppress coughs seems paradoxic and has led to the assumption that nonopioid receptors partially mediate the cough reflex.

Partial Agonists and Mixed Agonist/Antagonists

Opioids that have reduced efficacy at opioid receptors (partial agonists) or that possess efficacy at some opioid receptors but act as antagonists at others comprise a group of drugs that produce analgesia with a reduced attendant risk for dependence. This class includes pentazocine, nalbuphine, butorphanol, buprenorphine, and others. Their analgesic effects are partly a result of their actions at kappa and delta receptors and, where applicable, their partial agonist actions at mu receptors. As analgesics they are much less potent than morphine.

The prototypical drug in this group is pentazocine (Table 4–5). It is considered a weak, competitive antagonist/partial agonist at mu receptors and a full agonist at kappa$_1$ and kappa$_3$ receptors, with little affinity for delta receptors. Its weak-to-moderate analgesic potency is the result of its kappa actions and possibly its partial mu efficacy. As competitive antagonists or partial agonists at mu receptors, pentazocine, nalbuphine, and butorphanol can precipitate the withdrawal syndrome in patients dependent on full agonists at the mu receptor; addicts can discriminate the effects of these drugs from those of full agonists quite easily. Buprenorphine, on the other hand, is a more efficacious partial agonist at the mu receptor and addicts perceive it as morphine-like.

Since these drugs act primarily through kappa receptors, they do not cause significant respiratory depression. The respiratory depression that does occur exhibits a ceiling effect and fatal respiratory compromise is rarely seen. The mixed agonists/antagonists can induce psychotomimetic and dysphoric effects, however. At high doses these side effects can be accompanied by hyperexcitability and even hallucinations. These are thought to result from kappa-receptor activation, the effects of which are potentiated by inhibition of endogenous mu activity due to the mu antagonistic effects of these drugs. However, opioid antagonists only partially prevent the psychomotor actions of these drugs, so other receptor interactions may also be involved.

The ability of these drugs to induce potent kappa activation and block or reduce the activation of mu receptors markedly influences their effects on the cardiovascular system. As a group, these drugs do not produce hypotension but rather increase blood pressure and work performed by the heart. In the case of pentazocine, this effect may result from increased circulating catecholamines. Nalbuphine has little effect on the cardiovascular system and may be the analgesic of choice in patients with unstable cardiac disease. These agents can induce sedation and lightheadedness, but they have few smooth-muscle-related side effects such as constipation and biliary colic at doses that are equianalgesic with morphine.

Most of the mixed agonists/antagonists are absorbed readily from all sites and their generally good oral bioavailability makes them popular outpatient analgesics. Pentazocine tablets can be ground up and injected to engender euphoria. The coadministration of antihistamines such as tripelennamine potentiates the euphorogenic actions of pentazocine and

Table 4–5 Opioid Partial Agonists and Antagonists

Drug Generic (Tradename)	Analgesic Dosage Required Relative to 10 mg Morphine	Unique Actions
Partial agonists/antagonists		
Pentazocine (Talwin)	50 mg	Can precipitate withdrawal in full agonist users
		Respiratory ceiling effect
		Low dependence liability due to dysphoria
		Few smooth muscle effects
		Cardiovascular stimulant
		Formulated with naloxone to prevent i.v. abuse
Nalbuphine (Nubain)	10 mg	Not bioavailable orally
		Similar to pentazocine
		No cardiovascular effects
Butorphanol (Stadol)	2 mg	Very similar to pentazocine
Buprenorphine (Buprenex)	0.4 mg	Partial mu agonist
		Fewer psychotomimetic effects
Full antagonists		
Naloxone (Narcan)	Not analgesic	Full opioid receptor antagonist
		Precipitates withdrawal
		Short half-life (1 hour)
		Not bioavailable orally
		Used diagnostically for opioid overdose
Naltrexone (Trexan)	Not analgesic	Full opioid receptor antagonist
		Precipitates withdrawal
		Long half-life (24 hours)
		Orally active

smooths the dysphoric effects. (This combination is called "T's and Blues" by "street-drug" users.) To prevent this potential for abuse, pentazocine is available in formulation with the mu, kappa, and delta antagonist naloxone (see below) as Talwin-Nx. The bioavailability of naloxone following oral administration is extremely low due to first-pass metabolism. In its tablet form, the naloxone included in the formulation therefore does not influence the action of the pentazocine. However, if Talwin-Nx is ground up and injected, the naloxone will antagonize the actions of pentazocine and thereby prevent the euphoric effects.

Opioid Antagonists

The two major drugs in this group, naloxone and naltrexone, are full antagonists at mu, kappa, and delta receptors. Thus, they do not possess analgesic potency and are generally used to treat the opioid over-dose patient. They are capable of reversing virtually all of the deleteri-ous effects of the opioid class. Naloxone, the treatment of choice for opioid overdose, must be administered parenterally due to its ex-tremely low bioavailability following enteral administration. Its short half-life (one hour), its ability to rapidly reverse signs of opioid over-dose following intravenous administration, and its lack of adverse ef-fects (except for occasional seizures) make it an excellent diagnostic tool to confirm or dispute a diagnosis of opioid overdose. Thus, even if the drug responsible for the overdose is unknown, naloxone can be used aggressively in the emergency room because it will not potentiate the actions of any known coma-inducing drug. Because of its short half-life, however, it must be administered frequently to the opioid overdose victim in order to avoid toxic relapse. In contrast, naltrexone is highly bioavailable following oral delivery and its effects may last for 24 hours. Like naloxone, naltrexone can precipitate seizures in the dependent patient.

CHRONIC CONTROL OF PAIN

The chronic control of pain presents unique problems that are not associ-ated with acute therapy. Foremost is the development of tolerance (see Collin and Cesselin, 1991). Chronic use of opioids produces receptor-site down-regulation and a reduction in receptor–G-protein coupling. Be-cause of these changes, second-messenger-mediated effects are attenuated and pharmacodynamic tolerance develops. In addition, the actions of the opioids on other neurotransmitter systems produce physiologic toler-ance. Chronic use of opioids leads to increased activity of NE and at least some of the signs and symptoms of the withdrawal syndrome (tremor and anxiety) are effectively treated by the indirect-acting NE antagonist clonidine. Alterations in other neurotransmitters, especially DA and 5HT, likely contribute to physiologic tolerance as well.

Whatever the mechanism(s) involved, the development of tolerance makes it necessary to increase the dosage administered or reduce the dos-ing interval in order to maintain analgesic efficacy. In addition, the devel-opment of tolerance to the various effects of the opioids does not occur at the same rate. Miosis and constipation exhibit little, if any, tolerance while analgesic efficacy wanes. Fortunately, tolerance to the analgesic ef-fects of the opioids is accompanied by a similar rate of tolerance to the respiratory depressant and sedative-hypnotic effects of these drugs. Therefore, the administered dose of opioid can be increased to reinstate pretolerance analgesic effects without also increasing the risk of respiratory depression. Nonetheless, there is always an opioid dose high enough to produce fatal respiratory depression.

Several strategies have proven successful in maintaining analgesic efficacy in the face of tolerance (see Pasternak, 1993; Payne and Pasternak, 1992). Intermittent dosing, if tolerated by the patient, can usually extend the effective duration of analgesia without significant development of tolerance. The more continuous the dosing schedule, the faster tolerance to the analgesic effect develops. Switching drugs can also prove effective in maintaining analgesic efficacy since the various opioids described above have different patterns of receptor activation. The analgesic effects of a mu agonist do not exhibit significant cross tolerance to an agent with significant kappa activity. Switching back and forth between the two drug classes can therefore be an effective strategy for maintaining analgesic efficacy.

Since the opioids relieve pain in concert with nonopioid systems, manipulation of other neurotransmitters can potentiate their analgesic action. Cholecystokinin (CCK)-receptor antagonists such as proglumide (Watkins, Kinscheck, and Mayer, 1984), tricyclics such as amitriptyline (Spiegel, Kourides, and Pasternak, 1983), the noncompetitive antagonist to the NMDA receptor, MK-801 (Higgins, Nguyen, and Sellers, 1992), and inhibitors of nitric oxide synthesis (Kolesnikov et al., 1993) have all been shown to restore analgesic potency in animals made tolerant to the actions of morphine.

Alternate routes of administration can also be used in chronic pain management. Transdermal patches containing various opioid drugs are currently available and they represent a very convenient method of delivery outside the hospital setting. The continuous delivery of the drug produces tolerance more rapidly, however. Patient-controlled drug delivery utilizing implanted devices has proven effective. The patient depresses a button connected to a drug pump to deliver a preset amount of a drug when needed. The program controlling the drug pump prevents excessive use by setting an hourly administration limit. Studies have shown that patients who are able to control their drug delivery consume less drug overall than those administered drugs on request by traditional routes (Kerr et al., 1988). Apparently having control over delivery enables the patient to tolerate higher levels of pain in the knowledge that relief is available any time. The other advantage to this delivery system is that tolerance will develop more slowly owing to the reduced amount of drug administered.

Finally, spinal epidural or intrathecal (subarachnoid) delivery by a cannula attached to a refillable reservoir implanted subcutaneously is beginning to take its place in chronic pain management. The delivery of an opioid directly to areas of the spinal cord involved with pain in the periphery can yield CSF levels several hundred times higher than those obtained by traditional routes. The theory is that delivery to the site of need reduces the distribution of the drug to other sites where toxicity might occur. Depending on the drug, significant plasma levels can still be obtained, however, and systemic toxicity can follow. Drugs with reduced lipid solubility would not escape the CSF compartment and produce systemic effects as readily. Opioid peptides with high selectivity for receptors found predominantly in the spinal cord have been developed recently and will no doubt be used in this context.

5

Pharmacology of Headache

Prototypic agents: *Aspirin, ergotamine*
(Wigraine, Ergostat, Ergomar)

Prototypic prophylactic agent: *methysergide (Sansert)*

Headaches are the most common complaint of patients (Kurtzke et al., 1986). Each year 75% of the population will experience headaches of varying intensity and quality and at least 5% of them will seek medical advice for that head pain. A headache can be a symptom of a variety of conditions that are as innocuous as eyestrain or as life-threatening as intracranial hemorrhage. The vast majority of headaches are best treated with over-the-counter (OTC) medications such as aspirin. More severe forms, however, can be incapacitating and may be associated with additional neurological signs and symptoms warranting more aggressive pharmacotherapy.

Since there are many etiologies of headache that require different therapeutic approaches, the type of pain must first be ascertained before effective treatment can begin. No accepted physiologic measures or objective tests are available to assist the physician, so the diagnosis of headache depends almost exclusively on the medical interview. After tumor, temporal arteritis, tic douloureux (trigeminal neuralgia), meningitis, intracranial hemorrhage, and arteriovenous malformation are excluded, other more benign causes are then considered. The most common cause of headache is muscle tension. Tension headaches usually involve continuous, bilateral, nonthrobbing, posterior head pain occurring primarily during working hours, especially in the afternoon. This form of headache often responds to relaxation techniques, OTC analgesic medications, or benzodiazepines that reduce muscle tone and the anxiety that is likely responsible for the headache in the first place.

105

Headaches can also reflect eyestrain, increased ocular pressure, nasal congestion, ear infection, dental problems, and reactions to certain types of foods or beverages.

MIGRAINE HEADACHE

Unlike many milder headaches, migraine headache is unilateral in eight out of ten patients and characteristically has a pulsating or throbbing quality, the intensity of which can vary widely (Table 5–1). It is usually exacerbated by strenuous activity and often accompanied by nausea, vomiting, photophobia (light hypersensitivity), and phonophobia (sound hypersensitivity). It can be precipitated by birth control pills, menses, stress, several drugs (especially those affecting vascular tone), and pregnancy. Migraine headaches are three times more common in women than in men, and a genetic predisposition seems likely. The duration of the attack can vary from several hours to several days and, in some cases, can totally incapacitate the patient.

The symptoms that are most helpful in establishing a diagnosis of migraine headache are its throbbing quality, its unilateral location, and the presence of neurological symptoms. A premonitory phase lasting up to 36 hours and involving changes in mood and appetite may precede the headache. This phase may be accompanied by neurologic symptoms (auras), the most common being visual distortions (blurred images), scintillating scotomas (a dark or blind spot with highlighted fringes), zigzag-

Table 5–1 Migraine Classification[a]

Migraine Type	Symptoms
Migraine without aura (common migraine)	Unilateral in 80% of the cases Throbbing headache often associated with nausea and vomiting
Migraine with aura (classic migraine)	Same as common migraine but must be preceded by some form of aura that is most commonly visual
Complicated Hemiplegic	A sudden onset of hemiparesis (weakness or mild paralysis on one side) followed by a contralateral throbbing headache
Opthalmoplegic	Unilateral eye pain and ipsilateral opthalmoplegia (uncoordinated movement of the eyes)
Basilar Artery	Visual aura with alterations in consciousness that precedes the headache

[a]Adapted from Peroutka (1992)

ging lines in the visual field, or images that take on a mosaic-like appearance. Formerly called classic migraine, such headaches preceded by neurological symptoms are now called migraine with aura. Migraine without aura (formerly called common migraine) is the most common form of headache (90% of cases). It can have the same pain pattern as that seen in migraine with aura, but it does not have a prodromal phase. The other less common forms of migraine headaches are listed in Table 5–1.

Once a diagnosis of migraine headache is made, the most benign therapy should be tried first. Behavioral changes such as seeking a quiet, dark room to sleep in often produce a significant reduction or even complete abatement of symptoms. The development and use of drugs has been guided by several theories about the pathogenesis of migraine headache: the vascular hypothesis, the sterile inflammatory hypothesis, and the biobehavioral hypothesis.

PATHOGENESIS OF MIGRAINE HEADACHE

The Vascular Hypothesis

The vascular or ischemic theory of Wolff has long been used to explain the pathogenesis of migraine headache (Wolff, 1963). Some unknown action causes platelets to release serotonin (5HT) (Lance et al., 1989). Acting on vascular receptors, 5HT induces spasm in one or more of the major cerebral arteries (the vasoconstrictive or ischemic phase), producing cerebral ischemia (Fig. 5–1). The vasoconstrictive phase, if severe enough, causes localized ischemia leading to hypometabolism within brain tissue and the aura of migraine. Migraine without aura has the same pathogenesis, but the vasoconstriction is not pronounced enough to induce ischemia and associated neurologic symptoms. The eventual depletion of platelet 5HT removes all 5HT-mediated vascular tone, and the caliber of the atonic vessels waxes and wanes in response to pulse pressure. It is the stretching of the connective tissues by the pulse pressure that produces throbbing pain.

In support of this hypothesis, plasma studies have shown a depletion of 5HT with an associated increase in its acid metabolite 5-hydroxyindole acetic acid (5HIAA) during migraine. Moreover, blood-flow studies have documented reductions in brain perfusion during the aura and increases in perfusion during the pain phase (Lance, 1981). Vasodilators exacerbate headaches and vasoconstrictors alleviate the pain. However, several investigators have failed to observe alterations in cerebral blood flow (see Olesen, 1987) while others believe that such global vascular

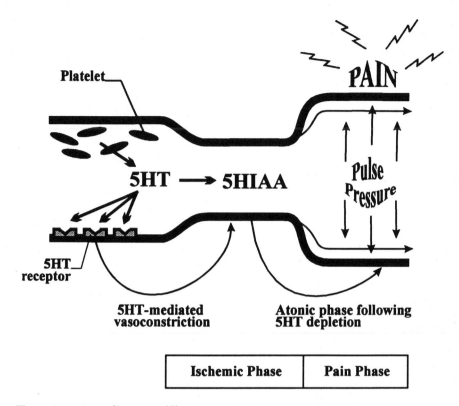

Figure 5–1. According to Wolff, migraine headache occurs when serotonin (5HT) released from platelets acts on vascular serotonin receptors to induce vasoconstriction, producing ischemia. Following the ischemic phase, loss of vascular 5HT leads to atonic arteries that respond to pulse pressure by stretching connective tissues to create the throbbing sensation of headache to produce the pain phase. Once it has acted, 5HT is oxidized to 5-hydroxy indoleacetic acid (5HIAA).

changes are inconsistent with the focal neurologic symptoms that occur during the prodromal phase (Sakai and Meyer, 1978). Thus, although vasoconstriction and vasodilation are probably involved in the pathogenesis of migraine, the vascular theory does not encompass all aspects of the disorder. Other hypotheses have therefore been advanced.

The Sterile Inflammatory Hypothesis

According to the neurogenic/sterile inflammatory hypothesis (Moskowitz, 1984), hyperactivity in the ophthalmic limb of the fifth cranial (trigeminal) nerve is responsible for migraine headaches (Fig. 5–2). Within the cranium, branches of the trigeminal nerve innervate the ipsilateral anterior, middle, and posterior cerebral arteries as well as the meningeal

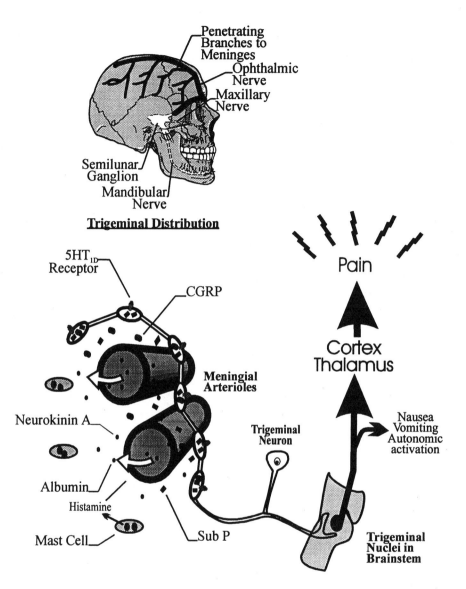

Figure 5–2. The relevant components of the sterile inflammatory hypothesis are depicted in this figure. An unknown process causes the release of substance P (Sub P), calcitonin-gene-related peptide (CGRP), and neurokinin from the trigeminal nerve, whose distribution is depicted in the upper left. These neuropeptides induce vasodilation as well as the release of histamine from mast cells. The combined effects of the peptides and histamine produce a sterile inflammation. The inflammatory response produces neuronal irritation that spreads throughout the ophthalmic limb of the trigeminal nerve to produce further inflammation as well as pain. This sensory activity is conducted into the trigeminal nucleus where it can also initiate nausea, vomiting, and autonomic activation.

arteries. Motor fibers in the ophthalmic limb are responsible for maintaining the vascular tone of these extracranial vessels (Goadsby and Edvinsson, 1993). Sensory C fibers surrounding the cranial arteries terminate in the nucleus of the tractus solitarius, a major relay station for autonomic function.

Through some unknown mechanism, the migraine trigger induces the release of Sub P, neurokinin A (a decapeptide), and calcitonin-gene-related peptide (CGRP, a protein with 37 amino acids) from the fibers of the trigeminal system. All three peptides are vasoactive and cause dilation of arteries, CGRP being the most potent. (The release of these neuropeptides is inhibited by 5HT acting through a heteroreceptor; Hartig, Branchek, and Weinshank, 1992.) In addition, Sub P and neurokinin A promote the leakage of albumin from the vessels producing edema and initiate a cascade of events that includes platelet aggregation and degranulation of mast cells that release histamine (a potent vasodilator). Consequently, a sterile (nonpathogen mediated) inflammatory response is initiated (Dimitriadou et al., 1992). This inflammatory response spreads to nervous tissue, initiating electrical activity in the ophthalmic fibers that spreads orthodromically (toward the terminal) as well as antidromically (toward the cell body; see Moskowitz, 1993) and increases the area of inflammation. C-fiber activation in response to pulse pressure in the inflamed areas leads to throbbing pain. Moreover, autonomic responses are initiated by the trigeminal fibers that project to the nucleus of the solitary tract. These fibers could also produce the nausea and vomiting that frequently accompany the onset of an attack. Support for this hypothesis is based on the numerous observations that agents effective in the management of migraine have been shown to alter 5HT or CGRP.

The Biobehavioral Hypothesis

The biobehavioral hypothesis (Welch, 1987) suggests that disorders of vascular tone are involved in migraine but are secondary to a process originating in the frontal cortex (Fig. 5–3). The involvement of the frontal cortex in this hypothesis explains why stress, menses, age, and genetic factors can precipitate a migraine, common observations of migraine sufferers not explained by the first two hypotheses.

The precipitating event originates in the orbitofrontal cortex. Once activated, it disinhibits the thalamus which in turn facilitates further activation of the frontal cortex. Activity in this circuit continues to cycle until a critical threshold is achieved in the orbitofrontal cortex that then activates the brainstem through a descending pathway. This pathway activates the locus ceruleus and the release of norepinephrine (NE) into the cortical mantle. The NE release induces a wave of slow depolariza-

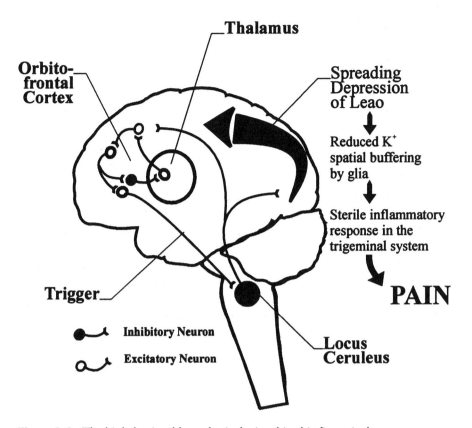

Figure 5–3. The biobehavioral hypothesis depicted in this figure is the most comprehensive in terms of its ability to explain the known pharmacology of migraine therapy. It proposes that the "perception" of stress in the orbitofrontal cortex initiates a feed-forward disinhibition within the thalamus that further increases activity in the orbitofrontal cortex. This upward spiral of activity eventually reaches a point where it activates the locus ceruleus. The subsequent release of NE acts through beta-adrenergic receptors on glia to inhibit K^+ spatial buffering. This leads to spreading depression (spreading depression of Leao) that initiates sterile inflammation in the trigeminal system with the subsequent production of pain. The involvement of the orbitofrontal cortex explains the efficacy of amitriptyline while the involvement of beta-adrenergic receptors explains the efficacy of propranolol.

tion in the cortical mantle, especially in the occipital cortex (spreading depression of Leao). This depolarization may result from increased extracellular K^+ caused by a beta-mediated reduction in K^+ uptake by glia, or from excessive cortical activity. (The former hypothesis is currently preferred.)

"Spreading depression" is an electrical phenomenon in which a focal reduction of electrical activity spreads across the cortical mantle at a rate of 2–3 mm/minute (Leao, 1944). It is initiated by depolarization that spreads to contiguous areas of the cortex at a rate of 3–6 mm/minute but that neither crosses the midline nor invades deep gray structures (Olesen, 1987). The rate and characteristics of this depression result in electrical anomalies similar to those seen in epilepsy, another disorder in which sensory auras can occur. In its wake, extracellular K^+ and glutamate concentrations are elevated, Na^+ is depleted, and blood flow declines (spreading oligemia; Lauritzen, 1994). Olesen and his colleagues have shown a spreading oligemia in patients during migraine with aura that started in the occipital cortex and spread anteriorly (Olesen, Larsen, and Lauritzen, 1981). This did not necessarily correspond to the distribution of major cranial vessels, but rather to the distribution of spreading depression. In the view of these authors, the symptoms of migraine with aura are initiated by spreading depression with an associated hypometabolism and decreased perfusion of the cortex. The fact that the spreading oligemia generally originates in the occipital cortex may explain the visual auras. Olesen (1987) argues that this spreading depression could also initiate a sterile inflammatory response in the trigeminovascular system that would induce pain. Thus, the spreading depression would be responsible for the aura while the sterile inflammation would be responsible for the pain.

PHARMACOTHERAPY OF MIGRAINE HEADACHE

Over-the-Counter (OTC) Medication

Aspirin-like compounds are the OTC medications most frequently used to treat migraine. These drugs are analgesic, antipyretic (reduce fever), and antiinflammatory to varying degrees and are called nonsteroidal antiinflammatory drugs (NSAIDs). The NSAIDs are a chemically diverse group of drugs including aspirin, acetaminophen, and ibuprofen (Fig. 5–4). They should be considered before prescription medication because of the low incidence of side effects associated with their use.

The analgesic properties of NSAIDs are thought to result primarily from inhibition of cyclooxygenase, a key enzyme in the prostaglandin biosynthetic pathway (Fig. 5–5). The NSAIDs differ in their mechanism of cyclooxygenase inhibition. Aspirin acetylates cyclooxygenase and new enzymes must therefore be synthesized to overcome the inhibition. In contrast, the other NSAIDs are competitive inhibitors of cyclooxygenase. All members of this group inhibit cyclooxygenase at concentrations that are clinically relevant. Moreover, their potency as analgesics is highly correlated with their ability to inhibit this enzyme. The NSAIDs may also prolong catecholamine and serotonin turnover that can produce analgesic effects (Bromm et al., 1992).

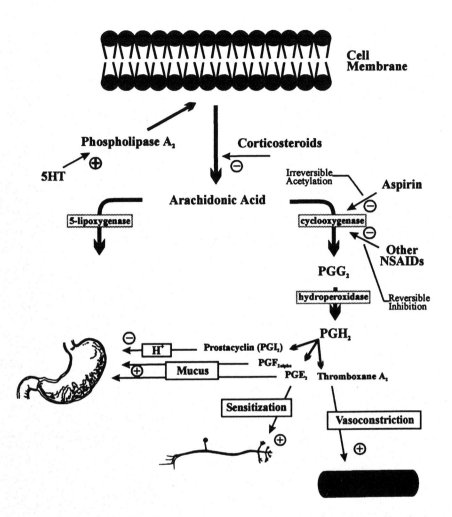

Figure 5-4. The prostaglandin pathway participates in the development of headaches by invoking vasoconstriction and sensitization of pain fibers as depicted here. Aspirin and other nonsteroidal antiinflammatory drugs (NSAIDs) inhibit the production of prostaglandin (PG) by irreversibly or reversibly, respectively, inhibiting the key synthesizing enzyme cyclooxygenase. Through this inhibition vasoconstriction is reduced and pain sensitization is attenuated. Since PGE_2-mediated sensitization involves an alteration in the phosphorylation status of the neuron terminal, aspirin-like drugs must be taken as early as possible in the pain phase. In addition, the various prostaglandins reduce acid secretion in the stomach as well as increase mucus production. The administration of aspirin-like drugs and the inhibition of cyclooxygenase leads to increased acid secretion and reduced mucus production, both of which contribute to GI pain.

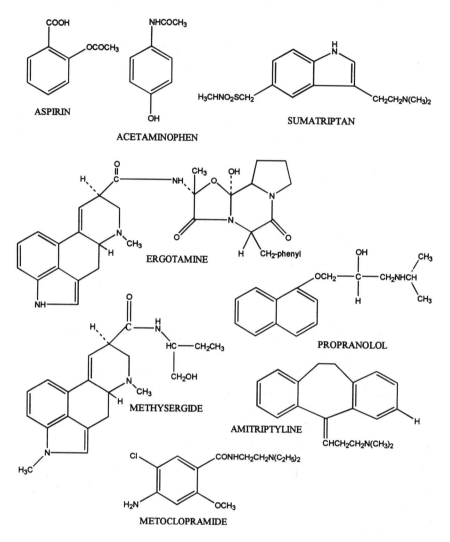

Figure 5–5. Structures of drugs commonly used in the management of migraine headaches.

Prostaglandins may play a role in migraine headaches by sensitizing pain fibers and producing inflammation. As described in Chapter 3, activation of phospholipase A_2 causes prostaglandin E_2 (PGE_2) to be produced which increases the sensitivity of pain fibers by altering the phosphorylation status of the neuron. In this way prostaglandins lower the threshold for activation in nociceptive fiber terminals and increase the likelihood that pain will be experienced. By blocking the production of prostaglandins, the NSAIDs prevent this effect. Of particular relevance to therapeutic management is the observation that the nociceptive sensitization induced by prostaglandins continues long after the prostaglandins have been biotransformed. Thus, once sensitization of a C fiber has occurred, it can only be reversed by phosphotases or by the fiber's gradual return to its original phosphorylation status over time. The clinical principle here is that the earlier in the pain phase the NSAID is taken, the greater the likelihood of its being effective.

All NSAIDs also possess antiinflammatory activity although acetaminophen is the least potent in this regard. (Acetaminophen's ability to block cyclooxygenase is prevented by the presence of peroxides that are generally very high in inflamed areas.) Since the prostaglandins increase membrane permeability and protein extravasation, blocking their production would reduce the sterile inflammation hypothesized to be a part of migraine pathogenesis. The NSAIDs thus may alleviate headache by reducing inflammation as well as sensitization. Although the prostaglandins are important regulators of platelet function and 5HT release (viewed as a critical step in the ischemic hypothesis) the involvement of this action in headache relief remains to be established.

Although it is true that the NSAIDs sold with or without prescription have properties besides cyclooxygenase inhibition that render some more effective than others in treating arthritis, one agent is not more efficacious than another at relieving head pain (see Tfelt-Hansen and Johnson, 1987). Thus, if the patient does not experience relief with one NSAID, it is highly unlikely that switching to another NSAID will prove beneficial although people often try this strategy. One possible explanation to this rule is the use of combination products. Agents combining aspirin, acetaminophen, and caffeine (Excedrin-like drugs) are often more effective. This may be because aspirin and acetaminophen inhibit cyclooxygenase via two different mechanisms while caffeine increases their absorption rate. Caffeine also stimulates adenosine receptors that may produce vasoactive effects. The combined effects of these actions can often prove effective in patients who do not find relief with single-formulation products.

Side Effects of NSAIDs

NSAIDs produce few side effects (those common to the NSAID class are summarized in Table 5–2). All of the NSAIDs can induce gastric bleeding and aggravate ulcers by inhibiting prostacycline and prostaglandin F_{2alpha} production, which normally inhibit acid secretion and reduce mucous production, respectively (Fig. 5–5). This problem can be overcome by coadministration of misoprostol (a PGE_1 analog). As acidic compounds, the NSAIDs also produce local irritation that leads to diffusion of acid into the gastric mucosa. This is a particular concern in migraineurs since

Table 5–2 Major Side Effects of Nonsteroidal Antiinflammatory Drugs (NSAIDs)[a]

Gastrointestinal upset and ulceration that may lead to blood loss and subsequent anemia

Inhibition of platelet aggregation reduces coagulation and increases bleeding

Inhibition of uterine motility that can extend gestation

Renal effects are minimal in normal patients but can profoundly affect special populations

  Decreased renal blood flow
  Reduced glomerular filtration rate
  Increased salt reabsorption
  Increased water retention (increased antidiuretic hormone action)
  Renal pathology (rare)

Hypersensitivity reactions

  Rhinitis
  Profuse watery secretions
  Various edemas
  Urticaria
  Bronchial asthma
  Bronchoconstriction
  Hypotension
  Shock

[a]All effects are thought to be related to the inhibition of prostaglandin synthesis including the hypersensitivity reactions. Even though hypersensitivity is generally considered to have an immunological basis, the fact that hypersensitivity reactions will continue even after the patient is switched to another member of the NSAID family indicates the involvement of prostaglandin inhibition

nausea and vomiting often accompany the attack. Moreover, the migraine attack is generally associated with a state of gastric stasis (see Tfelt-Hansen and Johnson, 1987). This stasis potentiates the gastric effects of the NSAIDs, which often leads to epigastric distress. Prokinetic drugs can be administered to combat this problem. As D_2 antagonists, prokinetic drugs such as metoclopramide and prochlorperazine enhance the passage of drugs into the duodenum by blocking D_2 receptors that, when activated, increase sphincter tone in the stomach. In addition, the D_2 antagonists are all effective antiemetic agents (see Chapter 10). If prokinetic drugs are not used, the NSAIDs should be taken with large amounts of water or with food to reduce G.I. upset and facilitate absorption. To circumvent these potential side effects completely, the NSAIDs can be administered as rectal suppositories since they are readily absorbed via this route.

Platelet aggregation is mediated by thromboxane A_2, the production of which is inhibited by NSAIDs. This results in increased bleeding time. Inhibition of platelet aggregation can reduce thrombus formation and the NSAIDs, in particular aspirin, are prescribed to reduce stroke and other thromboembolic disorders. Toxic reactions also occur. Salicylism is associated with a cluster of signs and symptoms that largely evolve from acid–base disturbances. The use of aspirin is contraindicated in the management of headache associated with viral infections such as influenza or chicken pox since Reye's syndrome may result (encephalopathy with hepatic injury). A small portion of acetaminophen is biotransformed to N-acetylbenzoquinone imine, a highly reactive toxic intermediate metabolite. Following overdose, this metabolite can deplete hepatic glutathione, facilitating sulfhydryl-mediated reactions that can potentially lead to hepatotoxicity.

Many migraine sufferers will say that the NSAIDs are not effective against their headaches. When specifically queried, patients often acknowledge that they do not take these medications until well into the pain phase, when the drugs are least likely to be effective. It is therefore critical to inform the migraineur of the importance of taking an NSAID as early after the headache starts as possible before abandoning their use. In addition, the acute suppression of headache is generally associated with rebound headache because of drug clearance. Because migraine headaches can last up to 48 hours, the migraineur must be informed of the possible need to take multiple doses of their NSAID to prevent rebound.

Ergot Preparations

Ergotamine and dihydroergotamine are the ergot alkaloids commonly employed in the treatment of migraine. They were long considered the treatment of choice for moderate-to-severe migraine and are still used widely in the outpatient management of migraine as well as in the emergency room. Historically, the ergots were thought to possess direct vasoconstrictive properties that would reverse the vascular atony responsible for the pain phase. Although the ergots have affinity for several neurotransmitter receptors including those for 5HT, DA, and NE (see Plosker and McTavish, 1994), recent studies suggest that their primary action in headache involves $5HT_{1D}$- and $5HT_{1B}$-receptor agonism (Deliganis and Peroutka, 1991). Activation of $5HT_{1D}$ heteroreceptors in the cranial vasculature has been shown to reduce the release of Sup P, neurokinin A, and CGRP, preventing the initiation of the sterile inflammation cascade. Activation of $5HT_{1B}$ autoreceptors reduces the release of 5HT that induces vasoconstriction through vascular $5HT_2$ receptors. The ergots are thus able to interfere with several components of the cascade of events thought to be involved in the pathogenesis of migraine.

When using the ergots, one must always consider the risk of ergot poisoning or ergotism (Table 5–3). Acute symptoms of ergot poisoning include vomiting, diarrhea, thirst, tingling (limb paresthesias), itching,

Table 5–3 Side Effects of the Ergot Alkaloids[a]

Phase	Side Effects
Acute	Nausea and vomiting
	Abdominal pain and cramping
	Paresthesias (tingling)
	Swollen fingers
	Leg cramps
	Tremor
	Diarrhea
	Confusion
	Unconsiousness
	Myocardial infarction
	Cerebral vasospasm
Chronic	Ergot-induced headache
	Ergot-withdrawal headache
	Intermittent claudication
	Gangrenous symptoms
	Constant nausea
	Ischemic neuropathy
	Dorsal column lesions
	Depression
	Hallucination
	Hemiplegia
	Fixed miosis

[a]Adapted from Tfelt-Hansen and Johnson (1987)

rapid and weak pulse, confusion, and unconsciousness. Chronic use can lead to gangrenous symptoms in the extremities, muscle pain, rebound headache, nausea, vomiting, diarrhea, and dizziness. In more extreme cases of toxicity, ergotism can even lead to confusion, hallucinations, depression, hemiplegia, and fixed miosis. Historically, the burning pain in the hands and feet associated with ergotism was called St. Anthony's fire. In addition ergotism and its associated hallucinations may have been responsible for many allegations of witchcraft. Townspeople suffering from ergotism because they ingested grains contaminated with ergot-producing molds may have perceived others as capable of flying and possessing mystical powers, a perception that was perhaps enhanced by the DA agonist actions of the ergots, which can induce paranoid ideation.

The ergots can be formulated with caffeine (Cafergot), which is thought to enhance their effectiveness by increasing absorption. Caffeine, acting through adenosine receptors (see Chapter 12), may also possess vasoconstrictive properties. Since the ergots can, by themselves, induce nausea and vomiting that is especially troublesome in migraineurs who experience these symptoms as part of their headache, the ergots are also formulated as suppositories. As vasoconstrictors, the ergots are effective in the treatment of postpartum intrauterine bleeding and are contraindicated in patients with coronary artery disease.

Sumatriptan

Sumatriptan was developed specifically for its 5HT agonist action since 5HT is thought to inhibit the release of neuropeptides which initiate sterile inflammation (see Plosker and McTavish, 1994, for review of sumatriptan). This new drug is a selective $5HT_{1D}$ agonist although it also has affinity for the $5HT_{1A}$ and $5HT_{1B}$ receptors. Unlike the ergots, however, it has very little, if any, affinity for the receptors of other neurotransmitters and therefore is associated with fewer side effects. Serotonin 1A, 1B, and 1D receptors are found in the CNS and mediate some of the neurotransmitter's interneuronal actions. However, sumatriptan does not readily cross the BBB and therefore, at normally administered doses, does not affect them (Dallas et al., 1989). Since the dural and cranial vessels thought to be involved in migraine are outside the BBB, the $5HT_{1D}$ heteroreceptors on the terminals innervating these vessels as well as the $5HT_{1B}$ autoreceptors located on 5HT terminals of vasoactive serotonergic fibers are accessible to sumatriptan. The mechanism of action of sumatriptan is therefore thought to be similar to that of the ergots.

Because the bioavailability of sumatriptan is extremely low (16%) and highly variable following enteral administration, the drug is available in a self-injectable form, its normal route of administration in both outpatient and inpatient settings. Absorption is rapid and bioavailability is high (96%) by this route. (An orally active formulation of sumatriptan was just released at this writing.) Although sumatriptan is effective in up to 77% of patients, its cost is very high. Because of its two-hour half-life, the drug clears the body rapidly, leading to rebound headache and the need for additional injections.

Sumatriptan's receptor-specific actions produce few side effects. However, patient complaints about "heaviness" in the chest, flushing and tingling, neck pain with stiffness, and pain at the injection site are common. Sumatriptan does constrict coronary vessels that might explain the chest heaviness. The associated pain can radiate to the left arm, which can be very disconcerting to the patient. Extensive studies revealed no relationship between chest pain and coronary ischemia, however (Hillis and MacIntyre, 1993). The mechanism of this side effect therefore remains unknown. Because of its ability to induce mild coronary vasoconstriction, sumatriptan should not be used with ergots or methysergide, both of which can exacerbate this vasoconstriction.

Combination Agents

Several drug combinations for headaches are available. Many of these formulations combine an analgesic with a sedative to assist the patient through an attack. Midrin is a combination of acetaminophen, isometheptene (a mild vasoconstrictor) and dichlorophenazone (a mild sedative). Other formulations include Cafergot P-B, which combines ergotamine, caffeine, belladonna, and pentobarbital.

Acute Emergency Management of Migraine

Despite the effectiveness of many drugs, migraine may not succumb to even aggressive home therapy. Intravenous dihydroergotamine is commonly employed for uncontrolled migraine although the safety of sumatriptan will undoubtedly lead to more widespread use of this agent in the acute emergency management of headache (see Raskin, 1986). Because of the risk of nausea associated with the ergots, metoclopramide or another DA antagonist such as prochlorperazine or chlorpromazine is generally given intravenously before the ergot. Metoclopramide may be particularly useful since it is also a weak $5HT_2$-receptor antagonist and would assist some of the actions of the ergots. Other less common therapies include intravenous aspirin, corticosteroids, and meperidine (Peroutka, 1992).

PROPHYLACTIC MIGRAINE MANAGEMENT

The best way to manage migraine headaches is to prevent their occurrence in the first place. However, prophylactic treatment is generally only indicated in patients who have frequent attacks (more than three a month). Even when it is effective, complete relief is seldom achieved. In addition, prophylactic treatment should be stopped periodically to determine if the need still exists since patterns of frequent headaches often wax and wane.

Methysergide is regarded as the prototypic agent for migraine prophylaxis (Fig. 5–6). As a $5HT_2$ antagonist, methysergide prevents the vasoconstrictive actions of 5HT released from platelets on vasoactive serotonin receptors and is clearly effective at reducing migraine frequency in many patients (Lance and Anthony, 1966). Although uncommon, several cases of retroperitoneal fibrosis have been associated with its use. This side effect is the result of a cumulative-dose phenomenon and can be avoided by four-to-eight-week drug holidays every six months. Methysergide, an ergot derivative, can also produce nausea, vomiting, and diar-

Prophylaxis   Acute Treatment   E.R. Treatment

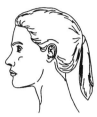
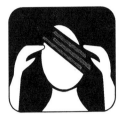
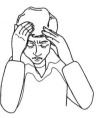

Methysergide
Propranolol
Amitriptyline
Ca^{++} Channel Antagonists

NSAIDs
Ergots
Sumatriptan

I.V. ergot with
metoclopramide,
sumatriptan, or an
opioid

Figure 5–6. Summary of drugs used to prevent and treat migraine headache (NSAIDs = nonsteroidal antiinflammatory drugs; ergots = ergot alkaloid agents; I.V. = intravenous delivery).

rhea. Cyproheptadine, an antihistamine/anticholinergic agent with 5HT-receptor-blocking actions, is effective in some patients.

Because of the risk, albeit small, for retroperitoneal fibrosis, methysergide has been replaced by beta blockers, especially propranolol, as the prophylactic treatment of choice (Weerasuriya, Patel, and Turner, 1982). The effectiveness of beta blockers became apparent when migraineurs reported reduced frequency and severity of their attacks while using these drugs for exertional angina (Wykes, 1968). It is assumed that propranolol blocks glial beta-adrenergic receptors which, in turn, increases K$^+$ uptake by glia, thereby preventing spreading depression of Leao. The main side effects are those traditionally associated with beta blockers, e.g., orthostatic hypotension and lethargy.

Amitriptyline is also useful in the prophylactic treatment of migraine (Couch, Ziegler, and Hassanein, 1976). Amitriptyline is an antidepressant of the tricyclic class whose potency as a 5HT-reuptake inhibitor is slightly greater than its ability to inhibit NE reuptake (see Chapter 11). As an antidepressant, amitriptyline may prevent the cyclic buildup of activity in the orbitofrontal cortex/thalamic loop that triggers the locus ceruleus to initiate the migraine cascade. Studies suggest that amitriptyline may also have 5HT$_2$-receptor antagonistic actions and its efficacy in the prophylaxis of migraine may therefore be similar to that of methysergide's (Fozard, 1982). Its side effects are mostly those associated with the tricyclic antidepressant drugs, which as a class possess potent antimuscarinic actions. The antimuscarinic side effects include dry mouth, urinary retention, dizziness, and blurred vision.

Several Ca^{2+}-channel antagonists are effective in some headache patients (see Greenberg, 1986, for review). Their ability to block different classes of Ca^{2+} channels may be effective in the prophylactic management of migraine because Ca^{2+} entry is the final mediator of vasoconstriction. Preventing Ca^{2+} entry would theoretically prevent the vasoconstrictive phase of headaches that is prevalent among most of the pathogenic hypotheses. Verapamil, nifedipine, flunarizine, and nimodipine have all been used with some success. Several of these agents possess a low affinity for $5HT_2$ receptors, and their ability to prevent migraine at low doses may therefore represent a combination of Ca^{2+}-channel and 5HT-receptor blockade. Their side effects are mild and include orthostatic hypotension and constipation.

6

Sedative-Hypnotics
and Anxiolytics

Prototypical agent: *diazepam* (*Valium*)

T he CNS depressants are a large and chemically diverse group of drugs that reduce the electrical activity of the brain. They are used clinically to facilitate sleep, reduce anxiety, produce anesthesia, promote muscle relaxation, and treat seizures. Drugs used to promote sleep (sedative-hypnotic agents) and reduce anxiety (anxiolytics) will be discussed in this chapter. The anesthetics and muscle relaxants are covered in the next chapter and the antiseizure drugs in Chapter 8. Ethanol, a drug abused for its depressant effects, will be discussed in Chapter 12.

CNS DEPRESSANTS AND CONSCIOUSNESS

Bloom and Lazerson (1988) define consciousness as an active "awareness of one's own mental and/or physical actions" (p. 272). Although their definition implies that we all know what consciousness is, it has thus far been impossible to come to any consensus regarding its neurobiology. What is known is that consciousness requires electrical activity in at least three brain regions: the reticular formation (RF), thalamus, and cerebral cortex. Reducing neuronal activity in any of these structures may disrupt an integration that apparently must be present among these three structures to maintain consciousness. Depressed activity in the RF, as when there is a sudden displacement of the brainstem from a fall or a punch on the jaw, can impair consciousness. Unconsciousness can also occur when increased pressure in the cranial vault compresses the brainstem,

123

compromising its function. On the other hand, bilateral cortical or thalamic depression is often seen in generalized epilepsy or when hypoxia follows asphyxiation or compromised vascular flow. Here, RF activity may be normal but the bilateral loss of cortical activity results in unconsciousness.

Between the states of being either fully alert or unconscious, there are several intermediate levels that have been characterized by behavioral and electroencephalographic means. Sedation is defined as a state of reduced alertness, decreased motor activity, and relaxation. It is a state of consciousness associated with bursts of sleep-like electrical activity during which the patient is neither asleep nor aroused. Hypnosis is a state of drowsiness that leads to sleep from which an individual is readily aroused. The electroencephalogram (EEG) associated with this state exhibits a generalized slowing of electrical activity compared with the awake state. Sedation and hypnosis represent different levels of consciousness that can be viewed as existing along a continuum (Fig. 6–1). As electrical activity in the CNS is depressed further, however, it becomes progressively harder to awaken patients and they become obtunded until a state of stupor exists from which they can be aroused only by painful

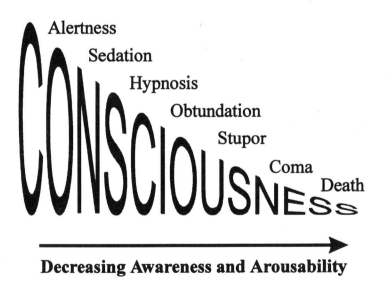

Figure 6–1. Levels of consciousness can be viewed as existing along a plane from a state of alertness through stupor, coma, and death. Distinct signs or symptoms that delineate the levels from one another exist only for stupor, coma, and death. Drugs that affect these levels of consciousness are therefore best viewed as altering levels of consciousness along an arbitrary continuum.

stimuli. Eventually, a state of coma develops from which the patient cannot be aroused by any stimulus. Such patients exhibit only primitive reflexes reflecting global CNS depression. At the final stage of CNS depression, medullary function is compromised to the point where control of respiration and cardiovascular function is lost and death occurs. Although such a continuum is an oversimplification suggesting that the progressive depression of electrical activity in the brain is associated with discrete behavioral patterns, it does help to characterize the various states of arousal. From a pharmacologic perspective it also implies that increasing doses of CNS depressants, with the notable exception of the benzodiazepines, will eventually reduce electrical activity sufficiently to produce coma and even death.

The sedative-hypnotics and anxiolytics share several common actions but also have notable differences. Their similarities and differences are a consequence of their pharmacodynamics. Unlike other chapters in this book, this one will therefore begin with the pharmacodynamics of these drugs and then discuss their use in the management of insomnia and anxiety.

THE SEDATIVE-HYPNOTIC AGENTS

The Benzodiazepines

The benzodiazepines are a large group of drugs whose structures are comprised of a benzene ring fused to a seven-membered diazepine ring (Fig. 6–2). The benzodiazepines currently available in the United States differ in their substitutions at various sites on the benzodiazepine moiety, which can confer dramatically different solubility and pharmacokinetic characteristics. These substitutions primarily determine the drug's onset of action and its duration of effect, which, under most circumstances, determine the choice of drug. In addition, these substitutions may also be responsible for certain subtle differences in CNS effects that are only now becoming apparent. Although such differences appear to be increasingly important, all the benzodiazepines share a common action at GABA receptors.

Benzodiazepine receptors and the Cl⁻ channel

GABA is the primary inhibitory neurotransmitter in the CNS and its effects are mediated by $GABA_A$ or $GABA_B$ receptors. The $GABA_B$ receptor is found predominantly in the spinal cord and is selectively activated by the drug baclofen (therefore the GABA "B" designation), a drug commonly used to treat spasticity. The $GABA_B$ receptor mediates neuronal in-

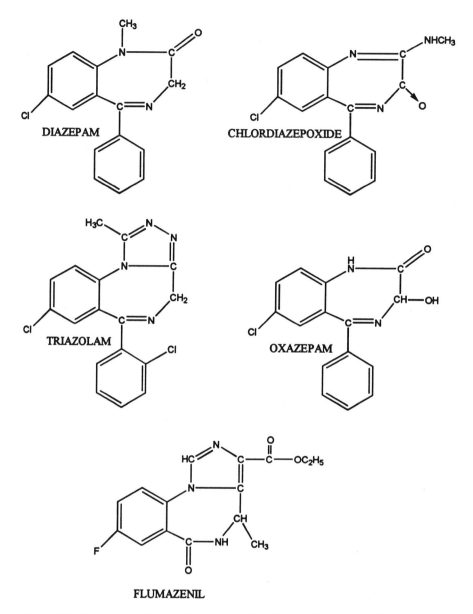

Figure 6–2. Structures of typical benzodiazepine drugs and the benzodiazepine receptor antagonist flumazenil.

hibition via a G protein and by opening K^+ channels that attenuate depolarization (Andrade, Malenka, and Nicoll, 1986). Benzodiazepines, and all other members of the sedative-hypnotic class, predominantly affect the $GABA_A$ receptor.

The $GABA_A$ receptor is a pentamer forming the Cl^- ionophore (Schofield et al., 1987; Fig. 6–3) by combining subunits from three families

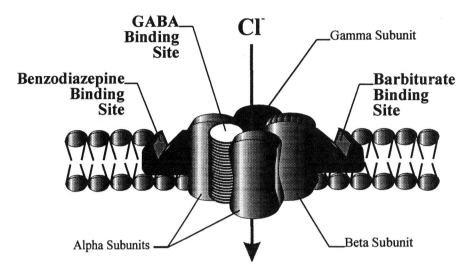

Figure 6–3. The $GABA_A$ receptor is a pentamer consisting of various combinations of alpha, beta, and gamma subunits. Together these subunits form the chloride (Cl^-) ionopohore (channel). In addition to the GABA biding site itself, the $GABA_A$ receptor also contains binding sites for benzodiazepines and barbiturates. These binding sites influence the frequency at which the channel opens and the duration of time the channel remains open in response to GABA, respectively.

designated alpha, beta, and gamma. It is a ligand-gated channel, so the binding of GABA to the $GABA_A$ acceptor moiety induces a conformational change in the pentamer, exposing positively charged amino acid side chains in the center of the protein. Cl^- ions can then bind to this site, causing further conformational change that, in a sense, collapses the extracellular domains of the pentamer and displaces the positively charged amino acid side chains in the channel. Cl^- then enters the cell. The resulting increase in Cl^- conductance neutralizes depolarizing current, attenuating the spread of current down a membrane. (Depolarization and hyperpolarization can also occur depending upon whether Cl^- leaves or enters the neuron, respectively. Which occurs will depend upon the chloride equilibrium potential across the membrane when the $GABA_A$ receptor is activated.) The benzodiazepines enhance the action of GABA at $GABA_A$ receptors by binding to a regulatory site on the ionophore.

One member of the GABA pentamer (the alpha subunit) was originally thought to be the site at which the benzodiazepines bind, but more recent evidence suggests that alpha, beta, and gamma subunits are needed (Pritchett et al., 1989). The site at which all benzodiazepines bind is called the benzodiazepine binding site or benzodiazepine receptor. When a benzodiazepine binds to the GABA pentamer it enhances the affinity of the complex for GABA, thus potentiating the GABA effect. When a benzodiazepine is bound to its site, GABA activates the channel more frequently (Twyman, Rogers, and MacDonald, 1989). The increased frequency at which the Cl⁻ ionophore opens in response to GABA in the presence of a benzodiazepine produces a greater degree of GABA-mediated inhibition. Since many neurons that have $GABA_A$ receptors are interneurons—especially collateral, recurrent, inhibitory fibers that synapse on the axon hillock of excitatory neurons—excitatory activity is reduced. Since GABA is widely distributed, the benzodiazepines reduce electrical activity throughout the brain.

Adenosine reuptake inhibition

In addition to their primary action on ligand-gated Cl⁻ channels, the benzodiazepines also inhibit the reuptake of adenosine (Phillis and O'Reagan, 1988). This action is consistent with the notion that adenosine reduces ACh release from the terminals of the RF's pedunculopontine nucleus (PPN), which is viewed as an important mediator of arousal. Thus, by potentiating the effects of adenosine, benzodiazepines will reduce the activity of the cholinergic PPN-thalamic projection that regulates cortical sensory trafficking (see below). Adenosine also has vasodilatory effects. The reduction in total peripheral resistance and the dilation of coronary vessels observed following systemic administration of benzodiazepines may reflect their effects on adenosine.

Effects on Na⁺ and Ca²⁺ channels

At very high blood levels, such as those seen in the overdose victim or in the patient being treated for status epilepticus, benzodiazepines can directly depress excitatory neurons through mechanisms independent of Cl⁻ conductance and GABA. This effect involves alterations in voltage-gated Ca^{2+} and Na^+ channels (see Haefely, 1989). Even though these effects primarily occur only at higher concentrations, a minor contribution to the overall actions of the benzodiazepines would be expected even at clinically used dosages.

Variation in action

Although all the benzodiazepines produce a similar action at the $GABA_A$ receptor, there are subtle differences in their mechanism of action. These differences contribute to the minor variations in side effects observed among the various benzodiazepines as well as to the ability of some of the agents to be more anxiolytic or antiepileptic than others. They can be summarized as follows: (1) There are known variations in the alpha subunit of the GABA receptor that may bind one particular benzodiazepine with greater affinity than others (Pritchett, Luddens, and Seeburg, 1989). (2) Some of the benzodiazepines are partial agonists at the benzodiazepine receptor site (Pellow and File, 1984). Depending on the dose administered and the relative degree of partial agonism, some agents would be expected to have different levels of activity even at high doses. In these cases, adequate anxiolytic activity may be achieved in the absence of profound sedation. (3) The agents vary in their adenosine actions. (4) There is evidence that certain endogenous steroids bind to the GABA pentamer (Harrison et al., 1987). This binding may account for certain behavioral effects of some glucocorticoids and steroids such as progesterone. Moreover, endogenous differences in the circulating levels of these hormones within a population would be expected to contribute to variations in benzodiazepine responsiveness. (5) There are variations in the relative ability of a given drug to alter voltage-gated Ca^{2+} and Na^+ channels. Although these differences may explain some of the subtle differences in the actions of benzodiazepines, that which most often dictates the choice of drug in a clinical situation is its pharmacokinetic characteristics.

Pharmacokinetics of the benzodiazepines
Even though the benzodiazepines are all moderately lipid soluble, their lipophilicity varies over 50-fold and contributes to the differences among these drugs in their rates of absorption, which determines their onset of action as well as their redistribution—which terminates the CNS effects. All the benzodiazepines are essentially completely absorbed following oral administration. However, clorazepate is decarboxylated in gastric juice to the active agent N-desmethyldiazepam while others, including prazepam and flurazepam, reach the circulation only as active metabolites after biotransformation in the liver.

Biotransformation is also a relevant pharmacokinetic consideration with the benzodiazepine compounds. The biotransformation of the benzodiazepines essentially occurs in three stages: N-desalkylation, hydroxylation, and conjugation. Not all drugs are biotransformed by each stage (Fig. 6–4) and many of the intermediate metabolites are active. Glucuronidation is always associated with loss of biological activity. Those agents that are dealkylated or hydroxylated in the liver exhibit significant first-pass metabolism. Other agents are simply conjugated and then excreted. Based on their method of biotransformation, their lipid solubility (which determines their rate of absorption and redistribution), and their half-lives, benzodiazepines are classified as short, intermediate, or long acting (Table 6–1). Thus, the choice of agent in a given situation is more a function of its pharmacokinetics than its mechanistic variations. If the patient needs a fast-acting drug to induce sleep because of situational anxiety, then a short-latency agent such as triazolam is indicated. Patients who wake up too soon or awaken frequently during sleep but do not have difficulty falling asleep would be more effectively treated with long-

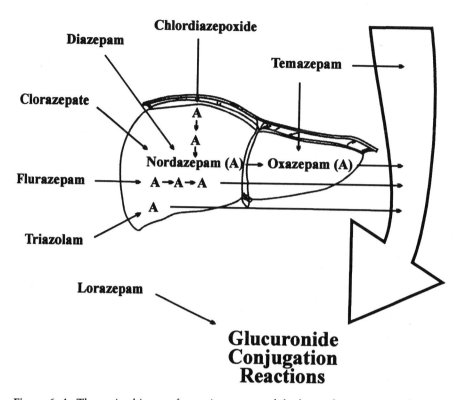

Figure 6–4. The major biotransformation routes of the benzodiazepines are depicted in this figure. Most of the drugs are biotransformed in the liver. In most cases, the product of biotransformation is active (A). However, temazepam, oxazepam, and lorazepam undergo phase II biotransformation only (conjugation with glucuronide), which can occur hepatically as well as extrahepatically.

latency, long-acting agents such as temazepam. Patients undergoing surgery that involves the liver or patients whose liver function is otherwise compromised would be better off using agents such as oxazepam, temazepam, and lorazepam that can be conjugated extrahepatically. (Note that the first letters of these three drug names—*o, t,* and *l*—yield the mnemonic "Outside The Liver.") These agents would also be preferred in young children and the elderly since liver function is generally lower than normal in these populations.

The benzodiazepines have long half-lives. Since they are lipid soluble and conjugated, most are enterohepatically recirculated. This recirculation effectively extends their duration of action. Because of their lipid solubility, benzodiazepines are also redistributed to skeletal muscle and then to body fat. It is this redistribution that curtails their action in the CNS and thus determines the duration of their sedative effects. Their deposition in muscle and body fat and subsequent slow release back into the cir-

Table 6–1 Duration of Sedative-Hypnotic Action[a]

Long Acting (1–3 days)	Intermediate Acting (10–20 Hours)	Short Acting (3–8 Hours)
Diazepam (Valium)	Lorazepam (Ativan)	Triazolam (Halcion)
Clorazepate (Tranxene)	Temazepam (Restoril)	Oxazepam (Serax)
Chlordiazepoxide (Librium)		Secobarbital (Seconal)
Flurazepam (Dalmane)		Amobarbital (Amytal)
		Pentobarbital (Nembutal)

[a]Trade names are in parentheses

culation contributes to the residual effects observed the next day (the drug hangover). Patients complaining of these symptoms should be switched to a shorter-acting drug that has lower lipid solubility. Another consideration in this regard may be that the agent prescribed is biotransformed to an active metabolite. Chlordiazepoxide and diazepam, for instance, are converted to the active intermediate nordazepam which is then converted to oxazepam, effectively extending the duration of sedative effects. Switching the prescription from diazepam to oxazepam may therefore reduce the severity of drug hangover.

Tolerance
Pharmacodynamic and physiologic tolerance accompanies chronic use of the benzodiazepines and reduces their ability to enhance Cl^- conductance (Yu, Chiu, and Rosenburg, 1988). No evidence for pharmacokinetic tolerance exists. The development of tolerance is the primary reason these drugs are not used as antiepileptic agents even though they are acutely effective as such (see Chapter 8).

The development of tolerance can be associated with a return of insomnia, increased muscle tone, and even anxiety while the patient remains on a fixed dosage of the drug. This leads to dosage escalation. A new series of partial agonists at the benzodiazepine receptor site does not appear to induce tolerance as readily (Garratt et al., 1988).

Toxic effects
The benzodiazepines are considered extremely safe drugs. At blood levels associated with suicide attempts or extreme abuse, and even in an occasional hypersensitive patient, they can produce side effects. These effects include light-headedness, lassitude, increased reaction time, ataxia, confusion, dry mouth, anterograde amnesia, bitter taste, nausea and vomiting, epigastric distress, diarrhea, paradoxical anxiety, euphoria, and even a rare hallucination. A wide variety of benzodiazepine-induced allergic, hepatotoxic, and hematologic reactions have been reported, but they are very rare. A significant interaction occurs with any other agent that pos-

sesses sedative-hypnotic actions, especially those drugs that facilitate GABA-mediated actions. Alcohol and barbiturates can thus readily produce additive and even synergistic toxicity. Patients must also be cautioned about the use of certain antipsychotics and antidepressants as well as over-the-counter drugs that, because of their antimuscarinic and antihistamine properties, can induce oversedation when taken with any of the benzodiazepines.

Emergency room treatment of patients resulting from benzodiazepine overdose is extremely rare. In contrast, patients with respiratory depression who are comatose as a result of combining a benzodiazepine with another CNS depressant such as alcohol or a barbiturate are quite common. In such cases, flumazenil (Romazicon), a benzodiazepine receptor antagonist, is often used successfully. Since it is impossible to antagonize the effects of alcohol or a barbiturate, antagonizing the contributing depressant effects of the benzodiazepine with flumazenil will often reverse symptoms adequately to sustain life while the nonbenzodiazepine depressant clears the system. Flumazenil is usually administered i.v. because oral administration is associated with a significant first-pass effect (25% bioavailability). Its short half-life (60 minutes) often necessitates continued administration to maintain respiratory drive. Flumazenil must be used cautiously, however, because a bolus injection, especially in patients who have ingested alcohol or tricyclic antidepressants, can precipitate seizures.

Benzodiazepine dependence
Although the effects of the benzodiazepines are relatively innocuous, chronic use can lead to dependence. This is especially true of their use as sedative-hypnotics. Patients become dependent on their "sleeping pills" to fall asleep. This dependence stems not only from tolerance and rebound insomnia but also from psychological factors. Since falling asleep is partly a ritual, disrupting that ritual (not taking the pill) elicits anxiety and prevents sleep. The individual may lie awake for hours thinking about the missed pill. In addition, withdrawal from the benzodiazepines induces signs and symptoms like those of an abstinence syndrome that can occur following long-term use at therapeutic doses (Owen and Tyrer, 1983). The abstinence syndrome develops gradually over several weeks because of the long half-lives of these drugs. Its signs and symptoms include insomnia, headache, anxiety, mild depression, subtle perceptual distortions, myalgia, and muscle twitches (see Ashton, 1984). This syndrome is not life-threatening and in most cases it is mild. Drug withdrawal symptoms are more pronounced when the drugs are abused at high dosages for recreational purposes (Griffiths and Sannerud, 1987). Although the presence of an abstinence syndrome contributes to contin-

ued use, it is unlikely that benzodiazepines produce compulsive drug-seeking behavior consistent with addiction. The likelihood for abuse and dependence is increased in individuals who have a history of drug abuse, especially when it has involved another CNS depressant.

The Barbiturates

Barbituric acid is 2,4,6-trioxohexahydropyrimidine, which lacks CNS-depressant activity (Fig. 6–5). Alkyl and aryl substitutions at position 5 confer CNS-depressant effects. Various substitutions at the 3' and especially the 5' position determine lipid solubility and therefore duration of effect.

Prior to the advent of benzodiazepines, barbiturates were the drugs most used as sedative-hypnotics. They are still used in various clinical settings (see Smith and Riskin, 1991, for review) but their pronounced ability to cause fatal respiratory depression and their greater potential to produce dependence should preclude their use as sedative-hypnotic agents. Today they are predominantly used as anticonvulsants and anesthetics. They can also be used to treat tremors, as diagnostic tools in epilepsy (Wada Test and others; see Chapter 8), and to aid in psychiatric interviews (the amobarbital interview). As is true of the benzodiazepines, all of these actions are a result of increased Cl^- conductance mediated by the barbiturate's ability to enhance $GABA_A$ activity. The mechanism through which this occurs, however, is distinct from that of the benzodiazepines.

Barbiturates and the Cl^- channel

Although it is unclear which subunit of the $GABA_A$ receptor the barbiturates bind to (see Ragowski and Porter, 1990), we do know that it is a site different from that of the benzodiazepines. An active site on the pentamer that regulates Cl^- gating is the most favored candidate (see Olsen, 1988). Like the benzodiazepines, the barbiturates enhance the binding of GABA to its receptor. While the benzodiazepines enhance the frequency at which the Cl^- channel opens in response to GABA, the barbiturates increase the amount of time the Cl^- channel remains open. Most important is the fact that the barbiturates (except the antiepileptic barbiturates such as phenobarbital) increase Cl^- conductance in the absence of GABA (MacDonald and Barker, 1979). This GABA-independent action is largely responsible for the toxicity of these drugs.

Barbiturates vs. benzodiazepines

The barbiturates such as secobarbital (Seconal) were the main "sleeping pills" until the benzodiazepines were developed. Unlike the benzodiazepines, the barbiturates depress respiration in a dose-dependent fash-

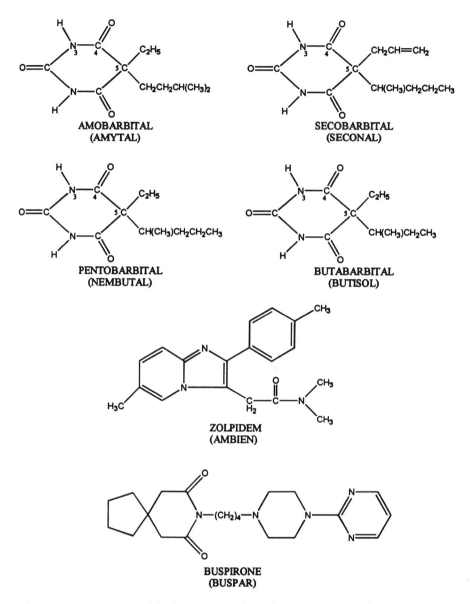

Figure 6–5. Structures of barbiturates used in the management of insomnia. Also shown are the utra-short-acting drug zolpidem and the anxiolytic agent buspirone. The trade names for the drugs appear in parentheses.

ion and can induce coma and fatal respiratory depression at high doses. Death due to a barbiturate overdose is not necessarily an intentional act and can occasionally be the result of a drug automatism. This involves patients who take their pills at 10:00 P.M., for instance, and for some reason awaken at midnight. Being awake and forgetting that they took their pills earlier because of the anterograde amnesiac properties of these drugs (see below), they take more. This cycle can repeat itself until enough of the drug has accumulated to produce toxic effects. A drug automatism is a behavioral pattern in which patients take drugs unnecessarily because the drugs themselves interfere with their ability to determine if the doses are really needed. Drug automatisms are commonly observed in street-drug abusers as well.

Whether intentional or unintentional, the barbiturates have the potential to cause fatal respiratory depression. When the benzodiazepines were developed and it was found that they do not produce respiratory depression when administered orally, they rapidly replaced the barbiturates.

Although both drug classes are sedative-hypnotics that influence Cl^- conductance via the $GABA_A$ receptor, one is safe while the other is potentially lethal. This paradox involves state-dependent action. The benzodiazepines can only enhance the effects of GABA when it is being released—a state-dependent action. When taken orally, the brain levels of the benzodiazepines rise slowly and progressively depress activity in the CNS. Associated with this CNS depression is a reduction in GABA release that eventually results in so little synaptic pool GABA that the benzodiazepine no longer has sufficient GABA to potentiate. As a result, the CNS-depressant effects of the benzodiazepines exhibit a ceiling effect: The ability of a drug to produce its action becomes limited as dosage increases. With the benzodiazepines, the ceiling effect occurs before respiratory depression develops. Thus, killing patients with benzodiazepines taken orally is virtually impossible unless they take so many pills that they literally choke on them. The benzodiazepines can induce respiratory depression when administered i.v., however, because they will be highly bioavailable to the brain when administered at high concentrations. As this high dose floods the brain it encounters normal levels of GABA whose activity is potentiated by the benzodiazepine. Even under these circumstances, however, the respiratory depression that does occur is short-lived due to the ceiling effect. Despite their safety, chronic high-dosage use of the benzodiazepines can lead to respiratory complications in patients with obstructive pulmonary disease since these drugs mildly suppress the ventilatory response to CO_2 (Harvery, 1985).

Although the barbiturates can increase the binding of GABA to the $GABA_A$ receptor, they can also open the Cl^- channel independently of GABA and herein lies the primary difference between these two drug classes. Since barbiturates continue to open the Cl^- channel in the absence of GABA, a ceiling effect will not occur. Even after GABA release is sharply reduced a barbiturate will continue to open Cl^- gates and produce further CNS depression, which can eventually lead to respiratory depression.

Tolerance, dependence, and side effects

Both pharmacokinetic and physiologic tolerance develop during treatment with the barbiturates. Pharmacokinetic tolerance develops first and dosage escalation may be required within a few days after the initiation of therapy. All barbiturates are inducers of the P-450 system that may necessitate a two- to threefold increase in dose within a month in order to maintain normal plasma levels. Shorter-acting barbiturates such as secobarbital are less likely to induce the P-450 system than longer-acting agents such as phenobarbital.

As with the benzodiazepines, continued use of barbiturates leads to dependence. Thus, the "need" to take the pill in order to fall asleep increases with time. In contrast to the benzodiazepines, however, chronic use of the barbiturates, especially if they are being abused for their euphoric effects, can lead to drug dependence associated with drug-seeking behavior—i.e., addiction (see Chapter 12). In addition to the side effects common to most sedative-hypnotic agents, the barbiturates produce several untoward effects. These will be described in detail in Chapter 8.

Other Sedative-Hypnotic Agents

Despite the widespread use of the benzodiazepines as sedative-hypnotic drugs, eight other sedative-hypnotic agents are still marketed in the

Table 6–2 Other Sedative-Hypnotics

Drug (Trade Name)	Half-Life	Distinguishing Characteristics
Zolpidem (Ambien)	2 hours	Benzodiazepine-like and does not disrupt sleep architecture
Meprobramate (Miltown)	6–17 hours	Approved for use in anxiety; overdose associated with hypotension and respiratory arrest
Chloral hydrate (Noctec)	5–10	Trichloroethanol is the active ingredient that produces synergistic effect with ethanol (the "Mickey Finn")
Paraldehyde (Paral)	4–10	Used in the treatment of delirium tremors
Ethchlorvynol (Placidyl)	10–20	Rapidly redistributed associated with early morning awakening
Glutethimide (Doriden)	7–15	Potent antimuscarinic actions
Methyprylon (Noludar)	3–6	Hepatic enzyme inducer
Ethinamate (Valmid)	2–3	Ultrashort acting

United States (Table 6–2). Zolpidem is a nonbenzodiazepine agent that has actions similar to the benzodiazepines. Its advantage over the benzodiazepines is its ultrashort half-life (two hours) and the fact that it does not produce alterations in sleep architecture (see below). All the other agents have actions similar to the barbiturates and although their pharmacodynamics have not been extensively studied, they are assumed to be similar to those of the barbiturates. They are included in this chapter because they are still encountered in the clinical setting, especially in older patients who have been using them for years.

GENERAL ACTIONS OF THE SEDATIVE-HYPNOTICS

Sedation

The neurobiology of sleep

Stimulation of the basal forebrain induces sleep (Fig. 6–6). The basal forebrain includes the nucleus of the diagonal band, the substantia innominata, and the preoptic area. Many fibers of this system are cholinergic. They bypass the thalamus and diffusely project to the cortex and hippocampus, but whether or not the ascending basal forebrain-cortical projections that induce sleep are indeed cholinergic remains to be established (see Jones, 1993, for review). Other regions of the brain, including some lower brainstem nuclei, also can induce sleep when stimulated (see McCarley, 1994, for review). However, the basal forebrain is the only region of the brain where a group of cells is active during slow-wave sleep (SWS) and quiet the rest of the time. In contrast, regions of the posterior hypothalamus have the opposite pattern of activity. They are always active during waking and shut off during sleep.

The induction of sleep is more complicated than simply turning one nuclear group on or off. Other systems are also involved, particularly those located in the reticular formation (RF). The brainstem RF used to be called the reticular-activating system since it was thought to be responsible for consciousness. Various poorly defined RF nuclei, called the pedunculopontine nuclear (PPN) group, project cholinergic fibers to the nucleus reticularis and other thalamic nuclei. This system, along with others in the RF, regulates the "trafficking" of sensory information through thalamic relays and into the cortex. It selectively converts the thalamic response to incoming sensory input from a phasic to a one-to-one relay system, permitting the accurate transfer of sensory information to the cortex. When it is inactive, the thalamus does not transfer sensory information efficiently to the cortex, facilitating sleep (see Steriade, Jones, and Llinas, 1990). Blocking activity of these projections is probably responsible for the sleep-inducing effects of antimuscarinic drugs while caffeine,

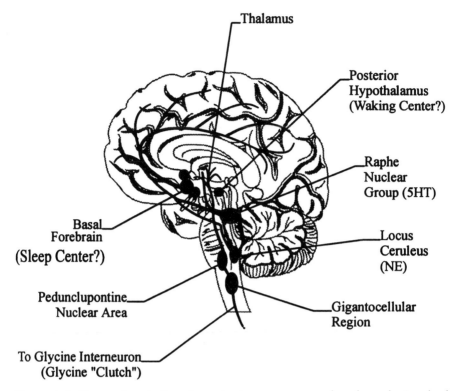

Figure 6–6. Two major cholinergic projection systems are thought to be involved with sleep. The so-called sleep center is in the basal forebrain while the waking center (noncholinergic) is located in the posterior hypothalamus. The pedunculopontine cholinergic group is centrally involved in regulating the flow of sensory activity through the thalamus. Both the raphe system and the locus ceruleus are involved with sensory processing as well as the dreaming cycle. The gigantocellular region is active during dreaming and, through its descending fibers, excites glycine interneurons to prevent motor activity. It may therefore be viewed as a motor function "clutch."

acting as an adenosine heteroreceptor antagonist, increases cholinergic activity and enhances arousal (Karacan, Thornby, and Anch, 1976; see also Chapter 12). In addition, ACh, NE 5HT, other neurotransmitters, and brain-active chemicals are thought to be involved with the sleep–wake cycle, including dopamine, histamine, glutamate, GABA, muramyl or sleep peptides (Brown, 1995), prostaglandins, and melatonin. Their respective roles are described and reviewed be Cabeza, Zoltoski, and Gillin (1994).

Sleep staging
Sleep is divided into five different stages according to their EEG wave forms (Williams, Karacan, and Hursch, 1974). The first four stages are

collectively called non–rapid eye movement sleep (NREM). The fifth stage is called rapid eye movement (REM) sleep. The high-frequency, low-amplitude activity that is indicative of the alert state gradually diminishes through stage I and II sleep until a low-frequency, higher-amplitude activity emerges during slow-wave sleep (stages III and IV). This activity suggests neuronal synchronization. Thus, numerous cortical neurons are firing simultaneously, yielding a high-amplitude, low-frequency waveform on the EEG during slow-wave sleep. In contrast, periods of low-amplitude, high-frequency activity during which ocular movements are seen characterize the EEG during rapid eye movement (REM) sleep. This type of activity is considered paradoxical during sleep since such an EEG waveform is characteristic of the waking state. The polysomnogram (an EEG recording pattern used to study sleep) reveals that the pattern of the sleep stages and also the time spent in each stage vary in a consistent and predictable fashion. Thus, one sleep cycle (REM episode to REM episode) averages 90 minutes (see Fig. 6–7). These patterns change with age as well as during certain pathophysiologic states and are readily influenced by drugs.

REM sleep, dreams, and the "glycine clutch"

The electrical activity of the brain in slow-wave sleep changes dramatically during REM sleep. Activity in the raphe group and the locus ceruleus is sharply reduced while activity in several regions of the RF increases (see Steriade, 1992). This increased RF activity facilitates thalamocortical trafficking, but "awareness" of that activity comes only in the form of a dream. Patients awakened during slow-wave sleep also report images, pictures, or feelings that are not considered dreams although some can be extremely frightening and lead to a condition called pavor nocturnes (night terrors) (Fisher et al., 1971).

The cortical activity that occurs during REM sleep would normally induce muscular activity. However, REM-stage EEG patterns include increased activity in and around the gigantocellular region of the medulla. The descending projections of this region excite glycine interneurons in the spinal cord that hyperpolarize alpha and gamma motor neurons in the spinal cord, effectively shutting off all muscle activity (Chase, Soja, and Morales, 1989). This condition is called REM atony. Thus, the gigantocellular region acts as a "clutch" to the motor-activation patterns that emanate from the cortex during dreaming. With the clutch engaged, the cortex can exercise any circuit without inducing movement that would awaken the sleeper. Abnormalities in this system may be responsible for narcolepsy or REM behavior disorders such as sleep walking. For example, cats with lesions in the pontine centers responsible for REM atony can be seen to act out behaviors as though they were dreaming (Jouvet, 1978).

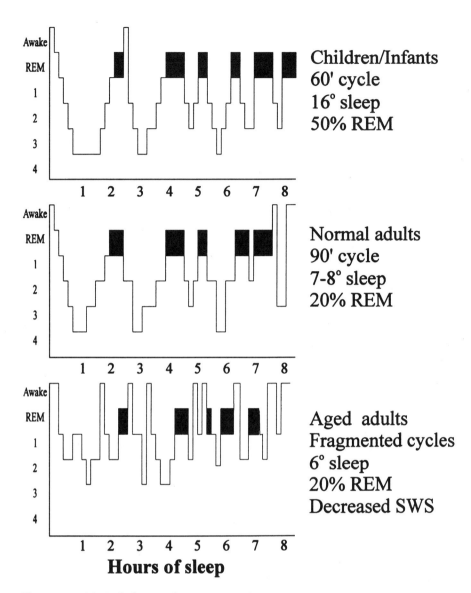

Figure 6–7. Typical sleep architecture in infants, normal adults, and aged adults is depicted. Children spend more time asleep than adults and disproportionately more time in rapid eye movement (REM) sleep. Their sleep cycles (REM burst to REM burst) are on average only 60 minutes. Normal adults have sleep cycles that are, on average, 90 minutes and REM sleep time represents only 20% of that time. Aged adults (>55 yo) require less sleep and spend disproportionately less time in slow-wave sleep (SWS) than do healthy adults. Moreover, their sleep cycles are fragmented.

Effects of the sedative-hypnotics on sleep

All the drugs described above reduce the time needed to fall asleep and extend the time spent in sleep. Increased sleep duration is mainly seen in individuals with sleep debt, not in normal sleepers. The sedative-hypnotics also reduce intermittent arousals during the night and reduce the amount of movement that occurs during sleep. When used appropriately for indicated purposes, the sedative-hypnotics usually induce a restful sleep from which the patient awakens refreshed.

Because they are so effective, however, the sedatives can mask sleep problems that are better managed with other methods or drugs (e.g., depressions, snoring, sleep apnea). In addition, some sleep disorders may be related to behavioral patterns that are best treated without drugs (e.g., late-night coffee, midnight pizza). Elderly patients often require less sleep than do adults and reassurance of this fact may relieve their symptoms.

Although the neurobiology of sleep is beginning to be understood, the mechanism(s) through which increased Cl^- conductance facilitates sleep is currently unknown. The effects of the sedative-hypnotics on activity in the PPN and basal forebrain have been poorly characterized. It is assumed that activation of $GABA_A$ receptors in the RF, thalamus, and cerebral cortex produce a generalized depression of electrical activity that is conducive to sleep. It is important to note, however, that with the exception of zolpiden and chloral hydrate, the sedative-hypnotics reduce the amount of time spent in stages III, IV, and REM sleep while increasing the amount of time spent in stage II. Thus, although these drugs facilitate sleep from a behavioral perspective, the normal EEG activity that characterizes sleep architecture is disrupted. It must therefore be assumed that the sleep induced by activating $GABA_A$ receptors does not mimic natural sleep. The disruption of sleep architecture produced by most sedative-hypnotics does have its clinical advantages, however. Decreasing the amount of time spent in stages III, IV, and REM sleep is often successful in reducing nighttime behavioral disorders such as night terrors, nighttime enuresis, sleep walking, and distressing vivid dreams that occur during these sleep stages.

The sedative-hypnotic agents are a highly effective drug class when used for indicated purposes for short periods (i.e., less than a week). When insomnia is expected, such as during situational stress (brain surgery in the morning) or intercontinental travel, these agents have a well-justified use. Unfortunately, sedative-hypnotic drugs are commonly overused in many of these circumstances. Since tolerance develops to the sedative effects of these drugs, dosage escalation is often seen in patients using these drugs for more than a week. If dosage escalation is not instituted, the alterations in sleep architecture produced by these drugs tend to normalize. As a result sleepwalking or nighttime enuresis, for example, may return. For this reason, the tricyclic antidepressants are considered better drug choices for the chronic management of nighttime behavioral disorders. Moreover, the normalization of sleep architecture with continued sedative-hypnotic use suggest compensatory processes within the brain are at work and such neuroadaptation can produce problems when the drugs are withdrawn.

A common problem with overuse of any sedative-hypnotic is rebound insomnia. After nightly use for only a week, a sedative-hypnotic will induce insomnia or restless sleep when it is withdrawn that can be worse than the problem that led the patient to ask for the medication in the first place. The REM suppression that is also an expected action of these drugs similarly leads to REM rebound when drug ingestion is stoped. Thus, the frequency of REM episodes will be increased and the latency to the first REM episode will be decreased in the nights following discontinuation of chronic use. REM rebound can be associated with bizarre dreams.

Respiratory Depression

The sedative-hypnotics all produce dose-dependent respiratory depression with the exception of the benzodiazepines. The respiratory depressant effects are a consequence of direct inhibition of all aspects of the respiratory cycle. Thus, the chemosensitive regions of the medulla become less sensitive to CO_2, resulting in a blunted neurogenic drive. As the depression increases, even the hypoxic drive generated by the carotid bodies is affected. The depression of the chemosensitive areas is accompanied by depression of the medullary centers responsible for the respiratory cycle. As a result, breathing can be compromised at doses that are only three times higher than those used to sedate. This is especially true when tolerance develops. Thus, tolerance to the sedative-hypnotic effects of these drugs develops more rapidly than the respiratory depressant effects. As the dosage is increased to ensure sedation, the therapeutic index associated with respiratory depression of the barbiturate-like drugs becomes smaller.

Muscle Relaxation

All CNS depressants produce some degree of muscle relaxation that contributes to their sedative-hypnotic effects. At higher doses, motor weakness and even motor incoordination will develop. All sedative-hypnotic agents depress the RF, reducing activity within the descending reticulospinal pathway that is partly responsible for maintaining muscle tone. As a result, gamma-motor-neuron activity in the spinal cord is decreased and muscle tone is reduced. Since the sedative-hypnotics induce muscle relaxation by depressing activity in the RF, muscle relaxation will usually occur only in the presence of sedation. Thus, these drugs neither reduce activity within muscle tissue nor selectively affect the reflex loops in the spinal cord without associated sedation. Consequently, they are not considered true muscle relaxants. The $GABA_B$ selective agonist baclofen (Lioresal) is a true muscle relaxant since it clearly reduces muscle tone at doses that do not significantly affect consciousness. Even with baclofen, if the administered dose is too high, sedation will occur.

Motor Incoordination

At moderately high doses of any of the sedative-hypnotics, many individuals exhibit motor signs similar to those seen when intoxicated from alcohol. These signs are likely a consequence of depressed cerebellar function resulting from $GABA_A$-receptor activation and include disequilibrium, various dysmetrias (e.g., finger-to-nose incoordination), general motor incoordination, slurred speech, increased reaction time, poor fine-motor coordination, and nystagmus. These side effects are not as pronounced following ingestion of the benzodiazepines because of the ceiling effect. In addition, all of the sedative-hypnotics can induce hyporeflexia. However, when plasma levels of the barbiturate-like drugs reach levels that induce stupor or coma, hyperreflexia, indicating global suprasegmental depression, will be seen.

Cognitive Effects

Normal cognitive processing is compromised by all sedative-hypnotics because of CNS depression. Thus, judgment, concentration, insight, and planning are all blunted as dosage is increased. This is particularly true of the barbiturates where toxic levels can severely decrease function at plasma levels that only mildly affect consciousness.

Disinhibition Release

All of the sedative-hypnotics can induce a pleasant feeling or mild euphoria accompanied by paradoxical excitement. Mood is elevated, motivation is enhanced, and behavior is less inhibited. This stems from disinhibition release, a neurobiological rather than a behavioral construct (see Speth, Guidotti, and Yamamura, 1980). Disinhibition release is defined as an increase in the brain's excitatory activity resulting from loss of inhibitory activity—disinhibition. Since inhibitory neurons are far more numerous than excitatory neurons in the CNS, global CNS depression produced by sedative-hypnotic drugs often reduces the activity of inhibitory neurons before the activity of excitatory neurons is affected. Thus, the probability of a drug interacting with an inhibitory neuron is greater. The tendency is also a consequence of the fact that inhibitory neurons tend to be small, unmyelinated interneurons whose large surface-area-to-volume ratio and lack of myelin render them particularly susceptible to the inhibiting effects of increased Cl^- conductance. As the dose of sedative-hypnotic is increased, excitatory neurons are disinhibited, which often translates into a euphoric-like effect. Disinhibition can, unfortunately, have another face, by inducing aggressive, antisocial behavior (Lader and Petursson, 1981). Thus, the pleasant euphoria experienced by most individuals can manifest as a significant personality change in others.

Disinhibition release may underlie, in part, the paradoxical excitement observed in patients medicated with barbiturates who have pain. Such patients exhibit increased motor restlessness, are hyperexcitable, and report increased pain sensitivity following the administration of a barbiturate. This is a unique characteristic of the barbiturates, and mechanisms in addition to the disinhibition release shared by all sedative hypnotics must be responsible.

Anterograde Amnesia

All members of the sedative-hypnotic class can impair memory and produce amnesia at some dose. This is especially true of the benzodiazepines, while the barbiturate-like drugs do so only at doses that are just below those needed to induce unconsciousness. Two forms of amnesia exist: retrograde and anterograde. In retrograde amnesia, the individual is unable to recall events that happened before a certain point in time. In anterograde amnesia, the individual loses the ability to recall events that occurred from a certain point onward. Automobile crash victims often experience anterograde amnesia such that they cannot recall how they got to the hospital or who visited them—events that followed their accident. The sedative-hypnotics and other CNS depressants such as anesthetics and ethanol primarily affect memory consolidation (i.e., the laying down of a new memory) and therefore produce anterograde amnesia. Events from the past that have already been placed into long-term memory are generally not affected.

Interestingly, the benzodiazepines are often used to induce anterograde amnesia. This practice is common in minor outpatient procedures or before major surgery (see Curran, 1986). Even if painful events occur during these procedures, the patient will have no recall of them, which in a sense results in a psychological anesthesia. Despite these indicated uses, anterograde amnesia is considered a negative side effect of these drugs. When used during intercontinental travel to induce sleep, susceptible individuals may function normally during an early morning meeting, recalling preparative work readily, but have no memory of the meeting's outcome. As a result of numerous complaints regarding anterograde amnesia following the use of triazolam (Halcion), a popular drug used for intercontinental travel, the FDA reduced the number of milligrams present in the formulation of triazolam (Halcion) and the United Kingdom banned its distribution altogether. Flunitrazepam (Rohypnol), a particularly potent benzodiazepine that is not marketed in the United States, has been recently abused for its anterograde amnesiac effect. Referred to on the street as "roofies," Rohypnol has gained fame as a "date-rape" drug. This formulation, which has no taste or odor, has been used to drug victims of subsequent sexual abuse. With no recall of the events that transpired the night before, it is difficult for the victim to allege rape.

Drug Hangovers

Several sedative-hypnotic drugs have long half-lives that result in residual effects the next day. These are often manifested as lethargy sleepiness, loss of motivation, and clumsiness and can be confused with the symptoms that led the patient to request a sedative-hypnotic in the first place. If drug hangover occurs, switching the patient to a shorter-acting agent is indicated. If the symptoms still persist, then a diagnosis other than insomnia should be considered. The general effects of CNS depressants are summarized in Table 6–3.

Table 6–3 General Effects of CNS Depressants

Induction of sleep
Lethargy
Sedation
Hypnosis
Obtundation
Stupor
Coma[a]
Death[a]
Anxiolysis
Respiratory depression[b]
Rebound insomnia
REM rebound[c]
Muscle relaxation
Motor incoordination (slurred speech, ataxic gait, and other cerebeller symptoms
Disinhibition release (paradoxic arousal)
Anterograde amnesia
Alterations in judgment, insight, and concentration
Drug hangover

[a]With the exception of the benzodiazepines
[b]Except with p.o. benzodiazepines
[c]REM = rapid eye movement sleep

ANXIOLYSIS

The sedative-hypnotic agents all posses anxiolytic properties to some degree. Anxiety is a normal emotional state involving changes in mood (apprehension, fear, or feelings of impending doom), physiologic arousal (increased heart and respiratory rates), and often increased perceptual acuity (hypervigilance). Anxiety occurs in all humans and anxiety-like behavior is thought to occur in many higher animals. Based on these observations the anxiety response is considered a "hardwired" neuronal circuit that is phylogenetically old. It is adaptive because it prepares the organism for a dangerous situation. In some people, however, anxiety is extreme, irrational, and disruptive enough to incapacitate them. Such persons are said to suffer from an anxiety disorder, which calls for treatment. There are three different forms of anxiety: generalized anxiety, panic disorder, and phobias.

The Amygdala and Anxiety

For anxiety to occur, the provoking stimulus must be interpreted as dangerous. Thus, cortical processing and memory systems must be involved. Increased vigilance and perceptual acuity suggest that sensory processing systems are involved as well. Since anxiety states also involve movement, such as the expression of fear on the face and freezing or flight behavior, specific motor pathways may be affected. Finally, anxiety is accompanied by autonomic activity that can increase blood pressure and respiratory rate and cause heart palpitations, gastrointestinal symptoms (nausea), dizziness, loss of libido, and tremor. Obviously, the neuronal connections mediating this diverse set of signs and symptoms must be extremely complex. Yet a large body of evidence suggests that one central structure, the amygdala, is crucial for this entire response (see Davis, 1992; Pratt, 1992, for reviews).

Electrical stimulation of the central nucleus of the amygdala in both animals and humans (Kuhar, 1986) induces the appearance of fear or reports of anxiety, respectively. Most anxiolytic drugs eliminate signs of anxiety when infused into the amygdalae of animals. In contrast, ablation of the amygdala appears to eliminate fear and anxiety. Mice with such lesions will walk over a cat. Perhaps most important for understanding the development of anxiety, the amygdala plays a central role in the acquisition of the conditioned-fear response. Consider, for example, an animal taught that an audible tone precedes the onset of a foot shock. During the anticipatory period, reliable changes in autonomic activity and "freezing" behavior are used as an index of anxiety. Lesions of the amygdala and anxiolytic drugs infused into the amygdala prevent the acquisition of the conditioned-fear response and the animal consequently does not express the overt signs of anticipatory anxiety (see LeDoux et al., 1988). Certain regions of the amygdala exhibit long-term potentiation so they may carry the memory that underlies the anticipatory anxiety. These are the lateral and amygdalostriatal regions of the amygdala. They are apparently responsible for the acquisition of conditioned fear while the central nucleus of the amygdala, through its connections, initiates the conditioned-fear response (Fig. 6–8). Support for this hypothesis comes from the studies of Reiman et al. (1989), who demonstrated that

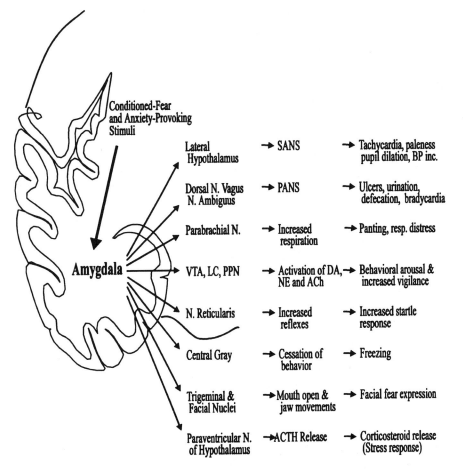

Figure 6–8. The amygdala is pivotally involved in the expression of fear and anxiety. Through the numerous efferent connections depicted in this figure it is capable of coordinating all of the signs and symptoms associated with the anxiety state. It is believed that anxiolytic drugs reduce anxiety by altering activity in this region, thereby disrupting the spiral of CNS activity thought to be involved with the induction of anxiety (VTA = ventral tegmental area; LC = locus ceruleus; PPN = pedunculopontine nucleus; ACTH = adrenocorticotropic hormone).

individuals with panic disorder had increased neuronal activity in the right temporal lobe where the amygdala is located. Moreover, this pattern of activity could be mimicked in normal volunteers anticipating a severe shock after the presentation of a light stimulus (conditioned-fear response).

Other Systems and Chemicals Involved in Anxiety

Although the amygdala plays a central role in the pathogenesis of anxiety, the locus ceruleus and the raphe system are involved as well. By releasing NE into the thalamus and cortex, the locus ceruleus probably helps produce the hypervigilance and heightened sensory acuity of anxiety. Moreover, activation of the SANS via the amygdala's projections to the hypothalamus and the subsequent interaction of NE and epinephrine with beta-adrenergic receptors in the periphery is responsible for the heart palpitations and other sympathetic signs of anxiety. The participation of the raphe system in anxiety is likely although the method is not clearly known (see Taylor, 1990; Charney et al., 1990, for reviews). Serotonergic projections enhance activity in the amygdala and may also mediate behavioral changes associated with the anxiety state through its projections to the frontal cortex and the hippocampus. In addition, raphe fibers increase activity of the locus ceruleus.

Many compounds have been shown to induce anxiety in humans with panic disorders. These include caffeine, several sympathomimetic agents, sodium lactate (product of increased muscle activity), CO_2, hyperventilation, and beta-carbolines (see Uhde and Taner, 1989, for review). The beta-carbolines are the most notable of this list since they are a group of anxiogenic (anxiety-promoting) substances isolated from brain and called diazepam-binding inhibitors (DBIs; Costa, Corda, and Guidotti, 1996). These endogenous substances and others synthesized since their discovery bind to the benzodiazepine acceptor site on the $GABA_A$ receptor, prevent access by benzodiazepines, and reduce the affinity of GABA for its receptor. They are often called inverse agonists since they bind to allosteric sites and reduce the affinity of the normal ligand (Braestrup et al., 1983). The implication of this discovery is that individuals who suffer from anxiety disorder may produce greater quantities of DBIs than does the normal population and consequently be more prone to anxiety attacks. From a pharmacologic perspective, it is especially important that $GABA_A$ receptors are highly concentrated in the amygdala. Thus, GABA-mediated inhibition would be expected to attenuate anxiety that was perhaps induced by excess activity of DBIs.

Based on current knowledge, anxiolytic agents should be effective if they (1) facilitate inhibition in the amygdala by increasing $GABA_A$ activity, (2) reduce SANS activation and especially beta-adrenergic receptor activity, or (3) block serotonin receptors. All of the drugs currently known to possess anxiolytic activity have one or more of these actions.

Anxiolytic Agents

All sedative-hypnotic drugs can alleviate anxiety at some dose. They have been extensively used but only with limited success since they generally reduce anxiety at doses that also produce sedation. Thus, they are not anxioselective. This is especially true of the barbiturates and the other barbiturate-like sedative-hypnotics even though meprobamate was originally approved for use as an anxiolytic agent. Whether or not benzodiazepines are anxioselective remains an open question. Eight agents have been approved by the FDA for the management of anxiety: chlordiazepoxide, diazepam, oxazepam, clorazepate, lorazepam, prazepam, alprazolam and halazepam. Since some benzodiazepines can produce regionally specific effects due to differences in their affinity for the various subtypes of benzodiazepine receptors as well as their varying ability to potentiate adenosine effects, the possibility exists that anxioselective actions can be produced. The evaluation of this notion is ongoing. It may be possible that tolerance develops to the sedative-hypnotic effect faster than the anxiolytic actions of these drugs. If such a differential tolerance occurs, the benzodiazepines would represent a very safe drug group for use in anxiety disorders.

The benzodiazepines are the drugs most commonly used for generalized anxiety. Alprazolam, clonazepam, and lorazepam are particularly effective in acute anxiety episodes where autonomic activity is pronounced (panic attacks). Phobias, however, are not effectively managed on a chronic basis with these drugs. Rather, when patients anticipate exposure to an anxiety-provoking cue, they are encouraged to take their benzodiazepine just before the attack. Continuously medicating such patients is much less efficacious. Other drugs can be effective in managing panic attacks and other anxiety disorders, including many of the tricyclic antidepressants (see Chapter 11). A new group of anxiolytic drugs, including buspirone, has pharmacologic properties differing from those of the sedative-hypnotics and tricyclic antidepressants and may represent a new type of anxioselectivity.

Buspirone

Buspirone (Buspar) and the related azipirones (gepirone and ipsapirone) are $5HT_{1A}$ agonists that reduce clinical measures of anxiety without causing significant sedation (see Taylor, 1990, for review). Moreover, buspirone does not have significant muscle relaxant or anticonvulsant properties and does not produce psychomotor impairment, potentiation of the effects of alcohol, anterograde amnesia, dependence, or tolerance. Its side effects are few—headache, dizziness, light-headedness, and nervousness. As a $5HT_{1A}$ agonist or partial agonist, buspirone reduces the firing rate of raphe neurons through its axodendritic feedback-inhibitory actions. This reduces 5HT release in the parahippocampal region, amygdala, and other limbic regions thought to be associated with anxiogenesis.

The anxiolytic effects of buspirone require three to four weeks to develop, which indicates that merely activating the $5HT_{1A}$ receptor and reducing 5HT release in target structures is not sufficient for anxiolysis. Charney and colleagues (1990) have proposed that the anxiolytic effect of buspirone results from increased serotonergic activity. They argue that the chronic reduction of 5HT release produced by buspirone leads to postsynaptic $5HT_2$ hypersensitivity. Since receptor-site hypersensitivity takes time to develop, this would explain the delay in the efficacy of buspirone.

Propranolol

Propranolol (Inderal) is the prototypical agent for situational anxiety such as stage fright. This nonspecific beta-adrenergic receptor antagonist reduces the actions of NE and epinephrine in the CNS as well as in the periphery where heart palpitations are thought to contribute significantly to the spiral of sympathomimetic effects that contribute to situational anxiety. Propranolol has few side effects and is therefore safe to use. The side effects that attend propranolol use are similar to those of any nonspecific beta-blocker and include bronchoconstriction, arrhythmias, reduced glycogenolysis, and glucagon secretion as well as impaired sexual function in some men.

7

General Anesthetics, Local Anesthetics, and Muscle Relaxers

Prototypic agents: *halothane* (*Fluothane*), *procaine* (*Novocaine*), *and curare*

Anesthetizing a patient for surgery is a complex pharmacological maneuver. According to Guedel's Stages of Anesthesia (Table 7–1), the anesthetized patient should be unconscious, have minimal muscle tone, maintain full cardiovascular and respiratory activity, and later have no recollection of the procedure and experience no side effects. This level of consciousness approaches a near-death state. General anesthetics administered alone, whether as volatile gases or as intravenous drugs, can induce such a condition only at dangerously high doses. But adjuvant agents, including muscle relaxers, analgesics, and sedative-hypnotics, administered before and after the general anesthetic allow the use of a lower dose of anesthetic and offer a wider margin of safety. Adjuvant agents also reduce the incidence of complications during and after surgery. They make anesthesiology a specialty involving extensive knowledge of the pharmacodynamics, pharmacokinetics, and interactions of several drug classes.

The use of local anesthetics, by contrast, is straightforward. These drugs are intentionally used to block nerve conduction only in specific regions of the central or peripheral nervous system. Since they do not normally affect consciousness, they have much higher therapeutic indices than the general anesthetics and produce fewer side effects. Although local anesthetics can be associated with systemic toxicity, the dosages that are generally employed produce negligible systemic effects even if the drug does enter the general circulation. Unfortunately, procedures involving large areas of the body for extended periods of time or those where extensive cutting of internal structures is required would necessitate nu-

151

Table 7–1 Guedel's Stages of Anesthesia

Stage	Phase	Characteristics
I	Analgesia	In this stage, analgesia is achieved without loss of consciousness with minimal or no loss of muscle tone
II	Delirium	This stage describes the transition from loss of consciousness to anesthesia during which excitement and involuntary muscle activity are present and increased muscle tone can occur; incontinence, hypertension, and tachycardia are also commonly seen
III	Anesthesia	This stage describes the transition from the end of delirium, when respiration smoothes and excitation wanes, to cessation of respiration; this stage is subdivided into four planes based on the character of respiration, eye movements, reflexes, and pupillary size; since many of the preanesthetic medications influence these features, respiration and blood pressure (BP) are the most useful indices of the various planes
IV	Medullary depression	During the stage of medullary depression, cessation of respiration and vascular collapse occur (no vascular smooth muscle tone)

merous injections of a local anesthetic and make their use impractical and potentially dangerous. In such operations, the general anesthetics, especially the volatile gases, are most often used.

VOLATILE (GAS) ANESTHETICS

The volatile anesthetics are a small group of drugs with simple molecular structures (Fig. 7–1). They are all CNS depressants since they reduce electroencephalographic activity globally in a dose-dependent fashion (Clark and Rosner, 1973). As CNS depressants, most of the discussion in the last chapter is applicable to these drugs. Thus, at some administered dose they can all produce unconsciousness, anterograde amnesia, motor incoordination, and depressed respiration. Unlike other CNS depressants, however, the volatile anesthetics have a profound effect on the cardiovascular system, making their use very dangerous. In addition, the principles that guide the delivery of volatile anesthetics are strikingly different because they are administered as gases. Dosing is therefore problematic and many anesthesiologists have adopted an entirely different unit of potency called the minimum alveolar concentration, or MAC.

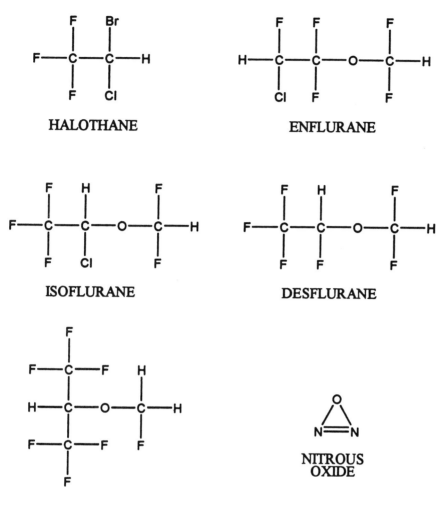

Figure 7–1. Structures of volatile anesthetics used in the United States.

Minimum Alveolar Concentration (MAC)

A MAC of 1.0 is defined as the amount (percent of 1 atmosphere) of an inhalation anesthetic administered at 1 atmosphere of pressure needed to prevent movement in response to a surgical skin incision in 50% of a general population of unparalyzed patients (Eger, 1974). MAC is thus an ED_{50} value. Its usage is based on the assumption that at equilibrium, the percentage of gas in the alveolar compartment is correlated with that in brain. Since alveolar concentration is readily measured, it serves as a convenient index of the brain's anesthetic concentration.

MAC is a measure without units although it is generally described in terms of volume percentage in the lungs. The potent agent halothane need occupy only 0.75% of the total pressure of gas in the lung compartment to attain a MAC of 1.0. The volume of gas needed to induce 1.0 MAC thus serves as a point of reference for comparing anesthetic potencies. It is important to note, however, that although MAC depicts the point on the dose-response curves where potencies are compared, the slopes of those curves can differ dramatically. Thus, the effects of 1.5 MAC for halothane may be very different from those observed at 1.5 MAC of enflurane (see Waud and Waud, 1970). Despite this problem, MAC is impressively stable from patient to patient and is not readily influenced by factors such as sex, duration of anesthesia, acid-base fluctuations, oxygen tension, or anemia (see Lerman et al., 1983; Quasha, Eger, and Tinker, 1980). Only patient age, time of day, thyroid function, and body temperature change it. Most anesthesiologists work at MACs between 0.8 and 1.2 and then ensure adequate anesthesia with adjunctive medications.

Administration, Distribution, and Elimination of Volatile Anesthetics

All currently used gas anesthetics are volatile liquids at room temperature. As such, they vaporize in the anesthetic apparatus and enter the lungs as a gas. Because they are gases, the term tension is used to describe their concentration in the blood or brain in the same fashion that concentration is used for drugs that are not gaseous. When administered as a gas into the alveolar compartment from an anesthetic apparatus they equilibrate with the blood. Excellent control over blood tension is achieved by adjusting the rate of gas flow. This is an important characteristic of these agents. Since the anesthetic gases have the lowest therapeutic indices of the commonly used drugs (TIs between 2 and 4) the ability to rapidly control blood tension enables the anesthetist to reverse a potentially dangerous overdose quickly. This characteristic is in marked contrast to the intravenous anesthetics that cannot be recalled once administered.

The distribution of an anesthetic is best described by using a three-compartment model: the alveolar, blood, and brain compartments. The drug must first pass from the alveolar compartment to the blood compartment, where one set of rate constants is in effect, and then from the blood to the brain, where a completely different set of constants is at work. During anesthesia, the anesthetist has significant control over the distribution of the drugs among these compartments because they are administered in a "closed system." Since the gases in common use today are not significantly biotransformed (except halothane) or excreted and less than 1% of a delivered gas diffuses out of the body across the skin, the drug has nowhere to exit the body and the system is said to be closed. The anesthesiologist thus controls the amount of drug entering the brain from blood by regulating the partial pressure in the alveolar compartment, which determines blood tension. This is markedly different from the kinetics affecting other drugs, where varying degrees of bioavailability, metabolism, and secretion, over which the physician has little control, dramatically affect brain levels. The solubility of an anesthetic in blood is therefore of paramount importance in determining the rate of induction of anesthesia. (Cardiac output and respiratory rate will influence induction but their contributions under normal circumstances are minor.)

Solubility of gas anesthetics in blood
Because volatile anesthetics are amphipathic (lipophilic and hydrophilic domains are present), they dissolve first in the aqueous phase of blood (unbound pool) and then equilibrate with the various components of blood forming the bound pool (albumin and membranes in blood cells). The amount of drug that dissolves into blood is determined by its blood : gas partition coefficient. (The blood : gas partition coefficient [designated by the Greek letter lambda] is a physical characteristic of a drug that describes the amount of drug present in blood in contact with a volume of the gas at 1 atmosphere of pressure.) Only the drug dissolved in the aqueous phase is free to leave the blood and enter the brain. Table 7–2 depicts the relative solubilities of the volatile anesthetics currently in use. The blood : gas partition coefficients for these agents vary more than fivefold while the brain : blood coefficients are virtually identical. This disparity reinforces the notion that the delivery of a drug to the blood is the driving force for anesthetizing the brain.

The relative solubility of the agent in blood and brain has a profound effect on the rate of induction of anesthesia. Halothane has the highest blood : gas partition coefficient and readily leaves the alveolar compartment to enter blood. In contrast, nitrous oxide is more soluble in air than in blood. One would therefore assume that the more blood-soluble agent

Table 7–2 Solubilites of Volatile Anesthetics in Air, Blood, and Brain

Anesthetic Agent	Blood : Gas Coefficient	Brain : Blood Coefficient
Nitrous oxide	0.47	1.1
Desflurane	0.42	1.3
Sevoflurane	0.69	1.7
Isoflurane	1.40	1.6
Enflurane	1.80	1.4
Halothane	2.40	1.9
Methoxyflurane	15.0	1.4

halothane would induce anesthesia faster than nitrous oxide, but the exact opposite is true. The induction of anesthesia is actually inversely related to a volatile anesthetic's blood solubility. Since the rate of entry from the blood into the brain is dictated primarily by its partial pressure in blood, it takes more time to raise the tension of halothane in blood than that of a less soluble drug such as nitrous oxide. Thus, the more soluble an anesthetic agent is in blood, the greater the quantity that must be dissolved in blood to raise its partial pressure there appreciably before it exits the blood to enter brain. A metaphor helps to better understand this apparent paradox.

In the three-compartment model of anesthetic delivery, consider the blood compartment as a bucket that must be filled with anesthetic (Fig. 7–2). In order for the drug to pass into the brain, the drug must fill the bucket and then spill over. Drugs with a large blood : gas partition coefficient such as halothane are very soluble in blood and the blood can contain a large quantity of the drug; i.e., the bucket is large. Nitrous oxide has a small coefficient so the bucket is small. The large bucket takes a long time to fill and overflow. Halothane thus induces the anesthetic plane slowly because it has high blood solubility. In contrast, the small nitrous oxide blood bucket fills rapidly, spills into brain quickly, and achieves the anesthetic plane more quickly. The notion that a drug with high blood solubility induces anesthesia slowly is counterintuitive unless it is remembered that blood represents only one compartment of a three-compartment model.

Brain concentration and elimination

The entry of the anesthetic gases into the brain depends on their partial pressures in blood and brain perfusion. For most anesthetics the brain: blood coefficient is around unity and the tension in blood is indicative of the concentration in brain. Highly perfused organs such as brain receive a disproportionate share of the total body load of the gas during the early phase of administration compared with the less perfused areas such as fat. Gas tension therefore preferentially builds up first in brain. Once in the brain, redistribution to muscle and then fat occurs (Eger, 1974). Such redistribution would normally cause the patient to awaken if anesthetic wasn't being continuously supplied to the alveolar compartment.

Once the flow of gas to the alveolar compartment is discontinued, the elimination kinetics for volatile anesthetics are governed by the same principles described above for induction but in reverse. (Liver biotransformation is a contributing factor only for halothane.) Redistribution from brain allows the patient to awaken. After redistribution, the drug is cleared from the system back out across the lungs. The rate of this elimi-

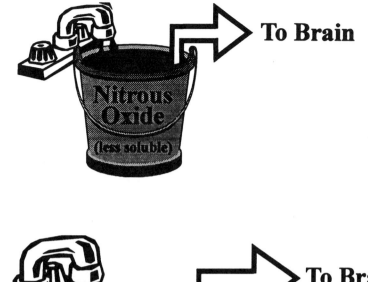

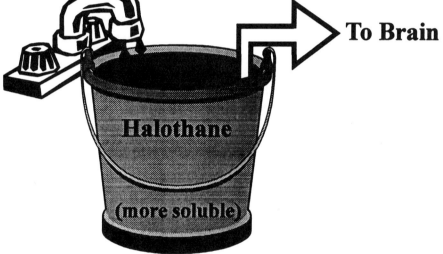

Figure 7–2. The rate of anesthetic induction is paradoxic in that agents with low lipid solubility induce anesthesia faster than do agents with high blood solubility. If it is assumed that an agent such as nitrous oxide has low blood solubility, it can be depicted as a small bucket. With low blood solubility, the bucket will fill quickly and spill over to induce anesthesia in the brain. In contrast, drugs with high blood solubility have large buckets that fill more slowly. A longer induction time is therefore needed before the bucket fills to overflow, when brain induction will occur.

nation is again controlled by the distribution coefficients of the particular drug. Thus, drugs such as nitrous oxide that are poorly soluble in blood, are eliminated into the alveolar compartment very rapidly. This rate of elimination into the lungs can be so rapid that anesthetic tension there becomes very high. As a result, high partial pressures of insoluble anesthetics prevent adequate amounts of oxygen from entering the lungs, leaving the patient hypoxic. This is called diffusion hypoxia and is prevented by slowly terminating the administration of such agents or by providing pure oxygen for the patient instead of room air. In contrast, drugs with high blood solubility such as halothane leave the body more slowly. This is especially true during long procedures. The fat : blood coefficient of anesthetics such as halothane is high, so despite its low perfusion, fat can represent a large reservoir for anesthetic. Large tensions can build up in fat during long periods of anesthesia, and halothane will continue to reenter blood long after anesthesia is terminated. The residual effects this blood tension will have on the brain will keep the patient groggy and lethargic after awakening—an effect similar to that described in the last chapter for the drug hangover.

Pharmacodynamics of Volatile Anesthetics

For almost 90 years it was assumed that volatile anesthetics destabilized the normal structure of neuronal membranes. As proposed by the Overton-Meyer hypothesis, anesthetic gases were thought to increase the fluidity of membranes and thereby disrupt the protein matrix sufficiently to interfere with the normal function of membrane proteins (Overton, 1990, translation; Meyer, 1906). Voltage-gated Ca^{2+} channels, for instance, are particularly sensitive to the effects of gas anesthetics. The Overton-Meyer hypothesis is supported by the fact that the MAC of an anesthetic correlates highly with its oil : gas partition coefficient at 37°C. (The oil : gas partition coefficient is a physical characteristic of a drug that determines the ratio of the amount of a gas that will leave air and dissolve in olive oil at 37°C.) This correlation implies that an anesthetic's efficacy depends upon its ability to enter a hydrophobic medium—the membrane.

It has been argued, however, that the concentrations of the anesthetics actually achieved in the membrane are insufficient to produce an appreciable effect (Franks and Lieb, 1981). This challenge was countered by the so-called critical volume hypothesis, which suggested that only a small concentration of anesthetic in lipid around embedded proteins would interfere with electrical conduction (see Miller, 1993, for review). However, single-unit recordings of sensory cells in an anesthetized animal revealed no attenuation of electrical spike density or character in response to sensory traffic, suggesting that generalized depression of neuronal conduction does not occur at tensions that can induce unconsciousness. Rather, the volatile anesthetics have been shown to reduce neuronal firing selectively in the thalamus and layer V of the cortex (reviewed by Angel, 1993). Layer V of the cortex gives rise to pyramidal neurons that serve as the primary outflow systems of the cortex which project to the basal ganglia, brainstem, and spinal cord. By acting on these selected neuronal networks, volatile anesthetics disrupt sensory processing in the thalamus and suppress motor output from layer V while leaving other major reflex systems unaffected. This specificity suggests specific binding sites.

More recently, the volatile anesthetics have been shown to induce anesthesia in a stereoselective fashion (Franks and Lieb, 1994). For instance, the dextrorotary isomer of isoflurane is much more potent than the levorotary isomer, suggesting a specific protein binding site. It now seems likely that volatile anesthetics bind to hydrophobic regions of specific proteins at membrane-spanning domains that interface with the surrounding lipid membrane (see Watts, 1991; Fig. 7–3). This binding site could only be reached if the agents first dissolve in the membrane, which would explain the high correlation between an anesthetic's partition coefficient and its MAC. Moreover, an action at a specific binding site would also explain the regional specificity of these drugs.

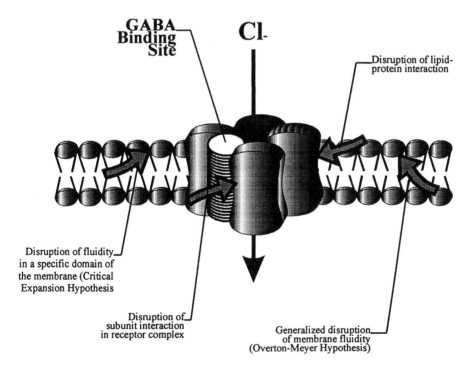

Figure 7–3. This figure depicts the possible sites at which volatile anesthetics may act on neurons. Both the critical expansion hypothesis and the Overton-Meyer hypothesis postulate that volatile anesthetics disrupt overall membrane fluidity. These hypothesis cannot account for the steroselective nature of anesthesia and, as a result, more recent hypotheses have proposed that volatile anesthetics interact with specific binding sites on the subunits comprising the GABA_A-receptor site or disrupt the interaction between the GABA_A-receptor complex and the surrounding membrane.

The Volatile Anesthetic Agents

The first gas anesthetic to be used was ether, and its introduction in 1846 revolutionized surgical procedures. The disadvantages of ether were its flammability (it could explode in surgical suites) and its propensity to increase respiratory secretions. Although care in its handling and in use of the adjuvant atropine markedly reduced these problems, ether was replaced by safer agents in the early 1960s. Chloroform and cyclopropane were introduced but had the disadvantages of hepatotoxicity and explosiveness, respectively. Today, several drugs are available that do not explode, induce only minimal airway secretion, and have relatively little toxicity. Of those agents in broad general use today, all are substituted ethers except halothane and nitrous oxide. Although the structure of halothane is atypical, it is still the industry standard and therefore appropriately designated the prototypic agent. The effects and side effects of halothane will be described below within the context of its prototypic standing. Unique characteristics of isoflurane, enflurane, desflurane, and sevoflurane will be described where appropriate and are summarized in Table 7–3. Because of its unique characteristics, nitrous oxide will be described separately.

Table 7–3 Common Effects of Volatile Anesthetics[a]

	Halothane	Isoflurane	Enflurane	Desflurane	Sevoflurane	Nitrous Oxide
MAC	0.77%	1.15%	1.7%	7.25%	2.05%	104.0%
Respiratory depression	++	+++	++++	++	++	—
Bronchial relaxation	Yes	Yes	Yes	No	No	No
Bronchial secretions	Yes	No	Yes	No	No	Yes
Reduced cardiac function	++	+	+	+	+	—
Catecholamine sensitization	+++	—	+	—	—	—
Decreased vascular tone	8%	32%	22%	~38%	~32%	Vasoconstriction
Analgesic potency	+/−	+/−	+/−	+/−	++	+++

[a]MAC = minimum alveolar concentration; — = none; +/− = minimal; + = slight; ++ = moderate; +++ = pronounced; ++++ = severe

Respiratory depression

The volatile anesthetics to varying degrees produce a dose-dependent reduction in respiratory drive typical of CNS depressants. Chemoresponsiveness (hypoxic and neurogenic) and motor coordination of the respiratory cycle are both attenuated. Oxygen transfer across the alveoli is also compromised. (The increase in membrane fluidity produced by gas anesthetics decreases the rate at which O_2 diffuses across the alveolar membranes.) Increasing the partial pressure of inspired oxygen overcomes this problem.

Many of the volatile anesthetics induce bronchodilation through their ability to reduce Ca^{2+} conductance in the bronchial smooth muscle, allowing their safe use in asthmatic patients. However, some of the agents including halothane and enflurane are mild bronchial irritants and reduce mucociliary flow that, together, contribute to increased bronchial secretions. These secretions can potentially compromise ventilation unless antimuscarinic adjuvant agents such as atropine are used.

Cardiac depression

The volatile anesthetics produce a dose-dependent reduction in cardiovascular efficiency by reducing Ca^{2+} conductance and by depressing the medullary cardiovascular centers. Halothane is most potent in this regard while isoflurane may actually increase heart rate. Halothane use is associated with a negative chronotropic, inotropic, and dromotropic effect on the heart. The negative chronotropic effect (decreased frequency of contraction) is a product of reduced sympathetic drive within the medullary cardiovascular centers resulting from CNS depression. Antimuscarinic adjuvants are often used to prevent excessive cardiac slowing. Negative inotropy (reduced strength of contraction) occurs when Ca^{2+} conductance becomes decreased following halothane's inhibition of voltage-gated Ca^{2+} channels. The negative dromotropy (slowed conduction rate through heart tissue) is also a consequence of reduced Ca^{2+} conductance that depresses the His-Purkinje system. The resulting slowed conduction velocity facilitates the emergence of arrhythmias, especially of the reentry type. This negative dromotropic effect can cause cardiac complications when epinephrine is released by the adrenals—a phenomenon called catecholamine sensitization.

Halothane is the most potent of the volatile anesthetics at inducing catecholamine sensitization. The term implies that the heart is overly sensitive to the effects of catecholamines and describes the increased propensity for arrhythmias to develop in response to epinephrine (Epi). These arrhythmias result from epinephrine's actions in a heart in which chronotropy and dromotropy are significantly depressed.

Epi is released during surgery in response to intact pain reflexes that activate the SANS stimulating the adrenal medulla. After many hours of surgery, increased plasma levels of Epi and NE are generally observed. Epi then binds to alpha- and beta-adrenergic receptors throughout the body including the heart, where it has a positive chronotropic effect. Normal electrical signals coming out of the His-Purkinje system travel around areas of preexisting cardiac pathology such as a subclinical infarct or area of reduced conduction. Normally, the electrical signal moving around one side of a tissue defect will enter the tissue on the other side of the defect and find that side already depolarized or in a refractory period (see Fig. 7–4). Reentry arrhythmias do not normally occur in cardiac tissue or even in tissue with preexisting pathology under the influence of halothane alone. However, if Epi causes a sudden increase in chronotropy in the presence of halothane, an electrical signal moving around one side of a defect can find the tissue on the other side of the defect nonrefractory and therefore excitable. This region then fires out of sequence with the rest of the heart. This depolarization then spreads to adjacent tissue, disrupting the normal pattern of synchronous depolarization, creating an arrhythmia. Electrical activity has thus reentered an area of tissue that should be refractory, and the resulting arrhythmia is called a reentry arrhythmia.

Vascular tone

The volatile anesthetics cause various degrees of vasodilation. These vasodilatory effects are a combined result of their direct actions on vascular smooth muscle (decreased Ca^{2+} conductance) and an indirect action caused by depression of baroreceptor reflexes and the SANS centers in the medulla. Anesthetics such as isoflurane and desflurane may require adjuvant vasoconstrictors to maintain adequate vascular flow during surgery. Despite the fact that most tissues exhibit reduced perfusion, autoregulatory function mediated by adenosine in the heart is not compromised and cardiac ischemia generally does not occur. The volatile anesthetics except for isoflurane also reduce the vascular response to CO_2 in the brain, making isoflurane the volatile anesthetic of choice among neurosurgeons.

Muscle relaxation

Skeletal muscle relaxation is needed in surgery to ease limb manipulation and allow for clean surgical incisions that can readily be apposed for suturing. At one time, the degree to which skeletal muscles were relaxed by volatile anesthetics was an important consideration in the choice of an agent. The dose of many volatile anesthetics needed to achieve this level of relaxation was dangerously high, however, and adjuvant muscle relax-

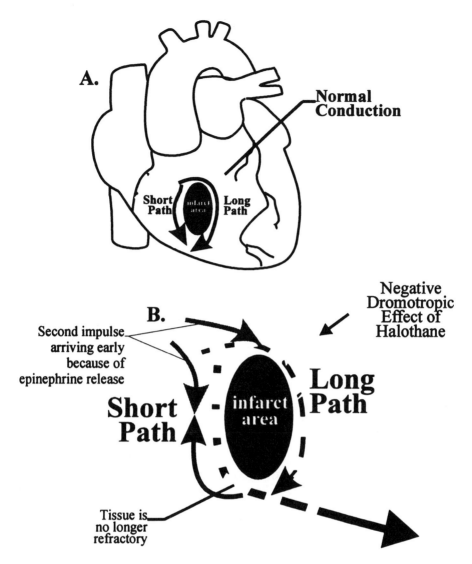

Figure 7–4. The mechanism for reentry arrhythmias following halothane administration is depicted in this schematic. In a normal healthy heart, excitability is transmitted through the His-Purkinje system. If a tissue defect such as an infarcted area exists, the excitation invading the area must travel around the area as depicted in A. Ectopic beats do not occur in the area of the infarct because the relative and absolute refractory periods preclude the initiation of a depolarization by the excitation of the long path that invades the area of the short path as it travels a longer distance. Under the influence of the negative dromotropic effects of the volatile anesthetics, however, conduction rate (dromotropy) decreases. This slowed conduction rate allows greater time for recovery from the refractory period. As depicted in B, the excitation traveling the long path can invade the area of the short path that is no longer refractory and initiate depolarization. The initiation of this depolarization would then interfere with the next (second) impulse traveling the His-Purkinje system, especially if it were to come earlier, as would be the case if epinephrine were present, preventing a normal pattern of contraction and a reentry arrhythmia.

ers such as gallamine are now commonly used. (Isoflurane is atypical among the anesthetics since it produces pronounced muscle relaxation at inspired tensions normally used during anesthesia.) Halothane actually potentiates the effects of muscle relaxers by enhancing their action at the neuromuscular junction (reduction of Ca^{2+} uptake by sarcoplasmic reticulum) and by reducing their biotransformation.

Analgesia

With the exception of sevoflurane and nitrous oxide, the general anesthetics do not produce sufficient analgesia at anesthetizing tensions to depress visceral pain reflexes during surgery. Consequently, adjuvant analgesics are often employed.

Liver function and biotransformation

Liver function is generally reduced by the volatile anesthetics to the extent that drug biotransformation by the microsomal system is impaired. This is likely a consequence of increased membrane fluidity which is thought to impair the activity of microsomal enzymes embedded in membranes. Biotransformation rates return to normal following anesthesia, however.

Of the volatile anesthetics in common use today, only halothane is biotransformed to any clinically significant extent (12 to 20%). This biotransformation is a factor during the induction and maintenance of anesthesia. Its biotransformation may also produce toxic metabolites that initiate an immunologic reaction, resulting in "halothane hepatitis" (Hubbard et al., 1988). The incidence of this hypersensitivity reaction is increased by continued exposure and has reduced the popularity of halothane, not so much because of the risk to the patient, which most often is minimal, but because of the risk to operating room personnel, who may be continuously exposed. Halothane hepatitis, if it is going to occur, will manifest in the days following surgery, can be progressive, but is rarely fatal. The biotransformation of high inspired tensions of enflurane can release adequate amounts of fluoride to compromise renal function in surgical patients with kidney disease and should therefore be avoided in this patient group.

Surgical and postoperative complications

Few postoperative complications are associated with the use of modern anesthetics. Recovery is generally rapid. Severe, postoperative tremors that could jeopardize surgical incisions, enhance bleeding, or interfere with patient monitoring are not a problem as they once were with ether. Nausea and vomiting, which were also common with older anesthetics, are minimal today. Enflurane will occasionally induce tonic-clonic spasms and a history of epilepsy is generally a contraindication for its use.

All volatile anesthetics can induce malignant hyperthermia—a potentially fatal condition that fortunately is very rare. It is manifest as extreme muscle rigidity (perhaps resulting from total lack of Ca^{2+} uptake by the sarcoplasmic reticulum) and can compromise respiration even when the patient is ventilated. Excessive heat production occurs in part because of central dysregulation of hypothalamic centers controlling body temperature and from excess heat produced by continued muscle rigidity. Malignant hyperthermia may occur in patients genetically predisposed although little is known about its cause. Anesthesia must be stopped immediately and dantrolene, a sarcoplasmic reticulum Ca^{2+} release inhibitor, is generally used to treat the symptoms.

Nitrous oxide

Nitrous oxide ("laughing gas") has been in use for a long time although it is not a good anesthetic, induces diffusion hypoxia, and is associated with considerable disinhibition release. However, it possesses many unique properties that ensure its continued use, the most important being its analgesic potency and its cardiovascular effects.

Analgesic Effects of Nitrous Oxide. Nitrous oxide is rarely administered alone as an anesthetic because it does not induce a level of anesthesia compatible with surgery. It is still commonly used, however, especially in dental offices, since its inability to induce anesthesia does not preclude analgesia. Of all the anesthetic gases it is the most potent analgesic. Thus, the dental patient may be semiconscious and still exhibit significant muscle tone and intact reflexes, but be unresponsive to dental-procedure pain or tolerate it well.

Cardiovascular Effects of Nitrous Oxide. Although nitrous oxide can induce vasodilation through its anesthetic effects on smooth muscle, it also causes Epi and NE release—a unique characteristic that distinguishes it from all other gas anesthetics. The release of catecholamines produces a net increase in vascular tone that is often a reason for its coadministration with anesthetics that induce vasodilation. However, nitrous-oxide-induced Epi and NE release can be dangerous when employed with other anesthetics that induce catecholamine sensitization such as halothane.

INTRAVENOUS GENERAL ANESTHETICS

The intravenous anesthetics currently used in the United States are a diverse group of drugs that include barbiturates, barbiturate-like sedative hypnotics, opioids, benzodiazepines, and DA antagonists. The higher therapeutic indices of the intravenous agents compared with the gases make them excellent choices for outpatient procedures. In addition, these drugs induce anesthesia rapidly and produce little cardiovascular depression and few postoperative complications such as nausea or vomiting, further enhancing physician comfort outside the inpatient setting. Historically, the intravenous agents were used primarily for specialized procedures of short duration (e.g., setting dislocations or changing burn dressings) or as inducing agents in general surgery. Since they all decrease intracranial pressure they are often used in neurosurgery. With the increased emphasis on outpatient procedures, however, they have become very popular and are now used for several generalized procedures. Their primary disadvantage is that unlike the gases, they cannot be readily recalled once administered. If problems arise during intravenous anesthesia, another drug must be given to counteract the undesired effects because effective antagonists are not available.

Thiopental, Etomidate, and Propofol

Thiopental, etomidate, and propofol are the most widely used intravenous agents. Despite their structural diversity, all three potentiate GABA activity at the GABA$_A$ receptor. Although all of the agents potentiate the action of GABA, the barbiturate thiopental (Schwartz et al., 1985), propofol (Hales and Lambert, 1991), and etomidate (Robertson, 1989) all open Cl$^-$ channels in the absence of GABA as well. Thus, as discussed in the previous chapter, this GABA-independent mechanism enables these agents to continue depressing CNS function until a level of consciousness compatible with surgical procedures can be achieved.

Thiopental and methohexital

Thiopental (sometimes called "truth serum") induces smooth, comfortable, and rapid anesthesia in 30 seconds. The patient tastes garlic and is then fast asleep. The anesthetic barbiturates, as thiopental and methohexital are called, are not only rapid inducers of anesthesia but are also very short-acting and thus classified as ultrashort barbiturates. They are not good muscle relaxers and can induce a state of paradoxic excitement in response to pain. Adjuvant muscle relaxers and analgesics are therefore often required. The anesthetic barbiturates decrease arterial pressure and cardiac output and can induce tachycardia that precludes their use in some patients but they do not sensitize the heart to catecholamines. Recovery from anesthesia is smooth with very little nausea or vomiting. Although the patient recovers quickly following discontinuation of infusion due to redistribution, the half-life of these drugs is such that psychomotor impairment may be present for at least two hours following surgery (Mackenzie and Grant, 1985).

Etomidate

The main advantage of etomidate is its negligible effects on cardiovascular function, making it the agent of choice in patients with cardiovascular compromise.

Propofol

Propofol is rapidly becoming the most widely used anesthetic agent for outpatient surgery because of its low incidence of side effects and its favorable pharmacokinetics. Like etomidate and thiopental, it induces anesthesia very quickly but redistribution as well as its short half-life of six hours renders the recovering patient impaired for only 30 minutes (Mackenzie and Grant, 1985). Furthermore, the latency to awaken following discontinuation of infusion can be as short as five minutes. Unfortunately, propofol can induce myoclonus, especially in children (Hannallah et al., 1991). Propofol has the fewest postoperative complications of this group of drugs and may actually possess antiemetic properties.

Ketamine

Ketamine was once a widely used agent for outpatient procedures but has fallen from favor because of its psychotomimetic properties. Ketamine has actions similar to those of phencyclidine (PCP), its parent compound, and produces a dissociative state (called dissociative anesthesia) that is compatible with many short procedures. Dissociative anesthesia leaves the patient semiconscious and in an analgesic state where discomfort experienced by the patient is reported to not be "associated" with the patient's body (*i.e.*, dissociated; see Murray, 1994).

Ketamine is a noncompetitive antagonist at the glutamate, N-methyl-D-aspartate (NMDA) receptor. The site where ketamine binds is called the sigma receptor. It is actually an acceptor moiety in the ion channel of the NMDA channel where ketamine prevents Na^+ and Ca^{2+} conductance produced by glutamate (Lodge et al., 1983). Blockade of NMDA receptors produces multiple actions within the CNS, disrupting neuronal processing throughout the neuraxis including the spinal cord and thalamus (see Murray, 1994). Although ketamine's excellent analgesic properties may be associated with its NMDA antagonism, its affinity for kappa and delta opioid receptors is also likely involved (Smith et al., 1987).

A unique property of ketamine that maintains its clinical use is its cardiovascular profile. It dramatically elevates SANS tone and may sensitize the heart to catecholamines (see Reich and Silvay, 1989). Although contraindicated in unstable coronary patients, this cardiovascular profile makes ketamine the agent of choice for procedures performed on patients with reduced coronary function secondary to hypovolemia or shock. Despite its unique advantages, ketamine induces muscle rigidity that must be countered with adjuvant benzodiazepines. Concurrent benzodiazepine administration also helps to reduce recall of bizarre, psychotic-like dreams or behavior that are especially prevalent during the long, postoperative recovery period of this drug.

Opioids

The opioid analgesics have had a gradual rise in popularity as intravenous anesthetics. While they remain widely used adjuvant agents because of their analgesic properties, the newer, more potent agents are sometimes used as the primary anesthetic agent although their ability to induce true anesthesia is controversial (see Bailey, 1994). The opioids are not associated with anterograde amnesia and benzodiazepines are generally coadministered for this purpose. Moreover, the opioids can produce muscle rigidity often requiring the use of adjuvant muscle relaxers. The major advantage of these agents, which include fentanyl, sufentanil, and alfentanil, however, is their excellent cardiovascular profile. Opioids produce few, if any, cardiovascular effects and, as a result, are excellent choices in patients with cardiovascular complications.

The opioid fentanyl is often mixed with the DA antagonist droperidol to formulate Innovar. This combination produces a "neurolept-analgesia." (Droperidol is also combined with the analgesic nitrous oxide to produce neurolept-anesthesia.) DA antagonists are often referred to as neuroleptic agents (see Chapter 10) and have a calming effect. Their alpha-adrenergic antagonist action also contributes to anesthesia. This alpha blockade is not pronounced enough to produce hypotension, however. As DA antagonists, the neuroleptics block the chemoreceptor trigger zone significantly, reducing the nausea and vomiting that often follows anesthesia—especially with opioids, since they possess emetic tendencies. Fentanyl is one of the most potent mu opioid agonists known. As such, it provides excellent analgesia. A major drawback to Innovar however, is the induction of chest-wall rigidity, which is common because both droperidol and fentanyl induce basal-ganglion-type rigidity. This rigidity can be severe enough to prevent mechanical ventilation, necessitating the use of muscle relaxers. Since droperidol has a long half-life relative to the opioid, (six vs. two hours, respectively), additional fentanyl must be administered by itself during prolonged procedures.

NEUROMUSCULAR BLOCKERS

Because most general anesthetics do not induce adequate muscle relaxation at the doses commonly used, adjuvant muscle relaxers are often needed. Reduced muscle tone is needed to facilitate physical manipulation during surgery (e.g., to enable appropriate retraction of the abdominal wall and to set fractures). The benzodiazepines are often used for this purpose. Their muscle-relaxing properties, their ability to induce anterograde amnesia, and their high therapeutic index make them popular drugs as adjuvants. Although effective, some procedures (e.g., microsurgery on the larynx or open-eye surgery) require complete muscle paralysis that can only be achieved using the neuromuscular blockers. Three drug classes are used to disrupt function at the neuromuscular junction (NMJ): nicotinic antagonists, direct-acting nicotinic agonists, and indirect-acting nicotinic agonists (Fig. 7–5).

Nicotinic Antagonists

The nicotinic receptor is a pentamer composed of two alpha subunits that each bind one ACh molecule. The alpha subunits found in nicotinic receptors on muscle and nerves are different, leading to the designations N_M and N_N receptors, respectively. Drugs specific for the N_M receptor bind the NMJ with negligible actions at other nicotinic sites. Specificity is possible because the active binding site on the NMJ is larger than at N_N receptors. Drugs with more carbons separating the two sites at which the drugs bind thus preferentially bind the N_M site.

Several N_M competitive antagonists are currently available. They differ in their latency to neuromuscular blockade and their duration of effect. The prototypic drug is curare. Curare is isolated from South American plants and used as an arrowhead poison to kill animals through respiratory paralysis. It is a large, bulky molecule that attaches to the alpha subunit thereby preventing access by ACh to the binding site. At higher concentrations it also blocks N_N receptors in the sympathetic ganglia, lowering heart rate and producing hypotension. Curare displaces histamine from mast cells that also contributes to hypotension. As a quaternary amine, it does not cross the BBB.

Pancuronium is a semisynthetic quaternary amine possessing greater specificity for the N_M receptor and therefore possesses few sympatholytic effects. Unfortunately, it has some affinity for muscarinic receptors and the resulting vagolytic effect produces tachycardia (Bowman et al., 1988). Rocuronium is closely related to pancuronium but is devoid of vagolytic effects and has a moderate duration of action. This profile makes it likely

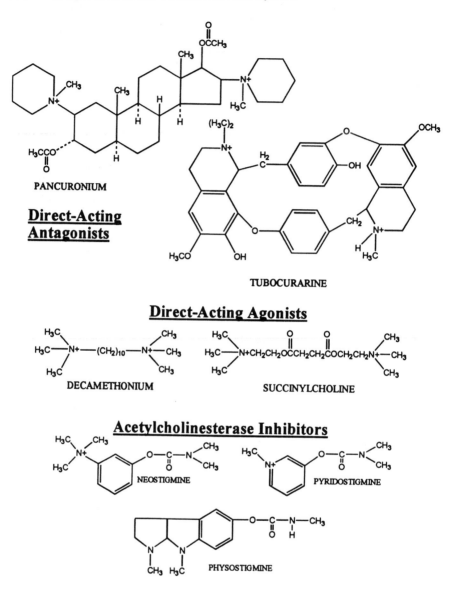

Figure 7–5. Structures of the various types of neuromuscular junction blockers.

that it will be a widely used muscle relaxer in the future. Gallamine is also used but, like many of the older agents, lacks specificity.

Direct-Acting Nicotinic Agonists

Succinylcholine and decamethonium are direct-acting nicotinic agonists used to induce muscle paralysis. As agonists with greater affinity for the

N_M site than has ACh, they bind to the receptor and lock it open. The muscle exhibits rapid but uncoordinated muscle twitches called fasciculations followed by flaccid paralysis. By locking the N_M receptor open, Na^+ continues to enter, K^+ continues to exit, and the channels cannot be reset. (They remain refractory.) Evidence also suggests that the physical size of the drugs enables them not only to bind to the receptor but also to prevent the ions from gaining access to the channel as well (a so-called open channel blockade; Lingle and Steinbach, 1988). Since the muscle is paralyzed due to continuous depolarization, this state is called depolarization blockade. Referred to as phase I blockade, the NMJ remains in a depolarized state as long as the drugs are present (Fig. 7–6). This occurs because ligand-gated channels remain open as long as a ligand is bound.

Phase I depolarization spreads to surrounding muscle membrane where voltage-gated channels are activated. The depolarization that develops there is called phase II. Activation of voltage-gated channels is transient and after a short period of time, the muscle can again be depolarized. However, since phase I blockade continues, a repetitive depolarizing signal cannot be transferred to the sarcoplasmic reticulum where the Ca^{2+} release necessary for muscle contraction occurs. As a result, the muscle is paralyzed.

In addition to depolarization blockade, succinylcholine is unique among the nicotinic agonists in that it also alters the sensitivity of the N_M receptor. The NMJ exhibits reduced sensitivity to ACh and is said to be in a state of desensitization block. The mechanism for this desensitization is unknown but may reflect a temporary transition of the receptor into a low-affinity state. Desensitization block will continue well past the time when succinylcholine has dissociated from the receptor, effectively extending the duration of NMJ blockade.

The main limitation to the use of the depolarizing agents is their affinity for ganglionic nicotinic receptors and muscarinic receptors. The combined effects of stimulation followed by depolarization blockade at these receptors can produce profound and unpredictable effects on cardiovascular function. Evidence also exists to suggest that succinylcholine contributes to the development of malignant hyperthermia (Hall et al., 1966).

Indirect-Acting Nicotinic Agonists

Depolarization blockade can be produced by overstimulation with direct-acting agonists as well as ACh. By blocking the catabolic enzyme for ACh using acetylcholinesterase inhibitors (AChEIs) both phases of depolarization blockade will develop although these drugs do not desensitize the receptor.

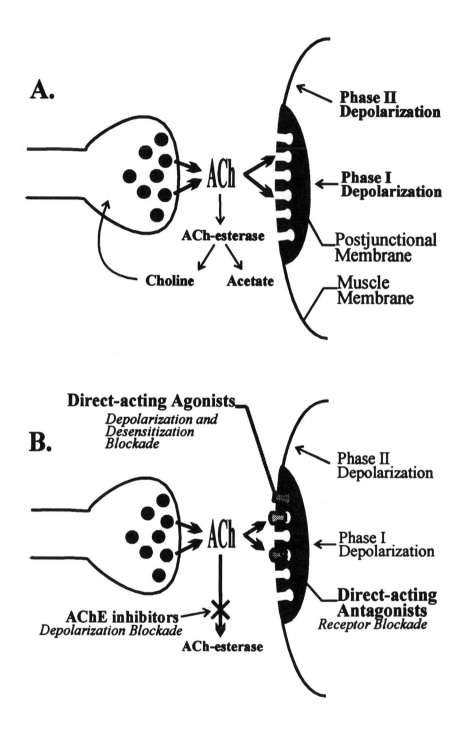

The short-acting drug neostigmine and the longer-acting drugs such as pyridostigmine and abenomonium, are all competitive inhibitors of acetylcholine esterase. They are not commonly used as NMJ blockers, however, because as AChEIs, they increase ACh at cholinergic synapses throughout the periphery producing both muscarinic and nicotinic toxicity. They do not produce CNS cholinergic effects, however, because only one member of this class, physostigmine, is a nonquaternary amine capable of crossing the BBB. In anesthesia these agents are primarily used to reverse the effects of NMJ blockade associated with the use of the competitive antagonists. They are also used clinically in the management of myasthenia gravis (MG).

THE LOCAL ANESTHETICS

Cocaine's anesthetic properties were discovered in the late 19th century but its autonomic effects and the eventual realization of its addictive properties precluded its use for most procedures. Other esters of benzoic acid were subsequently synthesized, resulting in the release of procaine in 1905. Since that time, several local anesthetic agents have been synthesized and today procaine is considered the prototypic agent. Because their effects were discovered as a result of cocaine, the "caine" suffix has been retained and the local anesthetics are often referred to as the "caine" drugs. They are a large drug class (Table 7–4) that now includes both ester and amide compounds. Their diverse chemical structures allow the local anesthetics to be delivered using several routes and used in a wide variety of clinical situations. Subcutaneous delivery is used to induce nerve block for dental work or small surgical procedures. They can be employed topically as salves and creams to treat sunburn or diaper

---

Figure 7–6. The various types of neuromuscular junction (NMJ) blockade used to achieve muscle relaxation are depicted. In normal transmission (A), the muscle depolarization occurs in two steps. The first involves the ligand-gated depolarization induced by the ACh released by the presynaptic terminal which simultaneously increases both Na^+ and K^+ conduction. Phase I depolarization spreads from the postjunctional region, depolarizing the surrounding muscle tissue. Phase II depolarization involves normal sequential activation of Na^+ and K^+ channels. Direct-acting nicotinic agonists such as succinylcholine produce phase I depolarization blockade by continuously keeping Na^+ and K^+ channels open. The muscle can recover from this blockade but a phase I desensitization continues after drug clearance, ostensibly as a result of receptor alterations. Depolarization blockade also occurs following the administration of an acetylcholine esterase inhibitor (AChE). This drug does not, however, produce a desensitization blockade. The muscle can also be paralyzed by directly antagonizing the nicotinic receptor.

rash or as powders for burn patients. They can be applied externally in solution for procedures involving the nose and eyes. Local anesthetics are also effective when inhaled as an aerosol for anesthesia of the trachea before intubation procedures. Although they are most commonly used for minor procedures, they can be delivered to the spinal cord in solution where they effectively anesthetize regions of the body below the site of administration. Although their diversity allows for use in a variety of clinical situations, they all share the same fundamental mechanism of action: blockade of voltage-gated Na$^+$ channels.

The Pharmacodynamics of Local Anesthetics

All of the currently used local anesthetics work through the same mechanism: They block Na$^+$ channels in a dose-dependent fashion (Frazier, Narahashi, and Yamada, 1970). Their structure is such that they can only enter the Na$^+$ channel from the cytoplasmic side of the membrane, bind inside the channel, and subsequently reduce Na$^+$ conductance. The local anesthetics, in effect, "clog" the Na$^+$ channel.

The Na$^+$ channel is a heterotrimeric complex comprised of four alpha domains which bind local anesthetics and a beta$_1$ and beta$_2$ subunit (Catterall, 1992). A voltage change across the membrane causes a conforma-

Table 7–4 Commonly Used Local Anesthetics

Drug	Chemical Class	Potency	Duration of Action	Normal Uses
Procaine	Ester	1	Short	Dental and infusion
Cocaine	Ester	2	Intermediate	Nasal procedures
Tetracaine	Ester	16	Long	Opthalmic and spinal
Benzocaine	Ester	—	Topical only	Sunburn, wounds
Proparacaine	Ester	—	Topical	Opthalmic
Lidociane	Amide	4	Intermediate	Broad general use
Prilocaine	Amide	3	Intermediate	Dental
Mepivacaine	Amide	2	Intermediate	Regional nerve block
Chloroprocaine	Amide	2	Intermediate	Broad general use
Bupivacaine	Amide	16	Long	Broad general use
Etidocaine	Amide	16	Long	Epidural and infiltration
Dyclonine	Ketone	—	Short	Nasal, anogenital
Pramoxine	Ether	—	Short	Nasal, anogenital

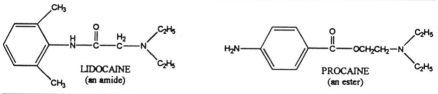

tional change in the alpha subunits that causes the channel to open. Once the channel is open, the drug can enter the channel, but only from the axoplasmic side. In contrast to the local anesthetics used clinically, tetrodotoxin (TTX; found in the puffer fish and the skin of certain newts) and saxitoxin (found in the dinoflagellate *Gonyaulax,* whose numbers can rise so high at times that they turn coastal waters red ["red tides"] and gain entry into humans through consumption of shellfish that feed on them) block Na^+ channels by entering the channels from the external surface of the membrane (Anderson, 1994). Tetrodotoxin and saxitoxin are frequently employed in research. The local anesthetics can also gain access to and block K^+ channels at higher concentrations, but this action is not thought to contribute to the "caine" effect.

Na^+ Channel Blockade and Ion Trapping

The "caine" drugs are all tertiary amines containing an amine, an aromatic ring, and either an amide or an ester linkage between the two. They are poorly water soluble and unstable but formulating them as salts reduces these undesirable properties. When injected, the salt ionizes according to equation 1.

$$R\!\equiv\!NH^+Cl^- \rightleftharpoons R\!\equiv\!NH^+ + Cl^- \qquad (1)$$
(Salt)   (Cation)

The local anesthetics are all weak bases. As predicted by their pKa's (generally between 8 and 9), the cation dissociates to the free base in body fluids (equation 2), the degree of which is predicted by the pH of the local environment and the Henderson-Hasselbach equation.

$$R\!\equiv\!NH^+ \rightleftharpoons R\!\equiv\!N + H^+ \qquad (2)$$
(Cation)   (Free base)

Only the cationic form is capable of entering the Na^+ channel and inactivating it. In its cationic form, however, the drug cannot cross the nerve membrane, and since the clinically used local anesthetics can only enter the channel from the inside, the cationic form does not have access to its site of action. In contrast, the dissociated free base readily diffuses through the membrane. Via diffusion, the free base passes down its concentration gradient into the axoplasm. Once inside the nerve, the dissociated base reionizes to the cationic form, the proportion of which is again determined by the Henderson-Hasselbach equation. The cationic form enters the Na^+ channel to produce blockade. As a greater proportion of the cation is incorporated (reversibly) into the Na^+ channel, the quantity of unbound, dissociated, free base in the axoplasm is reduced and more base diffuses into the nerve to maintain the equilibrium. Enough cation is eventually formed by the reionization of the dissociated base to block nerve conduction. The cation thus effectively becomes trapped in the nerve as it is being used to block the Na^+ channels—ion trapping (see Chapter 2). As the extraneuronal concentrations of the drug are eventually redistributed to the surrounding circulation or metabolized, the extracellular concentration of the free base decreases and the intracellular free base moves down its concentration gradient, out of the nerve, and into the extraneuronal space. This drives equation 2 to the right and effectively reduces the concentration of cation inside the nerve with an associated loss of conduction block. Four factors influence this process: extracellular pH, tissue perfusion, protein binding, and metabolism.

Effects of pH

The Henderson-Hasselbach equation determines the relative proportions of free base and cation at a given pH and therefore the amount of cation available for Na^+ channel blockade. At physiologic pH, most of an administered dose of a local anesthetic is in its cationic form and therefore unavailable for nerve block (Fig. 7–7). This is especially true in infected and inflamed areas (where these drugs are frequently used) since inflammation is associated with increased H^+ ion concentrations and a lower pH. A lower pH drives equation 2 to the left and increases the percentage of drug in the ionized, nondiffusible form. Buffer solutions (see below) or a larger administered dose must be injected to overcome this effect.

Tissue perfusion

The amount of local anesthetic available for blockade will be influenced by the extraneuronal concentration which, in turn, is dependent upon vascular perfusion. If an agent is injected directly into the specific location, the onset of nerve block will almost be immediate. If a field block is being induced by injecting drug into a region of a nerve trunk between the CNS and the area needing anesthesia, a certain degree of perfusion must occur in order for the drug to gain access to its site of action. Inflamed areas often have reduced perfusion and the spread of the drug is accordingly restricted. On the other hand, injection into a highly vascularized area can carry the drug away from the site of desired action and thereby reduce effectiveness. Vasoconstricting drugs such as epinephrine are often included in the formulation to prevent this redistribution.

Local Anesthetic pKa = 8.4

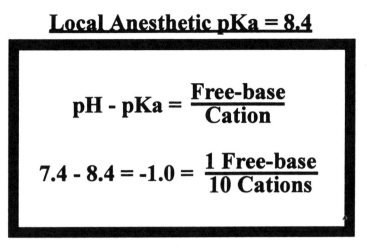

$$pH - pKa = \frac{Free\text{-}base}{Cation}$$

$$7.4 - 8.4 = -1.0 = \frac{1\ Free\text{-}base}{10\ Cations}$$

**Normal Extracellular Space
(pH =7.4)**

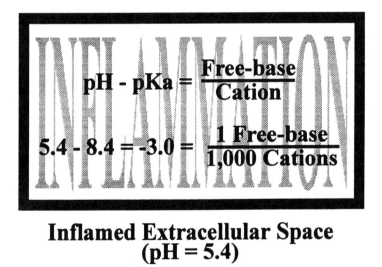

$$pH - pKa = \frac{Free\text{-}base}{Cation}$$

$$5.4 - 8.4 = -3.0 = \frac{1\ Free\text{-}base}{1,000\ Cations}$$

**Inflamed Extracellular Space
(pH = 5.4)**

Figure 7–7. Inflammation at the site of injection of a local anesthetic influences the amount of free-base available for diffusion into the nerve. Assuming a pKa of 8.4 for the drug, the ratio of free-base to cation in normal extracellular space is 1 : 10. Therefore, 10% of the drug is available for diffusion into the nerve. In an inflamed area where the pH can be as low as 5.4, however, the free-base to cation ratio becomes 1/1,000. Significantly less drug is available for diffusion, reducing local anesthetic efficacy.

Protein binding

As is true of most drugs, local anesthetics bind to plasma proteins as well as to other proteins that effectively reduce the amount of unbound drug available for diffusion (see Chapter 2). This is a major problem in inflamed areas where the influx of inflammatory proteins increases the number of potential nonspecific binding sites. Depending on the local anesthetic used, the amount bound to proteins varies between 40 and 95%. Agents that are highly bound have a smaller unbound pool available for biotransformation that effectively extends drug half-life. Thus, although protein binding reduces the amount of drug available for nerve block, it also serves as a reservoir for the drug, effectively extending its duration of action. This is especially advantageous in wound sites where inflammatory proteins will serve as reservoirs at the intended site of action.

Metabolism

The ester-linked "caine" agents (Table 7–4) are catabolized by nonspecific plasma cholinesterases that are found throughout the body, including the liver. High perfusion into the injection site supplies enzymes for biotransformation, effectively reducing the amount of drug available for conduction block. Since the amide agents are biotransformed almost exclusively by the liver, metabolism at the injection site is not a concern.

Formulation Considerations

The foregoing discussion suggests that several factors control the amount of drug that is actually delivered to the target site. Various strategies have been devised to limit the impact of these factors. Since pH is very important, the injection solution can be modified to limit the effects of pH. As weak bases, the local anesthetics will precipitate out of solution at a high pH. The injectable solutions are therefore acidified to lower the pH maintaining the drug in a protonated state so that it can form a salt and remain in solution during storage. When this acidic solution is injected, however, it will reduce the percentage of drug in the free-base form. Two strategies have been developed to circumvent this problem.

The first involves substituting carbonic acid for the hydrochloric acid normally used to acidify the solution. In a sealed vial, the carbonic acid effectively lowers the pH and keeps the drug in solution. When the vial containing the drug is opened just prior to use, it "fizzes" like any carbonated liquid because the carbonic acid forms CO_2 bubbles. When this solution is injected, the CO_2 diffuses away, effectively raising the pH and thereby increasing the amount of drug available in the free-base and diffusible form. Moreover, some of the CO_2 may diffuse into the nerve itself, thereby lowering the pH, facilitating ion trapping. A second strategy involves adding sodium bicarbonate to the solution just prior to use. Although inconvenient, this strategy does effectively increase the pH in the solution, resulting in a larger amount of free base available for diffusion. Sodium bicarbonate also raises the pH in the inflamed area, increasing the amount of free base for diffusion.

A number of local anesthetics are formulated with epinephrine (Epi) to limit perfusion. The vasoconstricting properties of Epi (alpha$_1$ action) reduce the influx of esterases that metabolize the ester-based drugs. Vasoconstrictors also reduce redistribution of all of the local anesthetic away from the injection site. Although this strategy effectively enhances the concentration of drug at the target site (Tucker and Mather, 1975) it has its disadvantages as well. Formulations which include Epi must be buffered to a more acidic pH to solubilize the Epi. The resulting acidic solution reduces the pH at the injection site and lowers the availability of the free base for penetration. In addition, circulation of the Epi away from the injection site, when it does occur, can induce peripheral toxicity in individuals predisposed to catecholamine toxicity (heart conditions, etc.). Formulations including Epi can also induce intense vasoconstriction, thereby increasing the possibility of ischemic damage and, in rare cases, gangrene, especially in distal portions of the limb. In cases such as the nasal mucosa where Epi would not be absorbed well, the alpha$_1$ agonist phenylephrine can be substituted.

Use-Dependent Channel Blockade

The voltage-gated Na^+ exists in three functional states: open-and-conducting, closed-and-not-ready, and closed-and-ready. When in the closed-and-ready state, activation by depolarization causes the tertiary structure of the channel to change. This alteration involves a "rotation" of the spirally configured alpha subunits and an associated shift in the polarity of the inside of the channel that exposes negative charge. This shift opens the channel and allows Na^+ to move down its concentration and electrical gradient into the channel. The entry of Na^+ into the channel neutralizes the negative charge of the channel, inducing further tertiary structural change. This reduces the affinity of the alpha subunits for Na^+ that then dissociates from the alpha subunits and enters the intracellular cytoplasm. Such passage and subsequent structural change result in the refractory period. The gate is now closed-and-not-ready. Repolarization is required to alter the structure from a closed-and-not-ready to a closed-and-ready state. This transformation is thought to occur in four steps (Joels, Yool and Gruol, 1989).

The fact that the "caine" agents only gain access to the channel while the channel is open-and-conducting has significant implications for effective nerve block. The greater the number of channels open at one time or the more frequently they open, the greater the potential number of binding sites for the anesthetic agent. A local anesthetic's ability to induce conduction blockade and the latency to full anesthesia is therefore influenced by the activity status of the fiber—a state-dependent action. Since the locale being treated is frequently infected, inflamed, or painful (as in stitching up a little boy's finger), those fibers that are most active will fall prey to anesthetic blockade first. The ability to block neuronal conduction is thus use dependent (Strichartz, 1973). Since pain fibers are the most active neurons in such areas, they are affected most.

Whether or not a fiber exhibits conduction block is also influenced by several factors in addition to those already discussed. The actual loss of conduction will depend upon the density of the voltage-gated Na^+ channels that contributes to a nerve's time and length constants. These cable properties determine the decay rate of the depolarization and how far a stimulus capable of inducing a depolarization will travel down a nerve, respectively. When a local anesthetic is administered, small, unmyelinated C fibers are affected first because they generally have faster time constants and shorter length constants. Even a slight decrease in functional Na^+ channel density brought about by a local anesthetic will effectively prevent conduction in these fibers. As the local concentration of the anesthetic increases, however, larger unmyelinated fibers and then myelinated fibers will also be affected.

Systemic Toxicity

Aside from their actions on nerve conduction, the local anesthetics have a variety of systemic effects that are consistent with their blockade of sodium channels. These effects can manifest during continuous infusion of a local anesthetic used in certain procedures or following bolus injection where the solution is inadvertently injected into a blood vessel and becomes available systemically. All excitable tissues are influenced to a greater or lesser degree depending on concentration, perfusion, and pH. In addition, cocaine is also a potent blocker of DA and NE reuptake. Its psychostimulant properties generally occur at plasma levels ten times lower than those that block Na^+ channels. Its indirect-agonist actions at NE synapses induce vasoconstriction, thereby obviating the need to formulate it with vasoconstrictors. This characteristic affords it some unique advantages, and it is still used for certain procedures. The toxic effects of the other local anesthetics are consistent with their mechanism of action. As Na$^+$ channel antagonists, these effects are best characterized as CNS depression.

CNS effects
The initial stage of toxicity is that of elation, euphoria, restlessness, tinnitus, and tremor that are likely the result of disinhibition release associated with progressing CNS depression. These signs and symptoms precede the lethargy and drowsiness that often herald the development of tonic-clonic seizures and eventual respiratory collapse. The seizure disorder is generally self-limiting, treatable with benzodiazepines, and rarely fatal.

Cardiovascular effects
The cardiovascular effects of local anesthetics are a direct result of the "caine" action on cardiac muscle, the smooth muscle of blood vessels (dilation), and the loss of autonomic reflexes. Cardiovascular complications can be fatal. Systemic toxicity induces negative inotropic, chronotropic, and dromotropic effects. These can combine to induce ventricular fibrillation and eventual vascular collapse. The negative dromotropic effect is a critical consideration if epinephrine were being coadministered due to the possibility of reentry arrhythmias secondary to catecholamine sensitization. Fortunately, the cardiac symptoms occur at significantly higher doses than do the CNS effects. The development of CNS effects therefore signals an impending and potentially fatal cardiovascular problem.

Respiratory effects
The local anesthetics interfere with all aspects of respiration in a dose-dependent fashion. This respiratory insult can be fatal and is most often the primary cause of accidental death.

Effects on skeletal muscle
The local anesthetics can inhibit phase I and II depolarization leading to paresis and eventually paralysis.

Biotransformation of Local Anesthetics

The ester-linked agents are hydrolyzed primarily by nonspecific esterases located in plasma. Hydrolysis produces paraaminobenzoic acid (PABA), a common allergen. The use of ester-linked agents in hypersensitive patients previously sensitized to PABA can lead to anaphylactic shock and possible vascular collapse. These patients should be anesthetized with the amide-linked agents that are dealkylated in the liver. The amide-linked agents have the letter *i* preceding the caine in their generic names. Thus, amides do not produce PABA following biotransformation and do not induce hypersensitivity. Another mnemonic my students have found useful in remembering which agents produce PABA is:

*"yester*day exposed—today die"

It is also important to note that some patients are hypersensitive to methylparaben, one of the common preservatives used in formulating both amide and ester-linked agents. This hypersensitivity is generally mild, produces a rash, and should not be confused with an anaphylactic reaction. Although the production of PABA can be dangerous in hyper-

Table 7–5 Types of Local Anesthesia

Type or Location	Characteristics and Considerations
Topical	A nonabsorbable form is preferred to prevent systemic toxicity; benzocaine is most often used; topical uses include sunburn, rash, irritation of mucous membranes, mouth, throat, tracheobronchial tree, esophagus, GI tract, and rectum
Opthalamic	Nonabsorbable and nonirritating; benoxinate and proparacaine are often used for tonometry
Local injectables	Lidocaine, bupivacaine, etidocaine, procaine, and prilocaine are most commonly used
Field block	Injection into the locale that will be affected; this procedure generally anesthetizes the terminal regions of a pain pathway and is commonly used in dentistry and acute traumatic injuries (*e.g.*, cuts to forehead or fingers)
Nerve block	Injection into locale of the nerve trunk resulting in anesthesia in a more distal area; this procedure yields a pattern of anesthesia that starts locally and spreads distally since local fibers enter the nerve trunk sequentially, will be most peripheral on the trunk, and are thereby affected first
Spinal anesthesia	Infusion into the subarachnoid space caudal to the cord; the solution is rendered hypo- or hyperbaric to regulate the spread of the anesthetic when the body is subsequently tilted; fibers are anesthetized as they enter or leave the spinal cord; sensory, autonomic, and then motor blockade is the pattern of anesthesia observed; complications due to autonomic dysfunction can develop
Epidural anesthesia	Infusion into the lumbar space where it penetrates the dura and subarachnoid space; this is the procedure commonly used for surgery involving the lower portion of the body or during labor (so-called saddle block)

sensitive patients, the esters can be used safely in spinal procedures since CSF does not contain esterases.

Although the majority of a delivered dose of an ester or an amide is metabolized, some portion is excreted unchanged in the urine, especially cocaine, which is excreted 20% unchanged. Acidification of the urine using ammonium chloride enhances excretion as predicted by their pKa's. This ion trapping would also occur to a limited extent in the gut.

The choice of local anesthetics depends upon the action being sought, the solubility of the drug, the potential for toxicity, and the ability of the drug to irritate local tissue. Drugs such as benzocaine are not very water soluble and are therefore impractical for infusion. However, this property makes them an excellent choice for topical anesthesia. Several anesthetics including benoxinate are used for ophthalmic anesthesia since they do not irritate tissues. Table 7–5 lists the various uses of local anesthetics relative to the type of local anesthesia used clinically.

Antiepileptic Drugs

Prototypic agent: *phenytoin* (*Dilantin*)

*E*pilepsy is the second most common neurologic disorder next to stroke. It is defined as a paroxysmal disturbance of CNS function that is recurrent, stereotypic in character, and associated with excessive discharge of a synchronous nature that is self-limited. Individuals who have only on episode of this type do not have epilepsy. A single episode of abnormal electrical discharge is called a seizure, or if it involves tonic-clonic motor activity, a convulsion. Only when seizures are recurrent is the patient appropriately diagnosed as having epilepsy.

Epilepsy is characterized by stereotypic seizures—various behaviors that are repeated in a fixed sequence. Since recurrent seizures are usually a consequence of the same pathophysiologic process originating in the same brain region (called the seizure focus), the abnormal electrical activity will spread along defined anatomic pathways, generating the same sequence of behaviors.

Although the behavior manifested during a convulsion suggests disorganized electrical activity in the brain, the opposite is actually true. A normal electroencephalogram (EEG) in an alert, conscious individual consists of 8 to 12 per second (cycles per second are measured as Hertz [Hz]) or 12- to 30-Hz low-amplitude, rhythmic, electrical patterns that are called alpha and beta rhythms, respectively (see Fig. 8–1). These rhythms reflect the electrical activity of tens of thousands of nerve cells in the cortical region underneath an EEG electrode. An alpha or beta rhythm therefore reflects a large number of cells firing at different times (high frequency) and in a "random" fashion so that any one peak reflects the activity of only a few cells that have fired simultaneously (low ampli-

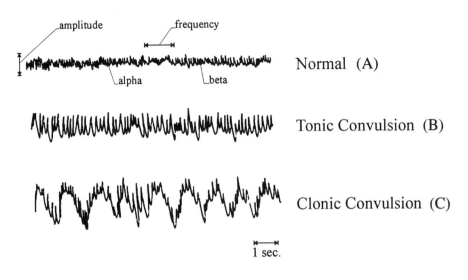

Figure 8–1. A: These excerpts of an electroencephalogram (EEG) depict the various types of rhythms found in normal healthy adults. Alpha rhythms (8–12 Hz) predominate in the activity of a normal brain. Occasional bursts of higher-frequency activity are called beta rhythms (12–30 Hz). Since the electrode is recording the activity of thousands of cells simultaneously, the high-frequency, low-amplitude activity reflects the asynchronous activity associated with normal activity. In contrast, the convulsive activity seen in the epileptic patient (B) is low frequency, high amplitude. This reflects the activity of hundreds of cells firing in a synchronous fashion. (C) During the clonic phase of a convulsion, the EEG activity oscillates in a rhythmic fashion.

tude). In contrast, the EEG of a patient undergoing a tonic-clonic seizure exhibits an initial phase of high-frequency, low-amplitude activity that quickly converts to a low-frequency, high-amplitude pattern during the seizure period. This electrical pattern during a seizure reflects a relatively large number of cortical neurons firing synchronously (high-amplitude) in a slow, rhythmic fashion (low frequency). EEG activity during a seizure is thus counterintuitive in that it exhibits a hypersynchronous or organized rather than a disorganized pattern of electrical discharge.

The final characteristic of a seizure is that it is self-limited; it does not continue indefinitely. Most seizures last for 15 seconds to five minutes. Due to metabolic factors (generally energy depletion) the brain cannot sustain this type of activity for extended periods and the abnormal electrical discharge reverts to normal. Just because the seizure (also called an ictus) is usually self-limiting, however, does not mean that abnormal electrical activity cannot be found in the interim. In fact, it is abnormal interictal activity that often characterizes the location and type of seizure. Since it is rare for an EEG recording to actually "catch" a seizure, neurologists must depend on the subtle EEG alterations during the interictal period to establish a seizure's focus. Under exceptional circumstances, however, the seizure may continue unabated for an extended period and require emergency treatment. In this case, it is called status epilepticus.

SEIZURE TYPES AND LOCALIZATION

Seizures are classified as partial or generalized depending on whether consciousness is retained (Table 8–1). If the patient remains conscious and is able to remember and report symptoms, the seizure is classified as a partial seizure. The symptoms may be progressive. In such cases the abnormal electrical discharge will spread out of the focus to other brain regions along defined anatomic pathways. If this activity spreads across the motor strip of the frontal cortex, it is called Jacksonian march after John Hughlings Jackson, who first described it. However, this term's meaning has broadened and an event is said to "march" across a strip of cortex regardless of whether or not it is in a motor, sensory, or some other region of the brain. Complex, partial seizures are a special category of partial seizures that involve a clouding of consciousness. These seizures are often

Table 8–1 International Classification of Seizures

Partial seizures (begin focally)
Simple partial (no loss of consciousness)
   Motor
   Sensory
   Autonomic-visceral
   Mixed
Complex partial, formerly called psychomotor seizures;
   consciousness is altered but patient is still responsive to simple
   commands and exhibits automatisms, stereotypies, and potentially
   bizarre behaviors
Secondarily generalized, a focal seizure that spreads to other regions
   of the brain and produces unconsciousness

Generalized seizure (immediate loss of consciousness)
Tonic-clonic, formerly called grand mal; periods of increased tone
   followed by clonic spasms
Atonic; sudden loss of all muscle tone
Tonic; increased muscle tone only
Clonic; clonic spasms only
Myclonic; rhythmic, jerking or flinging spasms
Absence, formerly called petit mal, involving a momentary loss of
   consciousness with eyeblinking or other minor muscle twitches
   during which postural tone can be maintained; EEG exhibits a
   characteristic 3–5-Hz spike and dome electrical pattern

associated with temporal lobe abnormalities (temporal lobe epilepsy or psychomotor seizures) in which the patient exhibits automatic or repetitive behaviors and is semiconscious. In generalized seizures the patient loses consciousness, indicating that the abnormal discharge has spread to envelop the entire thalamus or cortex (see Chapter 6).

Some seizures are preceded by neurologic signs and symptoms called auras that can range from a simple tingling in the foot to a heightened sense of well-being. Auras reflect the source of abnormal discharge in the brain and help identify a seizure focus. Following a seizure, especially if it is generalized and involves motor activity, the patient is often tired and confused. This syndrome is called postictal depression and reflects energy depletion in the brain.

THE NEUROBIOLOGY OF EPILEPSY

Several conditions can precipitate seizures. These include intrauterine and neonatal complications, stroke, head injury, uremia, hypo- and hyperglycemia, several types of drugs, heavy metals, toxins, and even psychiatric conditions (see Table 8–2; Engel, 1989). The fact that such a diverse set of conditions can lead to seizures suggests that there are several different mechanisms underlying epilepsy. Once initiated, however, the seizure process invariably provokes neurons in and around the focus to fire synchronously. This does not necessarily imply that the cells in the focus are abnormal. In fact, research now indicates that the cellular ensemble initiating the seizure discharge is normal but is abnormally regulated by its surrounding circuitry. Thus, epilepsy is probably a disorder involving faulty physiologic regulation of an ensemble of cells that leads to a bursting discharge. This bursting discharge, in turn, induces synchronized firing in other neurons that are connected to the organizing site.

The Paroxysmal Depolarization Shift (PDS)

Intracellular recordings reveal that cells in a seizure focus characteristically exhibit a paroxysmal depolarization shift (PDS). The action potential of a normal cortical neuron exhibits a rapid repolarization phase followed by an afterhyperpolarization (Fig. 8–2). In contrast, the PDS is characteristically a higher-voltage depolarization of extended duration during which "spikelets" are observed. An extended afterhyperpolarization then follows. It is called "paroxysmal" because it can occur all of a sudden, and the "shift" refers to the extended duration of discharge. This extended discharge is capable of synchronizing the activity of surround-

Table 8–2 Factors Affecting Seizure Threshold

Prescription drugs
Theophylline
Isoniazid
Tricyclic antidepressants
Phenothiazine antipsychotics
Diphenhydramine
Pseudoephedrine
Penicillin
Any potent antimuscarinic agent

Illicit drugs
Cocaine
Amphetamines
Substituted amphetamines

Withdrawal from chronic drug treatment
All anticonvulsant drugs
Alcohol
Barbiturates
Any sedative-hypnotic agent and CNS depressant

Heavy metals and other toxins
Mercury
Lead
Pentylene tetrazole
Alumina

Psychiatric disorders
Conversion disorder
Hyperventilation
Panic attack
Depression
Possession

ing cells, producing one of the hallmarks of an epileptic focus—hypersynchronous bursting.

The numerous electrical similarities between the PDS and the depolarization waveform associated with long-term potentiation (LTP; Bliss and Lomo, 1973) have led many to suggest that the two are related. LTP occurs in cells possessing NMDA receptors. If these cells are excessively excited by Glu, or conversely disinhibited while being activated by Glu, depolarizing current can alter the conformation of the Ca^{2+} channel such that it no longer is able to bind Mg^{2+} (Dingeldine, 1983). With Mg^{2+} displaced from its binding site, the ionophore is now able to allow Ca^{2+} to enter the cell (Nowak et al., 1984). Ca^{2+}, acting as a second messenger in conjunction with the intracellular Ca^{2+} binding protein calmodulin, turn on and off various intracellular processes that increase future excitability.

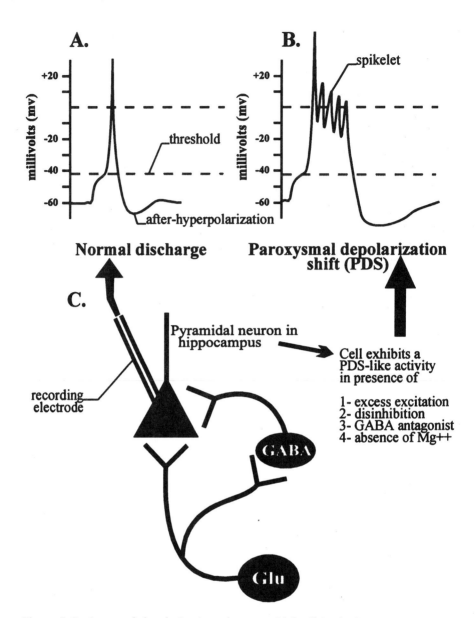

Figure 8–2. A normal depolarization of a pyramidal cell in the hippocampus (C) is shown in A. The depolarization develops rapidly after threshold has been achieved. These cells show a characteristic after-hyperpolarization that reflects the inhibitory activity of the GABA interneuron depicted in C. Thus, the excitatory impulse initiated by glutamate (Glu) is followed by an increase in Cl-conductance resulting from the action of GABA. The increase in Cl$^-$ conductance follows the excitatory impulse due to the synaptic delay associated with activation of the GABA interneuron. The depolarization found in the seizure focus (B) exhibits several spikelets and an even more pronounced after-hyperpolarization. This type of activity develops spontaneously within a seizure focus (paroxysmally) and the spikelets extend the duration of the depolarization (depolarization shift). This activity can arise if the cell is fired excessively such that Mg^{2+} ions are dislodged from their binding sites within the NMDA receptor.

The NMDA receptor is thus both a ligand-gated (Glu-mediated) and a voltage-gated (excessive depolarization) channel.

Several studies have demonstrated that LTP is also associated with increased presynaptic neurotransmitter release. Recent research suggest that Ca^{2+}-calmodulin in the postsynaptic cell activates the enzyme nitric oxide synthase which synthesizes the gas nitric oxide (NO) (Dawson et al., 1993; Fig. 8–3). NO diffuses to the presynaptic side of the synapse as a retrograde neurotransmitter where it activates guanylate cyclase to produce cyclic guanosine monophosphate (cGMP). The phosphorylation status of the presynaptic terminal is altered by cGMP producing increased Glu release in response to depolarization. Activation of the NMDA receptor thus produces both pre- and postsynaptic changes that enhance activity across the synapse for days, weeks, and even permanently.

Hippocampal cells exhibiting LTP produce effects similar to those observed in a seizure focus. First, because of the extended burst of firing produced by LTP, a neuronal ensemble will be excited more readily. Second, the duration of the burst synchronizes the activity of the ensemble. Third, other cells receiving this type of burst activity are more likely to dislodge Mg^{2+} ions from their NMDA channels, thereby facilitating LTP in other neurons. Such cells would possess lower thresholds for activation in the future and would therefore be more likely to fire in a synchronous fashion in response to increased activity in the original ensemble. Thus, in addition to their similarities in electrical discharge, PDS and LTP both possess the capacity to initiate and perpetuate synchronized activity in a group of interconnected cells.

Etiology of the Seizure Focus

The leading theory of epileptogenesis is the pharmacocentric hypothesis advanced by Prince (1969). Since most drugs used to treat seizures inhibit activity in the CNS, Prince suggested that seizure foci result from loss of inhibition, whatever the precipitating factor may be. The loss of input from inhibitory neurons releases excitatory neurons, leading to seizures. In a feed-forward hypothesis Engel (1989) proposed that a small group of cells, firing in unison, shut down a larger region of cells surrounding it by stimulating inhibitory neurons that pass through the area. A second excitatory burst, accurately timed, recruits other excitatory neurons and leads to synchrony. In the cell-packing hypothesis (Yaari, Konnerth, and Heinemann, 1986), traumatic injury to cells leads to increased Fe^{2+} that disrupts the function of the Na^+-K^+ATPase as well as the normal ion buffering that occurs in the brain. The influx of Na^+ is associated with the entry of obligatory water into the cell that swells them and thereby reduces the volume of the extracellular space. This reduction in extracellular fluid volume in-

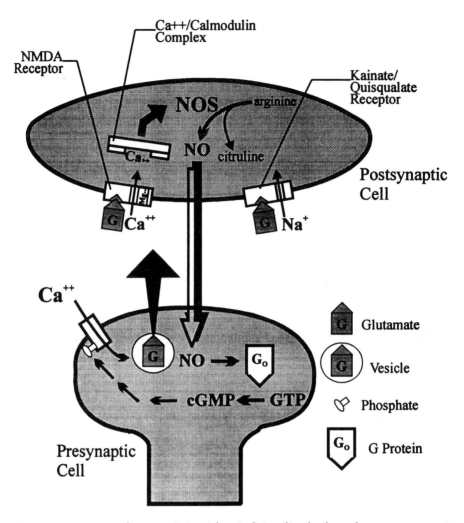

Figure 8–3. Retrograde transmission (chemical signaling backward across a synapse) is thought to involve gasses such as nitric oxide (NO). In the process of long-term potentiation (LTP; described in the text), excessive activation produced by the action of glutamate (Glu) on the NMDA receptor increases Ca^{2+} conductance. One of the actions of Ca^{2+} bound to its intracellular binding protein calmodulin activates the enzyme nitric oxide synthase (NOS), which acts on arginine to yield NO and citruline. The NO gas subsequently produced is free to diffuse and binds to the G_o protein in the presynaptic terminal, producing cyclic guanine monophosphate (cGMP). cGMP is thought to phosphorylate the voltage-gated Ca^{2+} channel (N-type), enhancing the Ca^{2+} conductance produced by an otherwise-normal depolarization. The presynaptic terminal will then release more Glu in response to normal neuronal activity then prior to the sensitization mediated by NO.

creases the effective concentration of ions such as K^+, which can induce further depolarization (see Schwartzkroin, 1994). Cell injury from trauma or other causes is common in epileptic brains (Meldrum and Corsellis, 1984) and the resulting dysregulation of neuronal circuitry could lead to abnormal electric discharge capable of initiating a seizure.

Theoretical Treatment of Seizure Disorders

Two fundamental strategies have been adopted to treat seizures: suppress the seizure focus or prevent the spread of electrical activity out of the seizure focus. The ideal antiepileptic drug (AED) would possess both actions without producing side effects. Such a drug has not yet been discovered.

Despite the diversity of mechanisms involved, there are several common features of seizure activity that would enable an AED to suppress a focus or prevent the spread of abnormal activity from it. Drugs that reduce Ca^{2+}, Na^+, or K^+ conductance, ions intimately associated with neuronal excitability, would likely be effective at suppressing the focus as well as the spread provided that these effects could be achieved at plasma levels that did not compromise normal neuronal function. Drugs that facilitate CNS inhibition would depress activity in the focus as well as reduce or prevent spread since seizure activity is enhanced by disinhibition. Drugs that block NMDA receptors would also be expected to prevent seizure development because Glu neurotransmission is so prevalent in the cerebral cortex and because NMDA-receptor-mediated LTP is so similar to the PDS. As described below, all of the AEDs currently in use exert their effects by these mechanisms.

THE ANTIEPILEPTIC DRUGS (AEDS)

Phenytoin

Before phenytoin, phenobarbital was the primary drug used to treat epilepsy. Sedation often interfered with effective therapy, however. Phenytoin resulted from an intentional effort to develop a less-sedating barbiturate structure with anticonvulsant properties (Merritt and Putnam, 1938). By the late 1930s, it was known that alkyl and aryl substitutions on the 5' carbon of the barbiturate nucleus were responsible for its sedating properties (Fig. 8–4). In general, the bulkier the alkyl substitution, the more sedating a barbiturate is. Substituting a phenyl group (*phe*nobarbital) at the 5' position reduced barbiturate-mediated sedation. At that time it appeared that the optimal antiseizure barbiturate structure was phenobarbital although it still possessed sedating properties.

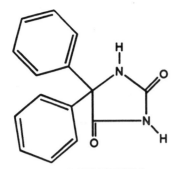

PHENYTOIN

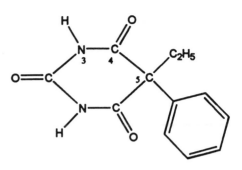

PHENOBARBITAL

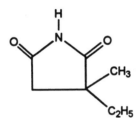

CARBAMAZEPINE

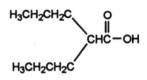

VALPROATE

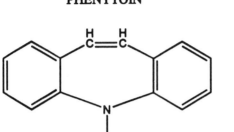

ETHOSUXIMIDE

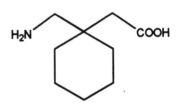

GABAPENTIN

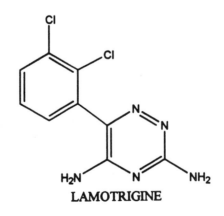

LAMOTRIGINE

Figure 8–4. Structures of antiepileptic drugs.

194

The structure–activity alterations were taken one step further by Merritt and Putnam, who substituted two phenyl groups on a chemically similar nucleus (the hydantoin nucleus) to formulate diphenylhydantoin (phenytoin). This substitution yielded a molecule that possessed potent anticonvulsive properties without significant sedation. Phenytoin soon became the industry standard against which all other AEDs were judged. (Other hydantoins used clinically include mephenytoin and ethotoin.) Although phenytoin's anticonvulsant profile was known to be distinct from that of phenobarbital, it was not until the 1980s that researchers discovered that the two drugs worked through completely different mechanisms.

Effects on voltage-gated Na$^+$ channels
A large and diverse literature strongly suggests that phenytoin acts by interfering with the normal cycling of the voltage-gated Na$^+$ channel (see Yarri, Selzer, and Pincus, 1986; Rogawski and Porter, 1990). Its effect is to reduce Na$^+$ conductance. Although molecular biological studies have demonstrated that the Na$^+$channel exists in a number of different states, only three are needed to explain phenytoin's action: closed-and-ready, open-and-conducting, and closed-and-not-ready (see Chapter 7). Phenytoin binds to the Na$^+$ channel in its closed-and-not-ready state, preventing the reinstatement of the closed-and-ready state, thereby reducing the ability of the neuron to respond to excitatory depolarization (Courtney and Etter, 1983). This action is well suited to suppress burst firing in the seizure focus and thus prevents the recruitment of other cells that normally leads to seizure spread.

Effects on voltage-gated Ca^{2+} channels
Phenytoin also blocks voltage-gated T-type Ca^{2+} channels (Twombly, Yoshii, and Narahashi, 1988) although this effect is minimal at therapeutic plasma levels (Coulter, Huguenard, and Prince, 1989). The T-type channel activates at moderately low voltage and exhibits time-dependent inactivation. In repetitively bursting neurons, this channel would therefore be expected to contribute significantly to depolarizing currents. By blocking this channel, phenytoin would prevent excessive discharge in a seizure focus.

Dosage considerations and use dependency
There is little doubt that phenytoin reduces Na$^+$ and Ca^{2+} conductance. However, controversy surrounds the relative contribution of these effects to antiseizure actions. Phenytoin is highly protein bound to plasma proteins (>90%) and its unbound concentrations in brain are similar to those measured in CSF (4–8 μM). Phenytoin's ability to block Na$^+$ and espe-

cially Ca^{2+} channels occurs at concentrations higher than those seen in CSF, implying that other mechanisms must mediate its antiepileptic action. However, its concentration in the seizure focus may be considerably higher than that observed in CSF for several reasons. First, the rapid cycling of the Na^+ channel that occurs in a seizure focus increases the number of channels to which phenytoin can bind, effectively increasing its concentration there (Willow, Gonoi, and Catterall, 1985). This use-dependent or frequency-dependent action of phenytoin is similar to that described for the local anesthetics (see Chapter 7). Second, the ability of phenytoin to block Na^+ channels is increased almost tenfold in the focus because extracellular K^+ concentrations are dramatically increased during the burst activity that characterizes the seizure focus (Adler et al., 1986). This increase reduces the concentration gradient for K^+, attenuates the afterhyperpolarization of the neuron, and induces neuronal depolarization. These effects combined prevent the Na^+ channel from cycling from the closed-and-not-ready state to the closed-and-ready state which appears to depend, in part, upon repolarization. As a result the number of Na^+channel binding sites available for occupancy by phenytoin is increased dramatically. Third, the increased metabolic activity that accompanies seizure activity increases CO_2 production, inducing vasodilation. The increased flow of blood into the focus delivers more phenytoin to the seizure focus. Taken together, these factors could effectively concentrate phenytoin in the seizure focus at levels that are sufficient to reduce Na^+ and Ca^{2+} conductance. Concentrating phenytoin in this way would explain why phenytoin's inhibition of Na^+ and Ca^{2+} conductance, which would normally be expected to depress neuronal activity globally and produce sedation, does not occur while abnormal discharge in the focus is reduced.

Pharmacokinetics and side effects
Phenytoin is not very soluble in water and the excipients used can influence its absorption rate (Bochner et al., 1972). Formulation differences do not alter the bioavailability of the various generic forms of phenytoin because of the bioequivalence requirement imposed by the FDA. However, the bioavailability of the original formulation (Dilantin) is different from that of generic formulations and can alter bioavailability (see Chapter 2). Care must therefore be taken when switching from Dilantin to a generic formulation and dosage adjustments should be anticipated. Regardless of the excipients used, phenytoin can precipitate out of solution when administered intramuscularly (causing sterile cysts) or intravenously (causing vascular inflammation) because of its low aqueous solubility. A new, more soluble form of phenytoin, phos-phenytoin, has recently been approved by the FDA. Its increased solubility significantly reduces the problems associated with i.m. or i.v. administration.

Phenytoin is absorbed slowly and erratically from the G.I. tract. Once absorbed it is biotransformed extensively in the liver via parahydroxylation, producing an inactive parahydroxyphenyl metabolite. This biotransformation can vary widely due to genetic polymorphism (Vermeij et al., 1988). Although phenytoin induces the P-450 system it does not induce its own metabolism because its metabolite inhibits the parahydroxylation process. This inhibition in conjunction with unmetabolized phenytoin saturates the biotransforming enzymes at plasma concentrations normally achieved clinically, at which point the biotransformation rate become zero order. Once saturation occurs the half-life can approach two days. When zero-order biotransformation kinetics have been attained, dosing becomes problematic and the risk of toxicity is high. Although phenytoin cannot induce its own metabolism, other drugs that affect the P-450 system can increase or decrease its biotransformation rate. Carbamazepine and phenobarbital increase phenytoin's biotransformation while chloramphenicol, isoniazid, dicumarol, sulfonamide, and cimetidine reduce the rate. Because phenytoin is highly bound to serum albumin (90–95%), drugs such as salicylate can displace it from its binding sites, increasing unbound concentrations. Under normal circumstances, this effect is inconsequential because the increased unbound pool will be biotransformed or excreted more readily. If parahydroxylation is saturated, however, such displacement can lead to toxicity.

Side effects attending AED *therapy*
In addition to the side effects unique to phenytoin that are described below the AEDs all produce cerebellar side effects at toxic doses (Table 8–3). The reason for this is unknown but may reflect the fact that the cerebellum fine tunes motor activity and is therefore sensitive to drugs that alter motor function. Intention tremor and nystagmus are characteristic cerebellar signs associated with AED use. As cerebellar function becomes depressed, the ability to generate smooth pursuit movements is compromised. Eyes or fingers following an object in space will not be able to pursue that object smoothly, exhibiting jerking movements that result in nystagmus and intention tremor, respectively. Compromised cerebellar function also produces an ataxic gait that is often described as "sailor's walk." Postural instability is compensated for by broadening the gait so that patients walk with their feet wider apart, as though they were walking on the rolling deck of a ship. Cerebellar toxicity is also associated with diplopia and hyperreflexia.

At toxic doses most AEDs induce seizures. This may reflect an inappropriate choice of drug and can often be confused with inadequate dosage. Abrupt termination of any of the AEDs can produce withdrawal seizures. This exemplifies a CNS drug-therapy principle reiterated through-

Table 8–3 General Side Effects Common to All Antiepileptic Drugs

Cerebellar signs and symptoms
   Intention tremor
   Nystagmus
   Ataxic gait
   Diplopia
   Hyperreflexia

Seizures
   High-dose seizure induction
   Development of absence seizures

Withdrawal seizures

out this text: The abrupt withdrawal of any centrally acting drug is associated with an exacerbation of the original condition the drug was used to treat. The likelihood of withdrawal seizures dictates slow withdrawal of a CNS drug (generally over a period of a month). The patient must be cautioned about the consequences of rapid withdrawal, such as might occur when forgetting to take medication. The development of seizures while a patient is on medication can thus indicate too low or too high a dose, inappropriate choice of a drug, drug interaction, or lack of patient compliance. It warrants an extensive interview with the patient to determine which of these possibilities is responsible.

Phenytoin-induced side effects
The microsomal enzyme induction produced by phenytoin contributes to several of its side effects and drug interactions. Steroid hormones and vitamin K are metabolized by this system. Phenytoin's induction of the P-450 system reduces the efficacy of birth control pills (leading to unexpected pregnancies) and lowers the circulating levels of all steroid hormones. The increased metabolism of vitamin K leads to hypoprothrombinemia and increased bleeding. This is circumvented with vitamin K supplementation.

   In addition to these side effects, phenytoin is associated with peripheral neuropathies in 30% of the patients on chronic therapy. Often these neuropathies are inconsequential but they can be bothersome to the patient and thus lead to noncompliance. Osteomalacia is another problem associated with phenytoin use. By decreasing Ca^{2+} absorption in the gut due to its effects on Ca^{2+} channels and by competing with vitamin D metabolism, phenytoin reduces Ca^{2+} utilization by bone tissue so that osteomalacia may develop, especially in the elderly.

   The use of phenytoin in young adolescent children should always be avoided if possible due to their risk of developing hirsutism and gingival hyperplasia. The latter may be a consequence of altered collagen metabolism secondary to alterations in Ca^{2+} metabolism and can be avoided with good oral hygiene (Diago, Sebastian, and Vera-Sempere, 1990). Adolescents developing these side effects exhibit an overt cosmetic defect that may contribute to the isolation of individuals already socially "special" as a result of their seizures. Phenytoin therapy can unmask subclinical absence seizures or potentiate those already present (Marescaux et al., 1984). In any patient exhibiting evidence of absence activity, phenytoin is therefore contraindicated. Like many AEDs, phenytoin can cause birth defects. This may result from the formation of a free-radical intermediate formed by the action of prostaglandin synthetase on phenytoin (Wells, Nagai, and Greco, 1989). The use of phenytoin is also associated with magaloblastic anemia and can produce a morbilliform rash.

Phenytoin is a well-known antiarrhythmic drug. At toxic levels it can induce arrhythmias and severe hypotension (Earnest, Marx, and Drury, 1983). At toxic levels it can also produce CNS depression. These effects are mostly seen during intravenous administration, as in the acute treatment of status epilepticus. Propylene glycol, a vehicle often used in the formulation of phenytoin for intravenous use, contributes to these effects as well. The need for this vehicle has been obviated with the release of phos-phenytoin.

Carbamazepine

Carbamazepine is structurally related to the antidepressant imipramine and has an antiepileptic profile like that of phenytoin. Unlike phenytoin, carbamazepine is biotransformed into an active metabolite (carbamazepine-10,11-epoxide) that probably contributes to its antiepileptic activity.

Effects on voltage-gated Na+ channels
Several studies corroborate carbamazepine's ability to block voltage-gated Na^+ channels in a voltage-and use-dependent fashion (see Schwarz and Grigat, 1989). In this regard, the pharmacodynamics of carbamazepine are the same as those of phenytoin.

Other effects of carbamazepine
Carbamazepine is an adenosine receptor antagonist and produces adenosine receptor site up-regulation with chronic use that correlates with antiepileptic activity (Daval et al., 1989). Its structural similarity with imipramine allows carbamazepine to also act as a NE reuptake inhibitor (see Chapter 11). Carbamazepine also binds to the so-called peripheral-type benzodiazepine receptor and Weiss et al. (1985) demonstrated that the ability of carbamazepine to prevent seizures could be

blocked with peripheral benzodiazepine receptor agonists. All these effects probably contribute, in part, to carbamazepine's side effects, although their relationship to its antiepileptic action is currently unknown.

Pharmacokinetics and side effects
Carbamazepine, like phenytoin, is an inducer of the P-450 system. Unlike phenytoin, it can induce its own metabolism, leading to reduced potency. This pharmacokinetic tolerance combined with its short half life (~7 hours) may require dosing frequencies of twice a day or more. The inconvenience of such schedules is a common reason for poor compliance. Overall, carbamazepine has significantly fewer side effects than phenytoin (Table 8–4) and, because of its similar antiepileptic profile, it is used in place of phenytoin in many clinical settings. Diplopia and respiratory depression can occur at high therapeutic levels and a transient leukopenia develops in many patients early in therapy. Like phenytoin, carbamazepine can increase the frequency of absence seizures.

Phenobarbital

Introduced as an anxiolytic agent, phenobarbital was serendipitously observed to be effective as an anticonvulsant agent. Before its introduction in 1912, sedative-hypnotic agents such as the bromides were the only drugs available for the treatment of epilepsy. Significant toxicity and profound sedation accompanied their use. With its markedly higher therapeutic index and its ability to provide antiepileptic benefit at dosages that did not induce significant sedation, phenobarbital became the first drug to provide selective antiepileptic activity.

Mechanisms of action
As a barbiturate, phenobarbital shares a similar pharmacology with the other barbiturates (Chapter 6). Thus, phenobarbital potentiates the action of GABA at the $GABA_A$-receptor site. In contrast to the benzodiazepines that increase the frequency at which the Cl^- gate opens in response to GABA, the barbiturates prolong the time the Cl^- gate remains open. However, unlike other barbiturates, phenobarbital and other antiepileptic barbiturates (primidone and others; see below) are significantly less potent in opening the Cl^- gate in the absence of GABA. This property is probably responsible for the ability of phenobarbital to provide antiepileptic activity without significant sedation (see Schulz and MacDonald, 1981).

Table 8–4 Antiepileptic Drug-specific Side Effects[a]

Phenytoin (Dilantin and others)	Increased bleeding Reduced steroid hormones and reduced birth control pill efficacy Peripheral neuropathy Osteomalacia Hirsutism Gingival hyperplasia Cardiac Arrhythmias Sedation Megoloblastic anemia Morbilliform rash
Carbamazepine (Tegretol)	Diplopia Respiratory depression Hyperirritability Nausea and vomiting Water retention with reduced plasma osmolarity
Phenobarbital (Luminal) Primidone (Mysoline) Mephobarbital (Mebaral)	Sedation Increased bleeding Reduced steroid hormones and reduced birth control pill efficacy Reduced renal blood flow and increased ADH production Hypothermia Muscle weakness Increased porphyrin synthesis Exfoliative dermatitis Eyelid swelling
Valproic acid (Depakene and others)	Fulminant hepatitis Lethargy Nausea and vomiting Diarrhea Weight gain Alopecia
Ethosuximide (Zarontin)	Gastric irritation, nausea, and vomiting Lethargy Dizziness Restlessness and anxiety Agitation Inability to concentrate Photosensitivity Parkinsonism-like syndrome Blood dyscrasias

[a]Side effects other than those common to all AEDs as summarized in Table 10–3

Ca²⁺ channels and neurotransmitter receptors

In addition to their effects on the $GABA_A$ receptor, the anticonvulsant barbiturates also block N- and T-type Ca^{2+} channels, nicotinic receptors, and Glu receptors of the non-NMDA type. The effects the anticonvulsant barbiturates have on Ca^{2+} channels are similar to those proposed for phenytoin and carbamazepine. However, the dosages required to block these channels are well out of the therapeutic range and these effects are probably relevant to the actions of phenobarbital only when it is used to induce coma in patients refractory to other treatment for status epilepticus. Blockade of nicotinic receptors in the CNS and especially their ability to block kainate and the quisqualate receptors probably add to the antiepileptic properties of these drugs because of the excitatory effects produced by Glu receptors in the cortex (Gage, McKinnon, and Robertson, 1986).

Antiepileptic action vs. sedation

Phenobarbital can produce antiseizure effects without significant sedation for several reasons. The relatively low potency of phenobarbital in opening Cl^- channels independently of GABA has already been discussed. In addition, tolerance to the sedative effect of phenobarbital develops in patients, especially children, much more quickly than it does to the antiseizure effect. Certain pharmacokinetic characteristics of phenobarbital contribute to its antiseizure specificity as well. Phenobarbital is a barbituric acid with a pKa of 7.3 that is much lower than the pKa's of barbiturates which are more sedating that anticonvulsant. During a seizure, the focus becomes more acidic, enhancing the percentage of phenobarbital in its protonated, active form. Thus, as a result of ion trapping (see Chapter 2), phenobarbital will achieve a higher concentration in the seizure focus than other barbiturates.

Pharmacokinetics and side effects

The pharmacokinetics and side effects of the barbiturates were discussed in Chapter 6. Only those effects that are relevant to its antiepileptic activity are described here.

Of the antiseizure drugs, phenobarbital possesses the longest half-life (80 to 120 hours). Many patients need to take the medication only once a day or once very other day. However, phenobarbital is an important inducer of the P-450 system. This induction can account for a two- to threefold increase in the biotransformation rate with an accompanying reduction in antiepileptic potency. This may require increased dosage or reduced dosing intervals in some patients. The pharmacokinetic tolerance that develops is an important consideration for toxicity. Fortunately, tolerance to the respiratory depressant effects of phenobarbital develops at the same rate as it does to the antiseizure effects. Since the former is produced at plasma levels that are significantly higher than those used for control of seizures, this side effect only occurs in overdose victims.

As a potent inducer of the P-450 system, phenobarbital produces effects on steroid synthesis similar to those of phenytoin. Thus, reduced steroid levels, reduced birth control pill efficacy, and increased bleeding time secondary to enhanced vitamin K metabolism have all been reported. In addition to the sedative-hypnotic, respiratory, and cerebellar effects, phenobarbital therapy is associated with several other side effects. It reduces renal blood flow, increases antidiuretic hormone release, and induces hypothermia. It increases porphyrin synthesis and is therefore contraindicated in patients with the genetic abnormality responsible for intermittent porphyria. Like phenytoin, phenobarbital can also elicit allergic reactions. The typical reaction is an exfoliative dermatitis and eyelid swelling, especially in patients with asthma or histories of allergies.

Primidone and Other Antiepileptic Barbiturates

Primidone and mephobarbital are barbiturates with favorable profiles for antiepileptic activity relative to sedation. Primidone administration is associated with the production of two active metabolites, phenobarbital and phenylethylmelanomide (PEMA; Bourgeois, 1989). The parent compound, primidone, and PEMA possess activity against myoclonic seizures, giving primidone a broader spectrum of action than phenobarbital. Mephobarbital is slightly more sedating than phenobarbital, however. All of these compounds are thought to work through the same mechanisms as phenobarbital.

Valproic Acid (Sodium Divalproate)

Valproic acid is a broad-spectrum AED. Of all the mechanisms advanced to explain the actions of the currently used antiepileptic agents, those proposed for valproate are the most controversial. As a fatty acid with low potency (hundreds of milligrams are usually administered), it is biotransformed to a number of metabolites, many of which have antiepileptic activity (Losher and Nau, 1985). The presence of these active metabolites may contribute to the overall action of the parent compound, and failure to consider their roles in the interpretation of pharmacodynamic studies may partially be responsible for this controversy.

Effect on brain GABA levels
Several studies in both animals and humans have demonstrated valproic acid's ability to increase the levels of whole-brain GABA (see Losher and

Siemes, 1984). This suggests an effect on GABA synthesis and/or degradation. GABA is synthesized from glutamate (Glu) by the action of glutamic acid decarboxylase (GAD; Fig. 8–5). If GABA is not taken back up by glia for reuse in the Glu metabolic pathway, or back into the GABAergic neuron, it is broken down by the enzyme GABA transaminase (GABA-T). GABA, as an amino acid, can also be incorporated into the Krebs cycle through a dehydrogenation pathway involving succinic semialdehyde dehydrogenase (SSA-DH). It has been proposed that at concentrations achieved in the brain, valproate stimulates GAD and inhibits GABA-T as well as SSA-DH (see Chapman et al., 1982). The result is an enhanced synthetic rate of GABA and a reduced rate of catabolism, producing increased CNS GABA levels. Although all of the enzymes responsible for GABA synthesis or inhibition are effected by valproic acid, these effects only occur at dosages that are at the high end of the therapeutic range, making suspect valproate's antiepileptic action in this regard. Interestingly, the synthesis of GABA, an inhibitory neurotransmitter, is inextricably linked to the degradation of Glu, an excitatory neurotransmitter. By reducing Glu and increasing GABA, valproate may change the balance of these two important and opposing neurotransmitters to a ratio that is not favorable for epileptogenesis. Despite these hypotheses, consensus regarding the role of GABA in valproate's action has not been achieved, and other alternative mechanisms, including an action similar to carbamazepine, have been proposed (McLean and MacDonald, 1986).

Pharmacokinetics and side effects

Unlike most other AEDs, valproate is very water-soluble, so 90 to 100% of an orally administered dose is bioavailable. Valproate is highly bound to plasma proteins and, because it is usually administered at such large doses, plasma binding saturation often occurs. Increases in the percent of unbound drug after saturation or after consumption of free fatty acids that readily displace valproate can lead to toxicity. Because of its affinity for plasma proteins, valproate also displaces phenytoin from its binding sites, leading to phenytoin toxicity (Perucca et al., 1980).

The most important side effect of chronic valproate therapy is fulminant hepatitis, a condition that can be fatal. Children are particularly prone to this problem. Hepatic function must therefore be monitored at least twice a year. The hepatotoxic effects of valproate are probably attributable to its metabolites. Because of the shift in the production of these metabolites that occurs when other drugs that induce the P-450 system are coadministered, such drugs increase the risk of hepatitis (see Dreifuss et al., 1987). Although several deaths have been reported, careful monitoring obviates this risk. Other side effects include lethargy, an increase in seizure activity or a change in its presentation, nausea, vomit-

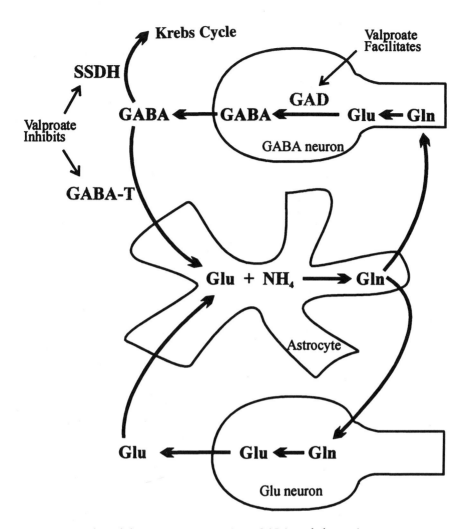

Figure 8–5. The inhibitory neurotransmitter GABA and the excitatory neurotransmitter glutamate (Glu) share a similar precursor pool in the biosynthetic pathways. In a GABAergic neuron glutamine (Gln) is converted to Glu that, in turn, is converted to GABA by the enzyme glutamic acid decarboxylase (GAD). Released GABA can enter the Krebs cycle through the action of the enzyme succinic semialdehyde dehydrogenase (SSDH) or be catabolized by GABA-transaminase (GABA-T) to Glu. The Gln can then be taken back up by GABA neurons or enter a glutaminergic neuron for subsequent synthesis of Glu. Valproic acid (valproate) is thought to invoke its antiseizure effects by enhancing the activity of GAD and by inhibiting the enzymes SSDH and GABA-T. The resulting increase in GABA levels increases CNS inhibition and deprives glutaminergic neurons of Gln.

ing, diarrhea, tremor, alopecia (hair loss), and weight gain. Although effective, valproate therapy requires very high dosages that approximate the plasma levels needed to induce motor toxicity in animals (TI for motor incoordination is 1.6); this side effect is rarely observed clinically. Because of valproate's very broad dose-response curve and the associated "wiggle room," the effective dosage is readily titered to achieve effective antiseizure control with minimal side effects.

Ethosuximide

Ethosuximide is the prototypic agent for the treatment of absence seizures. This special form of generalized seizure is associated with a characteristic spike-and-dome EEG pattern that is thought to reflect global recruitment originating in the thalamus (Vergnes et al., 1987). Recent studies suggest that ethosuximide is effective against absence seizures because it blocks Ca^{2+} T currents. A T current is characterized by its low-threshold, time-dependent activation. This pattern is highly effective at initiating rhythmic burst patterning. If thalamic neurons do initiate rhythmic burst activity, they could recruit cortical cells very rapidly and induce a generalized seizure. Ethosuximide has been shown to selectively reduce T currents in the thalami of animals as well as in culture at therapeutically relevant concentrations (Coulter, Huguenard, and Prince, 1989). Other drugs that can block these currents, include the active metabolite of trimethadione, methsuximide, phensuximide, as well as valproate, are all effective in treating absence seizures.

Pharmacokinetics and side effects

Ethosuximide does not have any unusual pharmacokinetics, is well absorbed orally, and is excreted approximately 25% unchanged. It can cause gastric irritation as well as nausea and vomiting. Other side effects include lethargy, dizziness, restlessness, anxiety, agitation, and an inability to concentrate. As with most AEDs that affect ion channels, several blood dyscrasias have been reported. Photosensitivity and a Parkinsonism-like syndrome may also occur.

Benzodiazepines as AEDs

Drug treatment for status epilepticus

Diazepam (Valium) remains the textbook treatment of choice for status epilepticus. Recall that status epilepticus is not self-limiting and can go on for extended periods of time. It represents a medical emergency. Intravenous diazepam has been the treatment of choice for status epilepticus because of its extremely high therapeutic index. (Its pharmacology was discussed in Chapter 6.) Its ability to increase the affinity of the $GABA_A$ receptor for GABA and thereby increase the frequency of Cl^- gate opening induces global CNS depression. Because this global depression is associated with such a wide margin of safety, the infusion rate of diazepam is gradually increased until the seizure has stopped.

As a benzodiazepine, diazepam's lipid solubility ensures redistribution, which may remove enough drug from the brain for the seizure to recur. Lorazepam (Ativan) is becoming the preferred drug for status epilepticus because it is as effective as diazepam but is redistributed much more slowly, reducing the recurrence of seizures. Because the risk of recurrent seizures is always present regardless of the benzodiazepine used, it is prudent to follow the acute treatment with a longer-acting antiseizure agent such as phenytoin or valproate so that antiseizure activity can be extended. If a patient does not respond to acute treatment, it may be necessary to induce a barbiturate coma. Phenobarbital or the fast-acting pentobarbital is generally used but only in the presence of full life-support capability.

Clonazepam

Although diazepam and lorazepam are very useful in the management of status, they are not effective AEDs because of their ability to induce rapid tolerance. In addition, their unfavorable ratio of sedative to anticonvulsant properties makes them impractical for routine use. But another benzodiazepine, clonazepam, is used to treat seizures. Its longer duration of action, relatively slow redistribution, and unique propensity to reduce the incidence of myoclonic seizures have led to its acceptance in the treatment of absence seizures and myoclonus.

Gabapentin

Gabapentin (Neurontin) is an analog of GABA. Although it was designed to increase GABA levels in the CNS, it does not appear to interact with GABA receptors, does not increase synaptosomal GABA levels (although it weakly inhibits GABA-T), and does not influence ion channels at therapeutically relevant doses (see Bartoszyk et al., 1986). Its mechanism of action against seizure activity is unknown.

Gabapentin has a number of desirable pharmacokinetic properties including very low protein binding. It is not extensively metabolized and does not induce liver enzymes. It is primarily used as an "add-on" drug in patients who are refractory to monotherapy with other traditional agents because its effectiveness as a monotherapeutic agent has not been established. Its favorable pharmacokinetic characteristics make significant drug interactions unlikely. It does have a short half-life (five to seven hours), however, necessitating administration several times a day. Because gabapentin is transported by the large neutral amino acid transport system, competition between other large neutral amino acids such as tryptophan and phenylalanine can reduce its absorption as well as its entry into the brain. (See Chapters 2 and 9 for further discussion of this form of competition.) Its therapeutic efficacy is often delayed, so patience is needed in determining its clinical usefulness.

Lamotrigine

Lamotrigine (Lamictal) has been recently approved by the FDA as an "add-on" drug for partial seizures. It reduces the incidence of partial seizures in patients refractory to monotherapy and it also possesses antiabsence seizure activity. Lamotrigine was initially developed as an antifolate drug because several AEDs reduce folate synthesis and high doses of folate can induce seizures in animals (see Gram, 1989). Its antiseizure activity is very similar to carbamazepine, however, and its mechanism of action is currently thought to resemble the Na^+-channel-blocking drugs phenytoin and carbamazepine.

Investigational Drugs

Because of the number of seizure patients in the world and the paucity of agents available to treat them, several drugs are currently under investigation. Felbamate binds at the glycine regulatory site on the NMDA receptor and allosterically hinders the action of Glu at this receptor. Such an action would be expected to reduce cortical excitation. Unfortunately, several cases of aplastic anemia were associated with its use, forcing the FDA to remove it from the market. Other drugs with a similar mechanism of action but a reduced ability to produce aplastic anemia are currently under development.

MK-801 is one of the most potent antiseizure agents known. Like phencyclidine (PCP) and ketamine, it binds inside the Ca^{2+} channel coupled to the NMDA receptor. It gains access to this binding site only when the channel is open and, like phenytoin, its antiseizure action is use dependent. The major problem with MK-801 is its toxicity. It shares many of PCP's negative effects on learning and memory and produces significant motor incoordination.

Gamma-vinyl-GABA (Vigabatrin) binds to GABA-transaminase (GABA-T) irreversibly and increases levels of GABA in the CNS by blocking the action of its primary catabolic enzyme. Following its administration, GABA levels increase significantly. The major characteristic of the drug that has slowed its widespread acceptance has been reports of dose-related microvacuolization of the outer sheaths of myelin. This effect is referred to as "intramyelinic edema" and is reversible. Although this is a known action of the drug, its clinical significance is suspect since it has only been reported in dogs, is not associated with clinically significant findings, and patients treated with this drug in Europe who came to autopsy did not exhibit evidence of it.

SEIZURE MANAGEMENT

Rationale

Aside from the social stigma that attaches to patients with seizures, the primary reason for treating seizures is that *seizures beget seizures*. If seizures are not brought under control, their frequency and intensity tend to increase. This increase may result from cytotoxicity leading to cytoarchitectural changes that further contribute to seizure development.

If it is assumed that seizing cells are hypermetabolic due to excessive excitation or reduced inhibition, then tissue damage could result directly from energy depletion. Indeed, the postictal depression that often accompanies generalized seizures is thought to reflect, in part, a state of hypometabolism in the brain secondary to depletion of what little energy reserve brain tissue has. The inability to maintain membrane potential, prevent the release of cytotoxic enzymes, or detoxify free radicals that would accompany significant energy depletion could contribute to cell loss.

As described above, seizure activity is also associated with excessive release of Glu from excitatory pathways. The release of Glu and its subsequent action on NMDA receptors can lead to excessive intracellular accumulation of Ca^{2+}. Excess levels of this ion inside cells is associated with the influx of obligatory water as the cells attempt to normalize osmotic pressure (see Zivin and Choi, 1991). This influx leads to osmotic swelling and can burst membranes, causing cell death. Calcium influx can also activate nitric oxide synthase, producing high levels of NO, a known membrane oxidant. Cell death produced by excess Glu activity is called excitotoxicity. If uncontrolled seizure activity kills neurons through excitotoxicity, new sites for the development of a seizure focus would arise.

Treatment Considerations

Table 8–5 lists the drugs most commonly used to treat specific seizure types. Although differences exist between the many seizure types, use of

Table 8–5 Drug Choice for Various Seizures

Seizure Type	First-Line Agent	Second-Line Agent
Partial (simple and complex)	Carbamazepine Valproic acid Phenytoin	Phenobarbital Primidone Gabapentin Lamotrigine
Generalized (tonic-clonic)	Carbamazepine Valproic acid Phenytoin	Phenobarbital Primidone Gabapentin Lamotrigine
Absence	Ethosuximide Valproic acid	Clonazepam
Atypical absence or myoclonic	Valproic acid	Clonazepam

one particular drug in a given seizure (with the exception of absence seizures), is generally not as critical as the ability of the patient to tolerate the drug. Since seizure therapy often means long-term drug treatment in many cases, a balance must be struck between effective seizure control and minimal compromise to the patient's activities of daily living. If administered in a high enough dosage, most of the drugs will prevent seizures but may incapacitate the individual. Thus, the dosage used in some patients may not completely prevent seizures but rather reduce their frequency or intensity to an acceptable level while producing tolerable side effects.

Generally, the dosage of drug should be increased gradually to allow time for adequate tolerance to the minor side effects to develop. A loading dose should be used only in emergency situations or when the patient is so incapacitated by the seizure that the side effects from rapid initiation of therapy are of little concern. Accepted practice is to try monotherapy first. If adequate seizure control is not achieved at the maximum tolerated dosage, then the drug should be tapered gradually and treatment with a second agent should be started again slowly. Because of the numerous pharmacokinetic interactions that occur among the AEDs, polypharmacy should only be considered after monotherapy has failed. The drug combinations should then be chosen so as to minimize anticipated interactions. Several of the newer agents such as lamotrigine and gabapentin have been developed specifically for this purpose.

Seizures that develop from a specific organic cause will often abate when that cause is treated. Even in the case of a tumor, however, the changes in the tissue that developed in response to the tumor may continue to invoke abnormal discharge after the tumor has been excised. If there is a reasonable chance that the seizures will abate after the cause has been healed, the patient should gradually be withdrawn from the AED to determine continued need. Many children who develop seizures early in life may "outgrow" their seizures. Other idiopathic cases also resolve spontaneously (albeit less often) and if a long seizure-free interval has occurred, therapy should be withdrawn slowly to see whether the drug is still needed.

Treatment of Movement Disorders

Prototypic agent: *levodopa/carbidopa*

*T*he movement disorders are a diverse set of diseases and syndromes resulting from dysfunction within the basal ganglia. This dysfunction leads to abnormal movements such as dyskinesias or choreiform movements in which muscles in addition to those needed to execute the movement become involved. Dyskinesias are jerky movements most commonly involving the face and limbs, as in tardive dyskinesia (TD), although the axial and even laryngeal muscles can also be involved, as in the "barking vocalizations" of Gilles de la Tourette syndrome (TS). The abnormal movements may also have a dance-like quality, as in Huntington's disease (HD), or may simply take the form of hyperactivity, as in attention deficit/hyperactivity disorder (AD/HD). In contrast to disorders characterized by excessive movement, dysfunction in the basal ganglia can also result in slow movement, abnormal posturing, or difficulty initiating movement. Representative examples of such disorders are Parkinson's disease (PD) and dystonia.

The basal ganglia are a group of highly interconnected subcortical nuclei that includes the caudate, putamen, substantia nigra, globus pallidus, and subthalamus (Fig. 9–1). Afferent fibers from the entire cortical mantle are integrated in the caudate and putamen, which together are called the striatum. Neuronal activity from these fibers is processed and fed back to the frontal cortex via the subthalamus, globus pallidus, and thalamus or sent to the brainstem via the substantia nigra. In either case it can modify the neuronal activity responsible for movement. Since the basal ganglia do not make direct connections with the spinal cord, dysfunction in the basal ganglia does not produce the paretic, paralytic, or

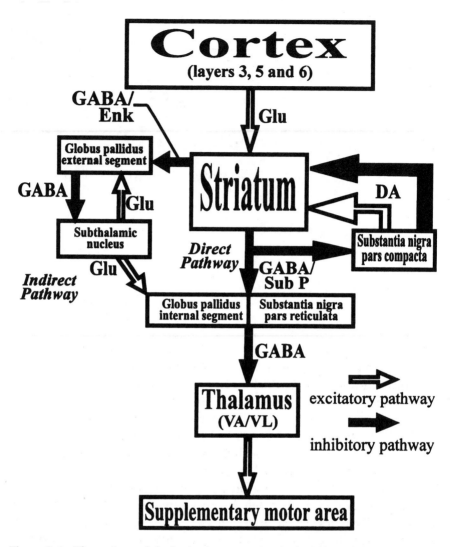

Figure 9–1. The regions of the brain that comprise the basal ganglia are depicted in this schematic. Where known, the neurotransmitters most associated with the pathways are designated. Dopamine has both excitatory and inhibitory effects on the striatum. Activity in the striatum is processed and influences the ventral anterior/ventral lateral (VA/VL) nuclei of the thalamus via the direct or the indirect pathway. These two pathways may have different roles in the expression of motor behavior. In Parkinson's disease, loss of DA reduces activity in the direct pathway while activity in the indirect pathway in increased. As a result, activity in VA/VL is reduced, leading to the reduced motor activity of Parkinson's disease. In contrast, Huntington's disease is characterized by early loss of striatal projection fibers containing GABA and enkephalin (Enk). As a result the external segment of the globus pallidus is less inhibited, leading to decreased activity in the subthalamic nucleus and the internal segment of the globus pallidus and pars reticulata. VA/VL is subsequently disinhibited, leading to increased activity in the supplementary motor area and to the expression of the choreatic movements which characterize Huntington's disease.

spastic types of movements that are characteristic of upper motor neuron disorders.

Although the basal ganglia are normally viewed as regulating motor function, it is becoming increasingly clear that dysfunction within this system contributes to cognitive and emotional problems as well. Thus, HD is associated with severe personality changes, PD is associated with slowness in thinking (bradyphrenia), and TS is associated with compulsive behaviors. The neuronal processing that occurs within the basal ganglia and within the interconnections this system makes with the rest of the brain therefore regulates more than just motor expression. It is integral to overall behavior. Whether the behavior expressed is motor, cognitive, or emotional, dopamine (DA) is, by far, the neurotransmitter most commonly associated with basal ganglia function. Although other neurotransmitter systems are clearly involved, most of the drugs used to treat movement disorders affect DA in some manner. In order to understand the pharmacotherapeutic management of movement disorders, therefore, a thorough understanding of the DA system is required.

THE DOPAMINE SYSTEM

The Dopamine Neuron

Dopamine neurons are found in the peripheral and central nervous systems. Their shapes and sizes vary markedly from the rounded glomus cells with short axons found in the carotid body to the large, multipolar cells possessing long, diffuse projections seen in the nigrostriatal pathway. Thousands of varicosities are found along the lengths of most DA axons (Fig. 9–2) and, because of this architecture, a single DA neuron with varicosities can influence the activity of thousands of postsynaptic target cells.

Dopamine is synthesized from tyrosine by the enzyme tyrosine hydroxylase (TH), which requires tetrahydropterin and Fe^{2+} for activity. TH is the rate-limiting enzyme in DA synthesis, and subject to end-product inhibition. Thus, excess intracellular DA prevents tetrahydropterin from binding to TH and thereby reduces its activity. In contrast, reduced intracellular DA increases TH activity. The synthesizing activity of TH is also regulated by the rate at which the DA neuron fires, by autoreceptors, and by heteroreceptors. These actions modify TH activity immediately by altering its phosphorylation status and, over a period of 12–48 hours, by altering the de novo synthesis of the TH protein (see Yebenes and Gomez, 1993; Zigmond, Schwarzchild, and Rittenhouse, 1989). Because TH is an extremely active enzyme, synthesizing very large quantities of levo-

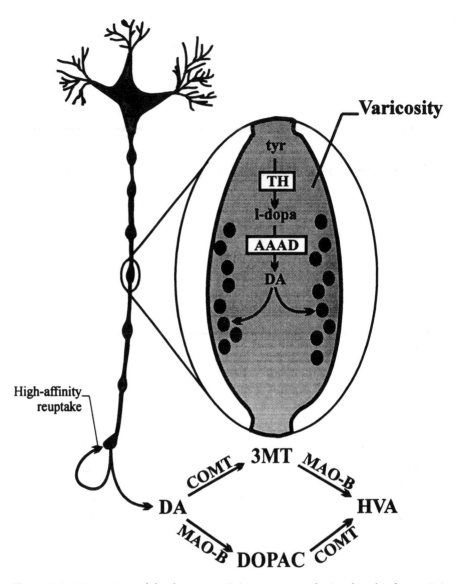

Figure 9–2. Varicosities of the dopamine (DA) neuron are depicted in this figure. DA uses tyrosine (tyr) as a precursor, which is converted to levodopa (l-dopa) by the enzyme tyrosine hydroxylase (TH). L-dopa is subsequently converted to DA by the enzyme aromatic amino acid decarboxylase (AAAD). Once released from a terminal bouton or varicosity, DA is taken back up into the neuron by high-affinity reuptake pumps. DA that is not recaptured is methylated by catechol-O-transferase (COMT) to produce 3-methoxytyramine (3MT) which is subsequently converted by monoamine oxidase type B (MAO-B) to homovanillic acid (HVA). Alternatively, DA is directly oxidized by MAO-B to 3,4-dihydroxyphenyl acetic acid (DOPAC) which is O-methylated by COMT to produce HVA.

dopa and dopamine in a very short time, drugs that affect dopamine profoundly affect the activity of TH. These alterations are always in the direction opposite to the acute action of the drug. Thus, DA agonists decrease while DA antagonists increase TH activity. Alterations in the rate
of dopamine synthesis that are opposite to the action of a dopaminergic
drug represent but one of the several compensatory responses of the DA
system and are an important aspect of the pharmacodynamics of dopaminergic drugs.

TH converts tyrosine into levodopa, which is subsequently converted
in the cytoplasm to DA by the pyridoxine-dependent (vitamin B_6) enzyme
aromatic amino acid decarboxylase (AAAD). AAAD is a nonspecific
amino acid decarboxylator found in several cell types within the brain
and throughout the body, including in serotonergic and noradrenergic
neurons, perivascular glial cells, the blood, the gut, the liver, and other
organs. Because of this broad distribution, the antiparkinson drug levodopa is converted by AAAD to DA in several areas outside the striatum,
which leads to reduced availability of the drug to the brain and to side
effects.

Following its synthesis from tyrosine by TH and AAAD, DA is sequestered in synaptic vesicles by a transport protein that is inhibited by
the drug reserpine. From the vesicular pool, DA is released from neuron
terminals and varicosities in a Ca^{2+}-dependent manner typical of small-
molecule neurotransmitters. Most of the DA released (~85%) is taken
back up into the DA terminal by a high-affinity reuptake pump called the
dopamine transporter (DAT). The DAT is relatively specific for DA although several drugs, norepinephrine (NE), and serotonin (5HT) can also
act as substrates, albeit with lower affinity. DA that is not taken up by
the DAT is O-methylated by the enzyme catechol-O-methyltransferase
(COMT) found on postsynaptic membranes (although see Westerink,
1985), yielding 3-methoxytyramine (3MT; Fig. 9–2). DA is also oxidized
to 3,4-dihydroxyphenylacetic acid (DOPAC) by monoamine oxidase type
B (MAO-B). 3MT and DOPAC are eventually converted to homovanillic
acid (HVA) by MAO-B and COMT, respectively, although intermediate
steps involving aldehyde dehydrogenase participate as well. Because of
the very short half-lives of the intermediate products of aldehyde dehydrogenase, however, the metabolites 3MT, DOPAC, and HVA are traditionally considered the major products of DA. All of these catabolic
products as well as DA can be nonspecifically conjugated with sulphate
or glucuronic acid in the brain. The conjugates and metabolites are present in extracellular fluid, blood, urine, and cerebrospinal fluid (CSF).
They are cleared from the CNS via the CSF. CSF levels of these substances, especially HVA, are often used as an index of DA activity in
the CNS.

The Dopamine Pathways

The diversity of dopaminergic drug action stems from the widespread distribution of DA projections in the brain. I can think of no other CNS system for which one's knowledge of the relevant neuroanatomy helps so much to understand the pharmacodynamics of a drug class. This system is described below, depicted in Figure 9–3, and summarized in Table 9–1.

Three important DA pathways project their axons to the forebrain from bed nuclei located bilaterally in the midbrain. In the ventral mesencephalon, DA cell bodies lie immediately superior to the crux cerebri (cerebral peduncles; Fig. 9–4). Although three nuclei have been described within this area, their borders are not well defined (Dahlstrom and Fuxe, 1964). They are commonly called the retrorubral area, the substantia nigra pars compacta (SNc), and the ventral tegmental area (VTA) (Bjorklund and Lindvall, 1984). The fibers from these cells course rostrally in the medial forebrian bundle along with other biogenic amine-containing fibers from the locus ceruleus (NE) and raphe complex (5HT). In general, the more laterally a DA cell body is situated in the mesencephalon, the more likely it is to control motor function, whereas cells found more medially influence limbic and cognitive function.

The nigrostriatal pathway
Most cell bodies of the nigrostriatal pathway are found in the SNc although some are interspersed within the substantia nigra pars reticulata (SNr; see Table 9–1). Ascending fibers from this area combine with other

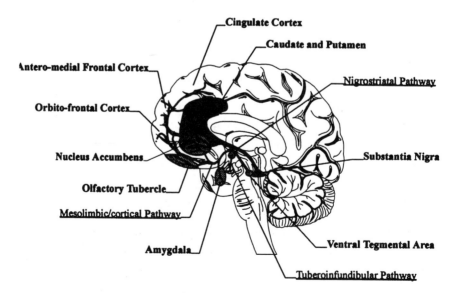

Figure 9–3. The DA pathways of the brain.

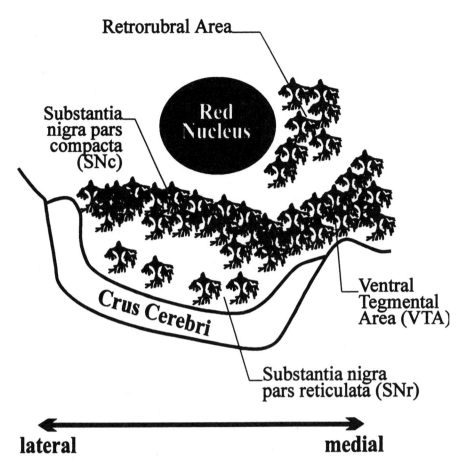

Figure 9–4. The bed nuclei of the primary dopamine (DA) neuronal projections in the brain lie in the ventral region of the rostral mesencephalon as depicted in this figure. Three primary cell groups have been identified including the substantia nigra, the ventral tegmental area, and the retrorubral area. The substantia nigra is further separated into two distinct areas called the pars compacta and the pars reticulata. The pars compacta contains the majority of the DA neurons whose projections form the nigrostriatal pathway. However, the pars reticulata, so named because of its reticulated or streaked appearance, also contains several diffuse fields of DA neurons.

ascending dopaminergic fibers, join the medial forebrain bundle, and project into the forebrain. The nigrostriatal pathway projects mainly to the striatum. This projection system is very diffuse and DA released from the varicosities of a single DA neuron can influence the activity of thousands of striatal target cells. The activity of the nigrostriatal pathway is regulated, in part, by the striatonigral pathway which contains GABA and substance P (Sub P) that functions as a long-loop, negative feedback system (see Fig. 9–1; Chapter 10). Fibers of the SNc project primarily to the same side of the brain although approximately 15% cross to innervate the contralateral striatum.

The nigrostriatal pathway is by far the largest DA projection subsystem in the brain, accounting for 80% of the brain's total dopamine. Degeneration of the SNc with subsequent loss of dopamine in the striatum is the key causal factor for PD. In contrast, hyperactivity in this subsystem is thought to be responsible for dyskinesias, choreiform movements, and the multifocal tics that characterize TS.

The mesolimbic pathway

The DA cell bodies whose fibers form the mesolimbic pathway are found in the medial regions of the SNc, the lateral regions of the VTA, and the retrorubral area. These cells project via the medial forebrain bundle to the nucleus accumbens (floor of the striatum), the olfactory tubercle, the hippocampus, the septal region, and the amygdala. The nucleus accumbens is important for locomotion and probably for the integration of motor activity with emotional state. Hyperactivity in this DA subsystem has traditionally been associated with psychotic behavior (see Chapter 10). It is also thought to contribute to the development of drug dependence (see Chapter 12). Limbic regions influenced by this pathway, especially the amygdala and septum, probably participate in the emotional response to environmental events.

The mesocortical pathway

The most medial cells of the ventral tegmental area, the retrorubral area, and some cells from the SNc project to the anteromedial-frontal cortex, the orbitofrontal cortex, the anterior cingulate cortex, the suprarhinal cortex, and other frontal cortical areas. As originally described by Bjorklund and Lindvall (1984) the mesolimbic and mesocortical projections were part of one pathway termed the mesolimbocortical pathway. However, it is likely that the two pathways mediate distinct functions and they are generally described today as separate pathways. DA released from mesocortical fibers is involved with cognitive processing and psychomotor stimulation. Hypoactivity in this system may be responsible for the slow thinking of PD patients and the reduced concentration abilities seen in patients with AD/HD, whereas increased activity is probably responsible for psychomotor agitation.

The tubero-infundibular pathway

The cell bodies of the tubero-infundibular pathway do not lie in the mesencephalon, but rather in the hypothalamus. DA neurons descend from the arcuate and periventricular nuclei of the hypothalamus into the neurohypophysis and pars intermedia to innervate the lactotrophs of the pi-

Table 9–1 Central and Peripheral Dopamine Systems[a]

Pathway	Origin	Target
Central pathways		
Nigrostriatal	Substantia nigra pars compacta, substantia nigra pars reticulata, ventral tegmental area, retrorubral area	Neostriatum (caudate and putamen)
Mesolimbic	Substantia nigra (medial) Ventral tegmental area Retrorubral area	N. accumbens Olfactory tubercle Amygdala, septum Hippocampus
Mesocortical	Substantia nigra Ventral tegmental area Retrorubral area	Anteromedial frontal, orbitofrontal, anterior Cingulate, suprarhinal, and other cortical regions
Tubero-infundibular	Zona incerta Periventricular nucleus	Pituitary
Incertohypothalamic	Zona incerta	Zona incerta Hypothalamus Spinal cord
Others	Periaqueductal gray n. tractus solitarius (?) Retina Olfactory tubercle Area postrema (CTZ) (?)	
Peripheral systems		
Carotid body	Glomus cells	n. tractus solitarius (?)
SIF cells	Paravertebral system	Postganglionic Sympathetic fibers
Renal system	(?)	Smooth muscle of renal arteries
Pyloric sphincter	(?)	Pyloric sphincter

[a]CTZ = chemoreceptor trigger zone (area postrema); SIF = small, intensely fluorescent

tuitary that secrete prolactin. Dopamine directly inhibits the activity of the lactotrophs and, as such, is called prolactin inhibitory factor (PIF).

Other central dopamine pathways

In addition to the four major pathways described above, several additional DA cell groups are found in the brain and mediate the actions of dopaminergic drugs (Table 9–1). The incertohypothalamic pathway has its cell bodies located in the zona incerta of the hypothalamus and projects to different regions of the hypothalamus and the septum. These cells may indirectly participate in the regulation of growth hormone secretion and temperature regulation. Dopamine is found in the n. tractus solitarius where it participates in respiratory drive. Dopamine is also one of the neurotransmitters that mediate central vomiting in the area postrema (floor of the fourth ventricle). Dopaminergic neurons in the retina mediate the center-surround phenomenon that enhances the contrast of visual images while periglomerular cells within the olfactory tubercle help translate odors into olfactory perception. In addition to its effects in the CNS, dopamine also regulates several peripheral nervous system functions.

Peripheral dopamine pathways

Dopamine is an important neurotransmitter in the carotid body. The DA-containing glomus cells in the carotid body, working in concert with the n. tractus solitarius, are involved in hypoxic drive (see Chapter 4). SIF cells (small, intensely fluorescent cells) are found throughout the paravertebral column and likely mediate some of the cardiovascular actions of dopaminergic drugs. Activation of DA receptors in the heart induces a positive inotropic effect. Dopamine neurons also innervate the renal arterioles where DA induces dilation. This action, coupled with dopamine's positive inotropic action on the heart, makes DA infusion the treatment of choice for hypovolemic shock. Finally, dopamine constricts the pyloric sphincter. Increased DA activity here induces sphincter spasms that can lead to epigastric distress and pain.

DA Receptors

As with all small-molecule neurotransmitters, several DA receptor subtypes exist. Dopamine receptors were traditionally divided into two major groups designated D-1 and D-2 on the basis of their positive or negative coupling with G proteins, respectively (Kebebian and Calne, 1979). Thus, D-1 receptors were coupled to G_S and increased adenylate cyclase activity, while D-2 receptors were coupled to G_i and reduced the production of cAMP. Although these two receptors antagonize one another, activation of both receptors is necessary to generate behavior. Thus, blockade of the D-2 receptor prevents the expression of behavior whatever the level of stimulation at D-1 and vice versa. This phenomenon is called cooperativity (Braun and Chase, 1986). That cooperativity exists in the basal ganglia suggests that either excess inhibition or excess excitation renders the circuit dysfunctional. Activity in the basal ganglia therefore operates within a functional range dictated by the excitatory and inhibitory actions of dopamine.

In the past few years, however, the genes for the DA receptors have been isolated and cloned. Molecular biologists then used gene libraries to identify five DA receptors designated D_1 through D_5 (see Palacios,

Landwehrmeyer, and Mengod, 1993). Because these receptors are thought to be positively or negatively coupled with adenylate cyclase, they have been divided into two families, called D-1 and D-2 (Table 9–2). Of perhaps greater importance was the discovery of the heterogeneity in DA-receptor distribution. This sparked the search for receptor subtype-specific agents to overcome the lack of target specificity that plagues this drug class.

Postsynaptic receptors differ in their affinities for dopamine. D-1 family receptors are activated by micromolar concentrations of dopamine while the D-2 family receptors are nanomolar sensitive. Therefore, low levels of DA release favor D-2 action while increased release will recruit the additional actions mediated by D-1 family receptors. Furthermore, DA autoreceptors (currently thought to be D_2 receptors) exist on the fibers of the nigrostriatal and mesolimbic pathways but are not as prevalent or are much less sensitive to the effects of released DA in the mesocortical pathway (Fadda et al., 1984). This has important implications for antipsychotic drug action since autoreceptor-preferring agonists that would reduce DA release in the striatum and nucleus accumbens would not be expected to do so in the frontal cortical fields where psychosis apparently originates (see Chapter 10). D_2 receptors are also found on the dendrites of DA-containing cells in the substantia nigra where dendritic release of dopamine may regulate the activity of DA neurons (Weiner et

Table 9–2 Classification of DA-Receptor Subtypes

Family	Subtype	Location	Action
D-1	D_1	Striatum N. accumbens Amygdala Olfactory bulb	Increases cAMP
	D_5	Hippocampus Hypothalamus	Increases cAMP
D-2	D_2	Striatum N. accumbens Substantia nigra Olfactory bulb	Decreases cAMP Opens potassium channels Closes calcium channels
	D_3	Striatal and n. accumbens Autoreceptors (?) Hypothalamus N. accumbens Olfactory bulb	Phosphoinositide cascade (?) Reduces cAMP (?)
	D_4	Frontal cortex Midbrain Medulla	Reduces cAMP

al., 1991). The functions of the DA released dendritically in the substantia nigra are currently unknown but may be relevant in the regulation of the endogenous rhythmic bursting activity of DA neurons.

Dopamine and Disease

Based on the previous discussion, it should be obvious that dopamine neurons, through numerous projection pathways, influence the activity of several regions of the brain. So it should not be surprising that drugs which affect DA are used in a wide variety of clinical settings that cannot be adequately described in one chapter. This chapter will deal with the use of dopaminergic drugs in the treatment of movement disorders while the next chapter will describe the use of DA antagonists in the management of psychosis. The pharmacology of the DA agonists cocaine and amphetamine, as well as the involvement of DA in drug dependence, will be discussed in Chapter 12. Because the vast majority of these drugs are neither receptor nor target specific, it should also not be surprising that dopaminergic drugs targeting basal ganglia dysfunction for the therapy of movement disorders, for instance, are associated with target-nonspecific effects including cognitive, hormonal, and emotional side effects. Such target-nonspecific effects are a predictable consequence of DA drugs acting on the various dopamine systems of the brain and in the periphery. By knowing the neuroanatomical distribution of the dopamine pathways and the actions of DA in their target structures, one can understand the numerous effects of the dopaminergic drugs.

PARKINSON'S DISEASE

Parkinson's disease (PD) is a widely known, extensively researched, and very treatable disease about which hundreds of books and thousands of research articles have been written. The pharmacotherapeutics of PD has been the central focus of my laboratory for 25 years, during which time it has become clear that the evolving knowledge of this disease contributes significantly to our understanding of the pharmacodynamics of the drugs used in its treatment. I can think of no other neurologic disorder where advances made in the laboratory have been transferred to the clinic as rapidly and effectively as they have been with PD (see Koller, 1992; Olanow and Lieberman, 1992; Jankovic and Fahn, 1993).

Clinical Features

Parkinson's disease (PD) is a movement disorder affecting approximately 500,000 patients in the United States. Its signs and symptoms result from the progressive loss of DA neurons in the substantia nigra. It is insidious in its onset and generally strikes older adults. (The average age of onset is 61.) The cardinal features of PD include (1) tremor ("pill-rolling" type), seen predominantly at rest, (2) hypokinesia or akinesia (slowed movement or inability to move, respectively), (3) rigidity (characteristic cogwheel type where the joints respond to passive range of motion as though they were drawn across the sprocket of a bicycle), and (4) postural instability (inability to respond to sudden changes in posture causing the patient to fall).

In addition to these cardinal features, many PD patients also suffer autonomic problems, slowness of thinking, excessive drooling, and depression. These associated features probably result in part from degeneration of other regions of the brain. Degeneration in the locus ceruleus likely contributes to autonomic dysfunction and depression. The cognitive slowing probably results from the loss of some of the DA fibers in the mesocortical pathway. The sialorrhea is a consequence of degeneration in the dorsal motor nucleus of the vagus.

Parkinson's disease is a progressive neurodegenerative disorder. The degree of DA loss increases with the duration of the disease, as do the deficits in motor execution. The progressive deterioration of motor function is staged by using the Hoehn and Yahr scale, which has six levels of disability ranging from 0 (no symptoms) to 5, where the patient requires full-time nursing assistance. Patients can progress rapidly or slowly through these stages with no known cause for either pattern. Death often comes naturally although pneumonia, complicated by the effects of excess rigidity (reduced ability to cough and chest wall rigidity), is often a major contributing factor. PD itself does not cause death.

Etiology of PD

Since its initial description by James Parkinson in 1817, numerous hypotheses have been advanced to explain the cause of PD. Although there is no consensus about its etiology, the various hypotheses advanced are important because they have fostered the development and use of many antiparkinson drugs. Because many patients who were afflicted and survived the encephalitis pandemic of the 1920s went on to develop parkinsonian features, a viral etiology was proposed but never verified. (These postencephalitic patients were the subject of the film *Awakenings*.) A genetic basis has also been proposed. Despite the few cases of familial PD reported, however, the vast majority of patients do not have a family history although many patients exhibit certain characteristics, such as a reduced capability to detoxify the drug debrisoquine, suggesting an inherited deficiency in liver enzymes which may be a predisposing factor.

Recent studies indicate that oxidative stress plays an important role in the neurodegenerative process. Of all the regions of the brain, the SNc has the lowest capacity to neutralize free radicals such as $O_2{}^-$ and OH^-. Deficiencies in superoxide dismutase in the SNc have been documented in some PD patients although it is not known if this deficiency preceded the neurodegenerative process or is a consequence of it. In addition, high quantities of free Fe^{2+} found in the SNc of PD patients can catalyze several reactions (e.g., Fenton reaction) that lead to the formation of free radicals.

The most popular hypothesis suggests that PD is a consequence of ingesting environmental toxins that selectively kill DA neurons. Several studies have observed a relationship between the incidence of PD and the consumption of well water in agricultural communities. The extremely high prevalence of parkinsonism on the island of Guam during the 1950s and 1960s is allegedly the result of ingesting a trace amino acid found in the cycad bean (beta-N-methylamino-L-alanine [BMAA]) indigenous to the island. Substance abusers in northern California who inadvertently ingested 1-methyl-4-phenyl-1,2,3,6-tetrahydropyridine (MPTP) developed a parkinsonian syndrome that is remarkably similar to PD. MPTP is a protoxin converted by MAO-B to the toxic metabolite MPP^+. MPP^+ is a selective substrate for the DAT and this uptake specificity may explain the selective DA neuron death observed in animals following systemic MPTP administration. Once in DA neurons, MPP^+ is further concentrated into mitochondria by high-affinity pumps present on the mitochondrial membrane. In mitochondria, MPP^+ uncouples oxidative phosphorylation at complex I, depletes DA neuron energy stores, and kills the cell. Since substituted pyridines are found widely in nature, the cumulative consumption of certain pyridines may be responsible for idiopathic cases. As proposed by the Calne-Langston hypothesis (Fig. 9–5) such toxic insults kill off only a portion of the DA neurons but the inexorable age-related loss of DA neurons reduces striatal dopamine to the symptomatic threshold.

In contrast to the lack of consensus regarding its etiology, it has been proposed and widely accepted that the clinical manifestations of PD do not occur until striatal DA (primarily in the putamen) falls to 20% of normal. This suggests that the striatum is remarkably capable of compensating for DA loss through such demonstrated mechanisms as increased neuronal firing, synthesis and release of DA, receptor-site proliferation, and possibly even terminal sprouting of remaining DA fibers. There comes a time, however, when the ability of these compensatory mechanisms to overcome the DA loss is overwhelmed and parkinsonian signs and symptoms develop. It is at this point when clinical symptoms of PD begin and when drug therapy starts.

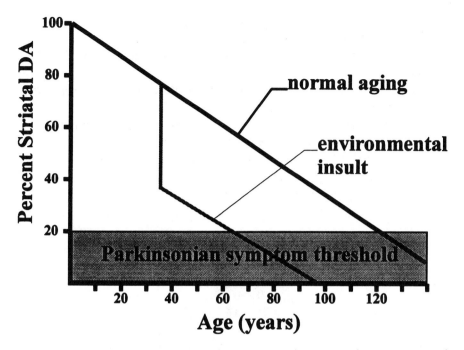

Figure 9–5. The Calne-Langston hypothesis suggests that some unknown toxic insult to DA neurons occurs in early life and kills DA neurons. The natural loss of DA that occurs as part of the aging process results in continued loss of DA until the symptomatic threshold of 80% loss is achieved.

Drug Treatment of PD

Based on the previous discussion, the primary therapeutic rationale involved in treating PD is the replacement of lost DA. Several indirect-acting DA agonists including selegiline, amantadine, benztropine, entacopone, tolcapone, and levodopa increase striatal DA through a variety of mechanisms. The direct-acting agonists bromocriptine, pergolide, pramipexole, and ropinirole are also effective. Since inhibiting ACh release from striatal interneurons is one of dopamine's primary actions, the increased release of ACh resulting from the loss of dopamine in PD can be effectively antagonized by the centrally acting antimuscarinic drugs trihexyphenidyl, benztropine, diphenhydramine, procyclidine, and biperiden. The use of direct-acting muscarinic receptor antagonists therefore represents a second strategy in PD treatment. The discovery that both dopaminergic and cholinergic agents were effective in the management of PD led to their use in other movement disorders and to the realization that dopamine and acetylcholine are integral to striatal function in general. As a result, the balance hypothesis of striatal function was advanced in 1967 and still guides the pharmacotherapy of PD and most other movement disorders today.

The balance hypothesis posits that the normal function of the striatum depends on a balance between DA and ACh (Fig. 9–6). The principle underlying the hypothesis implies that the absolute amount of either neurotransmitter is not as important to function as is the relative amount of the two. In the striatum, DA acting through a D_2 receptor inhibits cholinergic interneurons. Acetylcholine released from these interneurons excites GABAergic outflow neurons through muscarinic receptors. The dopaminergic and cholinergic neuron are thus in series.

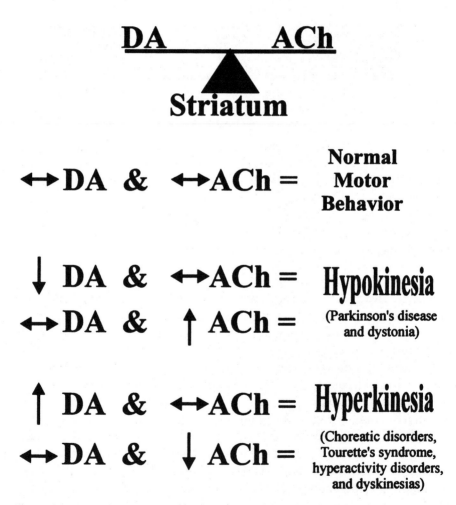

Figure 9–6. The balance hypothesis of striatal function is depicted. The principle is that the absolute amounts of the neurotransmitters DA or ACh are not as important as the relative amounts.

Because the dopamine projection neuron and the cholinergic interneuron are in series, the symptoms of PD can be treated by making the activity of DA equivalent to that of ACh, regardless of whether the DA and ACh levels are high or low. Since DA is low in PD, striatal balance can be reinstated by either administering an antimuscarinic drug to bring ACh activity down to that of DA or by increasing DA activity to bring it in balance with ACh. Theoretically the balance hypothesis is applicable to other movement disorders involving the striatum as well. According to the balance hypothesis, any movement disorder characterized by slowness or paucity of movement, such as dystonias, is associated with reduced DA activity relative to that of ACh. These disorders can be treated with DA agonists or antimuscarinic drugs. In contrast, increased DA activity relative to that of ACh is associated with excessive movements such as dyskinesias, choreiform movements, and tics. These disorders can be treated with DA antagonists or cholinomimetics. Moreover, as will be seen in the discussion that follows as well as in Chapters 10 and 12, the balance hypothesis of striatal function is not only very useful at guiding pharmacotherapy, it is also extremely helpful in understanding the development of side effects.

Treatment Strategy of a Progressive Neurodegenerative Disorder

Although a variety of drugs could be used (Fig. 9–7), the availability of physiologically appropriate DA release during the early stages of PD should be considered when choosing a drug. The remaining functional DA neurons present during the early stages of the disease are releasing DA into the striatum in response to ongoing brain activity. This release of DA is therefore "physiologically appropriate." A direct-acting agonist such as bromocriptine could be used and has been shown to be efficacious during this time. However, the increase in DA activity it produces is not predicated on the current dopaminergic requirements of the brain, but rather on the dosing regimen used and its pharmacokinetic parameters. The increased DA activity bromocriptine produces during the early stages of PD therapy are theoretically less physiological and therefore less likely to produce the best antiparkinsonian response. The use of an indirect-acting agonist such as selegiline, however, potentiates the actions of that DA released naturally by the nigral neurons in response to ongoing brain activity. The choice of such drugs is therefore more likely to produce a natural level of DA activity that is less associated with complications than the direct-acting drugs.

Treatment during early stages of PD
During stages 1 and 2, symptoms are mild and very manageable. Patients may still be working but are "inconvenienced" by their disease. DA levels

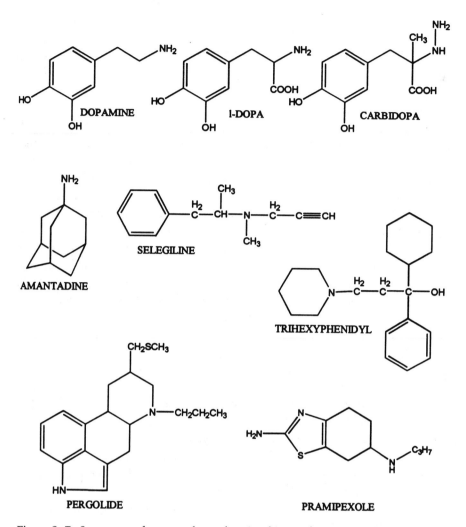

Figure 9–7. Structures of commonly used antiparkinson drugs.

have fallen to approximately 20% of normal and ACh is only slightly elevated. Once a tentative diagnosis of PD is made, most physicians are tempted to prescribe levodopa, the most effective and commonly used drug treatment. The use of levodopa, however, is associated with cumulative-dose side effects that complicate therapy and reduce its effectiveness in the later stages of disease when it is most needed (see below). Since striatal dopamine levels are only slightly lower than 20% of normal, other less potent indirect-acting agonists that do not exhibit cumulative-dose complications are used to raise DA activity above the symptomatic threshold.

Selegiline. As a competitive inhibitor of MAO-B, selegiline (formerly deprenyl—Eldepryl) reduces the oxidation of DA and thereby extends the duration of time released DA remains active in the synaptic cleft. Selegiline is also biotransformed to amphetamine, which increases DA release, inhibits reuptake, and blocks MAO (see Chapter 12). However, this effect may not be as clinically relevant as anticipated since the levorotary isomer of selegiline is used and the levorotary amphetamine resulting from its biotransformation is less potent as a DA releaser than the dextrorotary isomer (see Olanow, 1992). MAO-B inhibition by selegiline also leads to the accumulation of phenylethylamine (Paterson, Juorio, and Boulton, 1990). Phenylethylamine produces amphetamine-like effects and at high concentrations can stimulate DA receptors directly.

In addition to its actions as an indirect-acting DA agonist, selegiline is known to prevent the biotransformation of the protoxin MPTP to the DA neurotoxin MPP^+ (Heikkila et al., 1984). Speculation regarding the involvement of MPTP-like environmental toxins remains a popular hypothesis of PD etiology and two major studies were performed in an effort to support or refute it. Both studies clearly demonstrated selegiline's ability to delay the clinical progression of PD (LeWitt, 1991; Tetrud and Langston, 1989). Although it has been argued that these results support the notion that inhibiting MAO-B reduces the formation of MPP^+-like toxins thereby reducing the pathophysiologic progression of PD, this has never been proven. Selegiline's actions as an indirect-acting DA agonist are probably more responsible for the apparent delay in progression of symptoms than is an actual attenuation in DA neuron loss. Whatever its mechanism, when administered alone, selegiline is associated with few side effects (dry mouth is most common) and patients tolerate it well.

Antimuscarinic Agents. The antimuscarinic drugs trihexyphenidyl (Artane), benztropine (Cogentin), procyclidine (Kemadrin), and biperiden (Akineton) are often used in addition to, or instead of selegiline during the early stages of PD. Since these agents are competitive, direct-acting muscarinic antagonists, they effectively counteract the increased levels of ACh resulting from loss of DA. As competitive antagonists, the reduction in ACh activity produced by these drugs is physiologically compatible. Although they can be highly efficacious in early stage treatment, the antimuscarinic agents may not be well tolerated because of side effects that are especially prevalent in elderly patients. These include sedation, cognitive impairment, restlessness, tachycardia, constipation, urinary retention, and dry mouth. Delusions and even hallucinations may also occur at higher doses. Gradually increasing the dose results in tolerance to many of these side effects.

Of the antimuscarinic agents that could be used to treat early stage PD, benztropine should theoretically produce the greatest therapeutic benefit with the lowest incidence of side effects since it is also a potent DA reuptake inhibitor (Farnebo et al., 1970). As a competitive reuptake inhibitor, benztropine prolongs the residence time of DA in the synaptic cleft. From the perspective of the balance hypothesis, benztropine's dual action as an antimuscarinic drug and an indirect-acting DA agonist would simultaneously reduce cholinergic and increase dopaminergic activity. Working at the two primary sites of pathophysiology in the patient, this drug would effectively reinstate normal DA/ACh balance at dosages that are not likely to be associated with significant antimuscarinic side effects nor likely to enhance DA activity in nontarget structures.

Few pharmacokinetic studies have been done on the antimuscarinic drugs overall and benztropine in particular. Benztropine is assumed to have a short half-life (less than eight hours; see Cedarbaum, 1987). The antimuscarinic properties of benztropine would be expected to reduce gut motility and thereby reduce the absorption rate of other coadministered drugs such as levodopa.

Amantadine. Amantadine (Symmetrel) was originally developed as a prophylactic agent for type A viral influenza. In elderly patients who happened to have PD, it was shown to reduce parkinsonian symptoms and soon afterward became a widely used drug in the symptomatic treatment of PD (Schwab et al., 1972). Amantadine acts as a DA reuptake inhibitor and also stimulates the release of DA although the mechanism through which this action occurs is not known (Von Voigtlander and Moore, 1971). It is widely believed that amantadine possesses antimuscarinic properties based on functional studies. Competitive binding studies of amantadine at muscarinic receptors do not support this action, however (Gerlak et al., 1970).

Amantadine is well absorbed orally, is almost entirely excreted unchanged in the urine, and has a half-life of approximately 16 hours. It is widely used in the management of PD not only for its indirect DA agonist properties but also as a prophylactic agent against viral infection which can cause life-threatening respiratory infections in an elderly, late-stage parkinsonian patient. Amantadine is well tolerated and devoid of serious side effects although nausea and vomiting can accompany its use. Nervousness, insomnia, and dizziness have been reported as have ankle and leg edema and livedo reticularis. Unfortunately, amantadine has a limited duration of effectiveness (six to eight months) due to tolerance. It is therefore often used periodically during therapy.

Vitamin E (Tocopherol). Because of the popularity of the free radical hypothesis in the etiology of PD, the antioxidant alpha-tocopherol is frequently recommended for PD. Its effectiveness has been studied but not established (LeWitt, 1991). It is not harmful to the patient although extremely high doses (>2,000 IU/day) can cause GI upset in some patients. Interestingly, my laboratory has recently demonstrated that the administration of even high doses of alpha-tocopherol do not raise CSF levels significantly (Pappert et al., 1996). Thus, even though alpha-tocopherol has not proven effective as an antiparkinsonian drug, its lack of efficacy may be a result of its limited ability to enter the brain. Other free radical scavengers may prove effective and are currently under development.

Intermediate stage treatment with levodopa/carbidopa

At the end of stage 2 the drugs used earlier probably will not be effective enough to relieve clinical symptoms (Table 9–3). Levodopa/carbidopa (Sinemet) then becomes the cornerstone of therapy. The antimuscarinic drugs, amantadine, selegiline, and alpha-tocopherol are not necessarily discontinued, but rather levodopa is gradually introduced to the therapeutic regimen. Although levodopa would provide significant efficacy early in treatment, there are two reasons to withhold it as long as possible. First, levodopa has several side effects that may be a consequence of a cumulative-dose effect. Because reverse tolerance occurs in some DA systems, side effects such as dyskinesias and psychosis are more likely to develop the longer a patient is on levodopa. The use of levodopa during the early stages of the disease therefore increases the probability that dose-limiting side effects will occur at a time when levodopa is most needed. It also appears that a unique complication of therapy, the so-called on–off phenomenon (see below), may be a consequence of chronic intermittent stimulation of the glutaminergic corticostriate pathway where DA inhibits Glu release (Chase, Engber, and Mouradin, 1996). If true, this too would be a cumulative-dose phenomenon that would support the notion to withhold levodopa therapy as long as possible. Second, it has been argued that the excess amounts of dopamine that often accompany levodopa therapy lead to the production of cytotoxic free radi-

Table 9–3 Choice of Drug in Various Stages of Parkinson's Disease[a]

Drug	I	II	III	IV	V
Benztropine	+++	++	+	−	−
Other antimuscarinics	−	−	+	++[a]	++[a]
Selegiline	+++	++	+	−	+
Amantadine	+++	++	+	+	++
Levodopa/carbidopa	−	+	+++	++	+
Direct-acting agonists	−	−	+/−	+	+++

− = not generally used, + = seldom used, ++ = often used, +++ = generally used: [a]Provided that confusion does not interfere with efficacy

cals which might enhance disease progression. Despite the controversial nature of these arguments, most PD specialists withhold levodopa therapy as long as possible.

Levodopa is generally regarded as the prototypic drug among the DA agonists. Levodopa (L-dopa or simply dopa) is the levorotary isomer of the immediate precursor to DA. It is converted to dopamine by aromatic amino acid decarboxylase (AAAD). The overall effect of levodopa administration is to increase the available stores of dopamine for use by DA neurons. Administering the immediate precursor of a neurotransmitter to increase its activity in the brain is called a precursor-load strategy.

Levodopa is a poorly water-soluble substance that is usually administered orally. Because AAAD is present in the stomach, a significant portion of levodopa is converted to DA that is not absorbed, thereby contributing to the drug's low bioavailability. That levodopa which is not biotransformed in the gut is absorbed via facilitated diffusion into the portal circulation across the duodenum by the large neutral amino acid pump (LNAAP; Fig. 9–8). Other large neutral amino acids, including tryptophan and phenylalanine, compete with levodopa for access to this transport system. Protein-restricted diets reduce this competition and increase bioavailability. Once absorbed, levodopa undergoes significant first-pass metabolism due to the presence of AAAD in the portal vasculature and liver. A small proportion of levodopa is also converted by COMT in the liver to 3-O-methyldopa (3OMD). Levodopa is not significantly bound to plasma proteins and gains access to the CNS across the BBB via the LNAAP where it is again subject to competition by other large amino acids. Once it crosses the BBB, AAAD present in perivascular glial cells will convert levodopa to dopamine that is then subject to catabolism by MAO and COMT. Some of the levodopa will eventually gain access to brain regions rich in DA cells and terminals where it will be taken up by the high-affinity DA reuptake pump or the tyrosine transporter and converted by AAAD to dopamine for subsequent vesicular storage. The action of levodopa is terminated primarily by redistribution to muscle tissue although catabolism in the brain and the periphery contribute significantly as well. Five to 10% of an administered dose of levodopa is excreted unchanged and it has a half-life ranging from 50 to 90 minutes.

Because of competition by large neutral amino acids and biotransformation by AAAD and COMT, levodopa is poorly bioavailable (<30%) to the systemic circulation. Low bioavailability in combination with the various mechanisms that limit levodopa's access to the DA neuron terminal leaves less than 1% of an administered dose available for action. Very large quantities of levodopa are therefore needed to achieve clinically relevant levels in the CNS. In addition, the conversion of levodopa to dopamine in the periphery produces several side effects. DA action at the

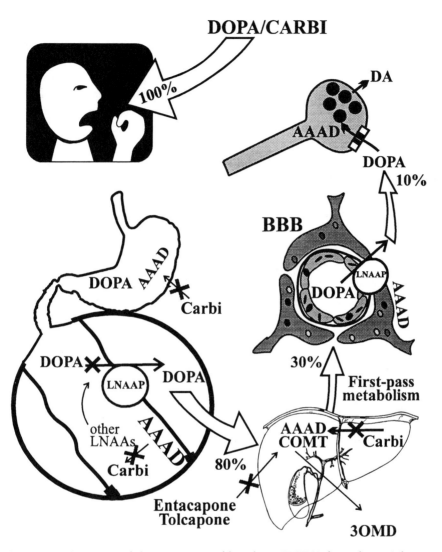

Figure 9–8. Summary of the movement of levodopa (DOPA) from the periphery to the CNS. The symbol "X" identifies points in that movement where carbidopa (Carbi) and catechol-O-methyltransferase inhibitors (entacapone and tolcapone) work. The percentages depict the approximate loss of levodopa in the presence of carbidopa achieved with a normal dosage (AAAD = aromatic amino acid decarboxylase; LNAAP = large neutral amino acid pump; LNAA = large neutral amino acids; 3OMD = 3-O-methyldopa).

pyloric sphincter can induce gastric stasis and sphincter spasm resulting in epigastric distress. These effects are not only uncomfortable to the patient but they also delay the delivery of an administered dose of levodopa to the duodenum, further reducing bioavailability. Circulating DA formed from the peripheral conversion of levodopa can also produce several side effects, including nausea and vomiting (stimulation of the D_2 receptors in the CTZ), increased renal blood flow, hypotension (potentially through SIF cells although a central action also participates as well), and enhanced cardiac contractility (positive inotropic action at DA receptors and levodopa metabolites that possess beta-adrenergic action). The potential for these side effects requires that the dose be gradually increased over a period of several weeks to allow tolerance to develop. Because of levodopa's low bioavailability and peripheral side effects, many strategies have been developed to increase its availability to the brain. These strategies not only increase CNS efficacy but also reduce the incidence and severity of peripheral side effects.

As a pyridoxine-dependent enzyme, AAAD's activity can be reduced by depleting vitamin B_6. This depletion is possible because of the large quantities of B_6 utilized in the conversion of levodopa to dopamine. Without vitamin supplementation, AAAD activity declines quickly, increasing central efficacy while reducing the DA-mediated peripheral side effects. Although useful, this strategy can produce B_6 deficiencies. The development of peripheral decarboxylase inhibitors increased the availability of levodopa to the CNS and reduced the incidence of peripheral side effects without producing vitamin B_6 deficiency. Today levodopa is almost universally administered with carbidopa as Sinemet in the United States or with benserazide as Madopar in other countries.

Carbidopa is a competitive antagonist of AAAD. The development of carbidopa was a result of an intentional drug discovery program whose goal was to identify an AAAD inhibitor that would not cross the BBB (see Bianchine and Shaw, 1976). Soon after its introduction, carbidopa was shown to increase the bioavailability of levodopa, increase the amount of levodopa available to the brain, and reduce peripheral side effects. In addition, the coadministration of carbidopa effectively extends the half-life of levodopa to one to three hours. Since carbidopa does not penetrate the BBB, it does not interfere with the conversion of levodopa to dopamine in the CNS, where the therapy is targeted. As a result, the antiparkinson potency of levodopa administered with carbidopa is increased approximately four- to sixfold compared with levodopa monotherapy. Although the levodopa/carbidopa combination significantly reduces the incidence and severity of peripheral side effects, the increased delivery of levodopa to the brain increases its central side effects.

Levodopa that enters the brain is converted to dopamine throughout the brain because of the ubiquitous presence of AAAD. Since the highest concentration of DA terminals in the brain is normally found in the striatum, much of the drug that crosses the BBB will be converted to dopamine in the striatum. Many of these terminals are lost in PD but even in a stage 3 patient, adequate numbers remain to take up levodopa, convert it to DA, and then sequester it in vesicles for future release. The DA terminal in a sense thus serves as a reservoir for the dopamine that has been formed from the administered levodopa. Once in the terminal the cycle of release and reuptake effectively extends the duration of action of an administered dose. This DA is released in a physiologically appropriate fashion, taken back up by the terminal, and released repeatedly. Thus, levodopa is probably most effective when an adequate terminal reservoir exists. As more terminals are lost, the drug's duration of action and efficacy wane, however. More frequent administration or higher doses are then needed. Less of the delivered dose is converted in the striatum while more is concentrated in DA terminals in nontarget structures such as the frontal cortex and nucleus accumbens, leading to side effects.

Levodopa Side Effects. Several side effects are associated with the conversion of levodopa to dopamine in the periphery (Table 9–4). Even in the presence of carbidopa, some levodopa is converted to dopamine, so the dose of levodopa should be increased gradually to reduce peripheral side effects. Although their frequency and severity are reduced by carbidopa, they are not completely abolished. This is probably because the usual coadministered doses of carbidopa do not reduce AAAD sufficiently. Newer formulations of levodopa/carbidopa have a 1 : 4 ratio of carbidopa to levodopa in contrast to the older 1 : 10 ratio and are therefore preferred.

The major dose-limiting side effects of levodopa are centrally mediated and include psychosis and agonist-induced dyskinesias that can potentially occur in all patients at some administered dose. Hallucinations and psychotic behavior probably arise from increased DA levels in the

Table 9–4 Levodopa Side Effects

System[a]	Without Carbidopa	With Carbidopa
Peripheral		
Pyloric sphincter	+++ epigastric distress	+
Area postrema	+++ nausea/vomiting	+
SIF cells/medulla	+ orthostasis	+
Heart	+ positive inotropy	+
Central		
Striatum	+	+++ dyskinesias
Striatum/basal ganglia	+	+ dystonia
Mesolimbic/mesocortical	+	+++ psychosis/hallucinations
Tuberoinfundibular	+	++ hypoprolactinemia
Incertohypothalamic	+	++ increased body temp.
Brainstem 5HT	+	+ myoclonus

[a]SIF = small, intensely fluorescent

mesolimbic and mesocortical systems, both of which are not targets of antiparkinson therapy. The development of psychosis necessitates a decrease in dosage that unfortunately usually results in an exacerbation of PD symptoms. Concurrent treatment with antipsychotic drugs has been used in an attempt to reduce psychotic symptoms without interfering with antiparkinsonian efficacy. Traditional antipsychotic agents such as haloperidol are contraindicated because they block DA receptors in the striatum and thus would exacerbate the patient's parkinsonism. The atypical antipsychotic drug clozapine has proven effective, however. It blocks D_4 receptors which are primarily located in the mesolimbic/mesocortical systems thereby effectively reducing levodopa-induced psychosis without significantly interfering with antiparkinsonian efficacy. Unfortunately, the use of clozapine is associated with agranulocytosis (see Chapter 12). Because of the potentially fatal consequences of this side effect, 5HT antagonists such as ondansetron which also possess antipsychotic activity (see Chapter 10) have been used and shown effective in some patients.

Agonist-induced dyskinesias secondary to hyperdopaminergic stimulation of the striatum is also a dose-limiting side effect of levodopa. They can occur at any point in the course of levodopa therapy but are much more common after several years of therapy. Levodopa-induced dyskinesias usually involve the lingual-facial-buccal musculature: Patients look as if they were chewing on large pieces of food while protruding their lips. Dyskinesias involving the arms and legs—writhing and flinging-like movements that accompany intended actions—are also common. Dyskinesias are thought to result from excess dopamine and are more commonly seen when levodopa levels in the brain are at their highest (peak-dose dyskinesias). Like the psychotic side effects, the severity and frequency of dyskinesias are readily reversed by reducing the levodopa dosage, but only at the cost of reduced antiparkinsonian effect. Although these choreic movements are visible and very disconcerting, most patients will tolerate them in deference to the rigidity and akinesia that accompanies a dosage reduction. Dividing the dosage or using sustained-release levodopa formulations may eliminate these side effects by reducing peak levels of the drug.

In addition to psychosis and dyskinesias, levodopa can also produce dystonia (an abnormal-maintained posture), hyperthermia, myoclonus (a rapid ballistic-like movement of a limb), and hypoprolactinemia and reduce growth hormone secretion.

Complications to Levodopa Therapy. In addition to the side effects described above, the wearing-off effect and the on–off phenomenon commonly develop during the course of therapy. They are more appropriately characterized as complications of therapy. The wearing-off effect describes the progressive reduction in the duration of action of an administered dose of levodopa that generally develops during the later stages of treatment. Thus, the antiparkinson effect of an administered dose of levodopa becomes shorter. It is thought to result from the loss of DA terminals in the striatum that results in a reduced capacity to store levodopa as DA in striatal DA terminals. Increasing the dosing frequency, switching to sustained-release levodopa/carbidopa formulations, or adding COMT inhibitors (see below) or low doses of direct-acting agonists to the therapeutic regimen have all been shown to extend the duration of clinical benefit from levodopa.

The on–off phenomenon refers to the rapid, almost instantaneous expression of the patient's underlying PD symptoms while still on medication. While the patient is responding appropriately to medication, the patient is said to be "on." Even with adequate blood levels of levodopa, however, this response can rapidly and unexpectedly switch "off," during which the patient appears to express the full constellation of symptoms associated with the unmedicated state. The inability to predict when an off phase will occur precludes the patient from performing normal activity such as driving a car. The on–off phenomenon is thought to be a consequence of daily increases and decreases in levodopa brain levels. This "sawtoothing" or "yo-yoing" of levodopa levels is a product of the drugs' short half-life and the frequent dosing that is more common later in disease when the loss of DA terminals reduces the residence time of levodopa and its product dopamine in the brain. It has been hypothesized that yo-yoing levels of levodopa sensitizes the GABAergic neurons in the striatum to the effects of Glu released from the corticostriate pathway and that this sensitization leads to intermittent excessive excitation of the GABAergic neurons that produces the off effect (Chase, Engber, and Mouradin, 1996). Continuous infusions of levodopa, sustained-release formulations, COMT inhibitors, and direct-acting agonists reduce the severity and frequency of the on–off phenomenon, but only temporarily. Glu antagonists are now being tested to determine if they are more effective.

Entacapone and Tolcapone. Entacapone is a peripherally acting, competitive COMT inhibitor that does not readily cross the BBB while tolcapone acts both peripherally and centrally. These drugs extend the duration of levodopa's effectiveness by inhibiting the O-methylation of DA. Both increase the bioavailability of an administered dose of levodopa by inhibiting peripheral COMT and extend the duration of its effectiveness. They are currently used as adjuvant agents with levodopa outside the United States and tolcapone is scheduled for approval by the FDA here in 1998. The chronic use of tolcapone is often associated with diarrhea.

Late-stage treatment

In the late stages of the disease, few DA terminals are left in the striatum. Indirect-acting agonists such as selegiline are no longer as effective and would be expected to contribute to DA toxicity in other regions of the brain. Amantadine is still used for its antiviral actions, however. Antimuscarinic drugs, if they are tolerated, are still effective because cholinergic activity remains elevated. Levodopa treatment has many side effects and complications that compromise its use by this time. Theoretically, it is now time to use the direct-acting agonists. Usually, the daily dosage of these drugs is gradually increased while the doses of the indirect agents are being reduced. Rarely are the indirect agents completely stopped, however, so that it is not unusual to find late-stage patients on several antiparkinson drugs. The possible antiparkinson drug choices are summarized in Figure 9–9.

Pergolide (Permax) is a partial agonist at the D-1 and D-2 receptor families. Bromocriptine (Parlodel), an ergot derivative, is a D_1 antagonist and a partial agonist at the D-2 receptor family. Several studies suggest that the incidence of dyskinesias is lower with bromocriptine than with levodopa or pergolide. The incidence of psychotic side effects associated with both direct agonists is, however, higher. Other side effects include those associated with DA agonist action. Hypotension is pronounced with pergolide and especially bromocriptine and probably results from a combination of DA agonist actions in the periphery and a central action in cardiovascular regulatory centers in the brainstem. Because of the risk of severe hypotension, the dose of these drugs must be increased gradually. The relative merits of bromocriptine vs. pergolide have not been clearly defined.

Bromocriptine is well absorbed orally, exhibits an extensive first-pass effect, and possesses a biphasic elimination curve of 50 hours. It is excreted in the bile and feces. Pergolide shares a similar pharmacokinetic profile but possesses a much longer half-life (Rubin, Lemberger, and Dhahir, 1981). Pergolide and especially bromocriptine are also used in the management of hyperprolactinemia and in neuroleptic malignant syndrome (see Chapter 10).

Pramipexole and ropinirole are two recently released direct-acting DA agonists. Both drugs preferentially bind D_3 receptors, have significant affinity for D_2 and D_4 receptors, and do not bind to the D-1 family of receptors. Their antiparkinson effect is probably a consequence of their actions at D_2 and D_3 receptors, both of which are present in the striatum. They are the first drugs to be approved by the FDA for PD monotherapy since levodopa and their increased efficacy relative to bromocriptine and pergolide reflects their ability to act at D_2 receptors with full intrinsic activity. Their side effects are typical of those seen with the other DA agonists. They are both readily absorbed from the GI tract. Pramipexole's

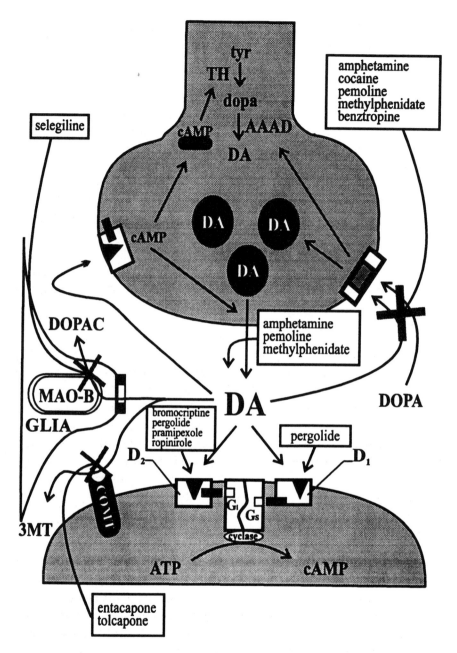

Figure 9–9. Summary of the synthesis and biotransformation of dopamine (DA) and the sites of action at the DA synapse where the various drugs possessing antiparkinsonian efficacy work.

half-life (12–16 hours) allows once-a-day dosing while ropinirole ($t_{1/2}$ = 4 to 6 hours) must be administered several times a day.

Depression management

As many as a third of PD patients may have "endogenous" depression and still others will have a "reactive" depression to their illness. Depression is most often seen in the later stages of the disease although it can appear earlier and even be the presenting symptom. If an antidepressant is needed, a tricyclic with antimuscarinic actions is theoretically an excellent choice. Many first-generation antidepressants such as imipramine and amitriptyline possess significant antimuscarinic activity which, according to the balance hypothesis, would provide antiparkinson benefit. Choosing one of these agents would likely require the discontinuation of any adjuvant antimuscarinic agent. Interestingly, selegiline was first introduced to PD therapy as an antidepressant for late-stage disease. Its efficacy in this regard has never been well established, however.

Other Treatment Strategies for PD

Although the drugs currently available possess dramatic antiparkinson effects, the inexorable progression of the disease coupled with the numerous complications associated with multiple drug therapy results in diminished therapeutic benefit. The now-established efficacy of surgical treatment can offer the end-stage patient treatment options.

The transplantation of embryonic fetal nigral tissue into the striatum of patients with PD has proven effective in many patients. Hyperactivity in the internal segment of the globus pallidus has also been effectively managed through ventral pallidotomy. The primary outflow target of the striatum is ablated using an electrode that destroys the tissue. More than a thousand of these surgical procedures have been performed with many producing remarkable success. Deep-brain stimulation has also shown promise in relieving disabling tremor poorly controlled by usual drug therapy. Implantation of an impulse generator attached to electrodes that are fixed in predetermined loci in the ventral intermedius nucleus of the thalamus is reversible as well as adjustable. All of these procedures involve brain surgery and the benefits to the patient must be carefully weighed against the risk of surgical complications.

HUNTINGTON'S DISEASE

The paucity of movement associated with PD contrasts sharply with the excessive movement that characterizes patients with Huntington's disease

(HD). This is an autosomally dominant, inherited disease involving neuronal degeneration of GABAergic neurons in the striatum, other basal ganglia structures, and to a lesser degree the cortex (Roos, 1986). Both Sub P colocalizing and enkephalin colocalizing GABAergic neurons degenerate in the striatum while cholinergic cells are only marginally affected. Clinically, the disease has an average age of onset in the late 30s and is characterized by choreoathetoid (dance-like) movements of the limbs and rhythmic movements of the lingual-facial-buccal musculature. Saccadic eye movements are also seen. Personality disorder often precedes the movement disorder and develops into psychosis and dementia (Young et al., 1986). Afflicted patients often succumb to the disease process within ten to 15 years and die of respiratory complications. The HD gene has been identified on chromosome 4 although the function of its product (Huntingtin) is unknown (Gusella et al., 1983). Based on the similar pattern of neuron loss in patients with HD and animals receiving intrastriatal injections of excitotoxins such as quinolinic acid, Young et al. (1986) proposed that glutamate-induced excitotoxicity may be responsible for the cell loss: High levels of glutamate initiate a cascade of events that leads to excess intracellular Ca^{2+} and an influx of obligatory water, causing cell swelling and rupture. Elevated intracellular Ca^{2+} also activates nitric oxide synthase, increasing the synthesis of nitric oxide, which kills cells through oxidation (see Chapter 8).

The excess movements of HD suggest an increased ratio of DA to ACh. This would imply that DA agonists should worsen while DA antagonists should improve symptoms, and this is the case in the early stages of the disease. But, the efficacy of DA antagonists (haloperidol is generally used) wanes with disease progression as the striatal cells with DA receptors are lost. The antipsychotic actions of haloperidol, however, are useful in reducing the psychotic behavior that often emerges in late stages. Benzodiazepines may also be useful in reducing excess movement since they potentiate the actions of GABA released by those cells remaining in the basal ganglia. As the disease progresses, however, the larger dosages needed are too sedating to be effective.

GILLES DE LA TOURETTE SYNDROME

Tourette syndrome (TS) is an extrapyramidal movement disorder characterized by multifocal tics (tics in various muscle groups) that are often associated with obsessive-compulsive behavior (counting and arranging things symmetrically), attention deficit hyperactivity disorder, sleep disorders (insomnia, somnambulism), rituals and stereotypical movements (touching, squatting, hitting), coprolalia (spontaneous swearing) and copropaxia (lewd gestures), and echolalia (repeating words or phrases) and echopraxia (mimicking gestures; Robertson, 1989; Lees and Tolosa, 1993). The average age of onset is invariably before 15 and most often between the ages of six and nine. The incidence of TS is much higher in males than in females.

Tics are rapid, brief jerks most often affecting muscles in the face and head. They can also involve the laryngeal muscles and lead to tic-like vocalizations. Tics wax and wane and are exacerbated by stress. Many children outgrow them (Robertson, 1989). TS patients describe an urge to tic that precedes the actual motor expression and a feeling of relief after the act.

Few postmortem studies of TS brains have been conducted and most of what is known about the underlying pathology has come from functional imaging studies of children with the syndrome. The nucleus accumbens is thought to be hypofunctional in TS (Stoetter et al., 1992). This disinhibits the superior frontal cortical regions that project to the striatum and the resulting increase in striatal activity produces the excessive movements or tics.

DA antagonists such as haloperidol or pimozide are the treatment of choice for TS, but they are only partially effective at controlling the obsessive-compulsive disorder and coprolalia. The DA antagonists can produce several overt side effects (see Chapter 10) that can lower the self-esteem of a clinical group that already suffers from social stigma because of their movement disorder. Although DA antagonists are most often used, tricyclic antidepressants and alpha-2 noradrenergic agonists such as clonidine are also effective in some patients.

OTHER MOVEMENT DISORDERS

Tremor

The 3–5-Hz tremor at rest characteristic of PD is but one of many tremor types. The saying, "all that shakes is not parkinsonism," is quite true. Most patients seeking medical attention for their tremors are not parkinsonian. Recognizing the various tremor types is therefore crucial to the therapy prescribed.

Benign essential and familial tremor

In contrast to the rest tremor of PD, "benign essential and familial tremor" has a higher frequency (9–12 Hz) and is continuous. (Since patients with severe tremor do not consider their disorder benign, this adjective is fast disappearing from the literature.) A family history of tremor suggests a genetic basis (familial tremor) although tremors can also occur idiopathically (essential tremor). The cause of these tremors is thought to involve an exaggeration of physiologic tremor which results from reciprocating muscle tone in antagonistic muscles produced by the muscle spindle and gamma motor loop. This form of tremor can be severe enough to preclude activities of daily living. Unlike the tremor of PD, which disappears during sleep, essential tremors may interrupt sleep. Receptor-subtype nonspecific beta-blockers such as propranolol are often very effective at reducing symptoms, but alcohol will work as well. Selective beta-1 antagonists such as metaprolol are also effective. Many drugs, including indirect-acting DA agonists, lithium, and phosphodiesterase inhibitors such as caffeine as well as stress and hyperthyroidism worsen essential tremors.

Intention tremor

Intention tremor describes a tremor that becomes more exaggerated as the target of an intended movement is approached. Patients with intention tremors may have no tremor at rest but exhibit severe oscillations of movement when they attempt to touch their nose, for instance. Intention tremor is a sign of cerebellar pathology and no effective drug is currently available to reduce it.

Dystonia

Dystonia is a neurologic syndrome (as well as a symptom seen in movement disorders) characterized by involuntary, sustained, patterned, and often repetitive muscle contractions of opposing muscles that cause twisting or spasmodic movements or abnormal postures (Jankovic and Fahn, 1993). A common example is spasmodic torticollis, in which the neck and shoulder muscles are dystonic as though the patient were looking over his or her shoulder. The muscles groups involved in dystonia can be focal, segmental, multifocal, or generalized. The severity of the dystonia may have a diurnal pattern (worse in the afternoon) or it may be unvarying. Dystonia can be induced by several drugs including DA agonists, DA antagonists, and anticonvulsants. It can also be a complication of several diseases including metabolic disorders. Generalized dystonia more often presents in early childhood and is the more debilitating form while focal dystonias generally presents in adulthood.

Little is known about the etiology of dystonia although the fact that bilateral surgical thalamotomy can dramatically relieve symptoms in some patients hints at a basal ganglion origin. That dystonia can be induced by both DA agonists and antagonists similarly suggests that it is a basal ganglion disorder. If dystonia is secondary to another disorder, effective treatment of the primary disorder often resolves the dystonia. In mild to moderate idiopathic generalized dystonia, GABA agonists such as baclofen and the benzodiazepines can be useful (Ziegler, 1981). In moderate to severe cases, the antimuscarinic agents are most effective although the side effects related to the high dosages used are troublesome (Greene, Shale, and Fahn, 1988). Unfortunately, most generalized dystonia patients do not respond well to any drugs. In contrast, patients with focal dystonia can receive considerable benefit from localized injections of botulinum toxin.

The administration of botulinum toxin, the endotoxin produced by bacteria of the genus *Clostridium,* usually induces a flaccid paralysis of muscle by blocking the release of ACh from the terminals of motor neurons. The botulinum toxin protein has three distinct subunits that are responsible for (1) binding specifically to cholinergic nerve terminals, (2) allowing the toxin to cross the membrane via the endocytotic/lysosomal vesicle pathway, and (3) releasing a proteolytic subunit of the toxin into the cytosol of the nerve terminal which enzymatically cleaves the vesicle-associated membrane protein, synaptobrevin. This latter action prevents the synaptic vesicle from docking with the membrane, thereby blocking Ca^{2+}-dependent vesicular release (Schiavo et al., 1992).

Because of its nonspecific action at motor neuron terminals, systemic injection of botulinum toxin (BoTox) can cause respiratory paralysis. However, focal dystonia can be effectively although temporarily (three to four months) relieved by local botulinum toxin injections into the muscles involved. This therapy is in wide clinical use and, because of the focal injection of the toxin, is rarely associated with systemic side effects. An overdose can, of course, lead to muscle weakness and respiratory collapse. Occasional patients have developed immunity against the toxin, precluding further therapy.

Wilson's Disease

Wilson's disease (hepatolenticular degeneration) is a hepatic encephalopathy with CNS features that are parkinsonian. These CNS features result from copper deposition in the striatum and other brain regions secondary to a recessively inherited deficiency in ceruloplasmin, the copper-transport protein. Cu^{2+} is not bound sufficiently to its transport protein and free circulating Cu^{2+} deposits arbitrarily in many organs. Deposition of Cu^{2+} in the cornea leads to the formation of copper-colored rings that are pathognomonic for the disorder. Wilson's disease often presents with hepatitis but can present initially with CNS symptoms. Besides the parkinsonian features, patients can exhibit tremor, dysarthria, dysphagia, emaciation, spasmodic contractions, and emotionalism (Wilson, 1912).

The hepatitis and encephalopathy are consequences of the cumulative buildup of Cu^{2+} in the body. Thus, patients will have had the ceruloplasmin deficiency since birth but will not have accumulated sufficient Cu^{2+} to induce toxicity until their teens or 20s.

The parkinsonian signs of the disease are not responsive to levodopa therapy when high levels of Cu^{2+} remain in the body because the symptoms are the result of reduced responsiveness of striatal neurons to DA. Wilson's disease can, however, be effectively treated by chelating free Cu^{2+} with penicillamine or trientine, a less potent but better tolerated agent. Penicillamine can induce nausea, vomiting, diarrhea, dyspepsia, nephrotic syndrome, and a variety of blood dyscrasias. Chelation therapy requires abstention from foods rich in Cu^{2+} including chocolate, nuts, shellfish, liver, mushrooms, broccoli, and certain cereals. The house tap water should also be screened to detect its content of Cu^{2+}. Zinc acetate consumed with meals can reduce copper absorption for those who have difficulty controlling Cu^{2+} intake. Zinc acetate induces metallothionein production in the gut that chelates copper allowing it to be passed in the feces. Following chelation therapy, patients may exhibit residual parkinsonian features after the body copper load has normalized. They often respond favorably to antiparkinson medication at this time.

ATTENTION DEFICIT/HYPERACTIVITY DISORDER (AD/HD)

Attention deficit with or without hyperactivity is a common childhood problem characterized by an inability to remain focused on a task that may or may not be associated with increased motor activity (hyperactivity). The hyperactivity commonly seen in children or adults with attention deficit is probably a consequence of abnormal cortical control of basal ganglia function. The apparent increase in the incidence of AD/HD over the last decade probably reflects the fact that only children with hyperactivity were formerly diagnosed as having the disorder. Now children with attention problems without hyperactivity are thought to represent a subpopulation of those with AD/HD and the primary deficit is seen as the inability to sustain attention at a task. This is associated with several symptoms including easy distractibility, interrupting others incessantly, inability to follow instructions, and loquacity.

A common lay perception was that AD/HD children were eating too much sugar and that removing sugar from their diet would improve their behavior (Feingold Diet). Significant dietary changes were often associated with behavioral improvement but carefully controlled studies demonstrated that the clinical improvements observed were the result of the extra attention the children were paid by their families. Contrary to popular opinion, sugar does not lead to hyperactivity and may actually reduce motor activity. This excludes the consumption of chocolates or colas that contain high quantities of caffeine, a known CNS stimulant.

The indirect-acting DA agonists amphetamine, methylphenidate, and pemoline are the drug treatments of choice for AD/HD. The rationale for using these central stimulants is that they increase attentiveness. Well-controlled studies indicate that the DA agonists improve academic performance in most children with AD/HD (see Calsi, Grothe, and Elia, 1990, for review) and that playtime activities are improved as well (Swanson et al., 1991).

Amphetamine, Methylphenidate, and Pemoline

Amphetamine, methylphenidate, and pemoline are CNS stimulants that increase DA and to a lesser extent NE activity. These three drugs have proven to be equally effective in AD/HD. Amphetamine induces a Ca^{2+}-independent release of DA and NE, blocks their reuptake, and at high concentrations inhibits MAO (see Chapter 12). Methylphenidate possesses amphetamine-like properties and is the most widely prescribed drug for AD/HD. At normally administered doses it has a higher ratio of central to peripheral side effects than amphetamine, ostensibly reflecting a preference for the DA neuron relative to the NE neuron. As a result, methylphenidate produces fewer autonomic side effects than amphetamine. The mechanism of action of methylphenidate is different from amphetamine's in that the two drugs release different terminal pools of DA (see Clemens and Fuller, 1979). The nature of this difference has never been fully characterized although the fact that methylphenidate primarily releases vesicular pool DA suggests an effect on the vesicular release process. Regardless, the reduced effects methylphenidate has on NE make it the drug of choice in the management of AD/HD. Methylphenidate (Ritalin) is rapidly absorbed following oral administration, has a half-life of two to three hours, and as much as 80% of an administered dose is converted to the active metabolite ritalinic acid. Because of methylphenidate's short half-life, which often requires multiple daily doses, sustained-release formulations are available although erratic absorption can complicate efficacy (see Chapter 2).

Pemoline is an indirect-acting agonist with amphetamine-like properties although it is structurally dissimilar to amphetamine and methylphenidate. It is much less potent than is methylphenidate or amphetamine although its efficacy in AD/HD is similar. Like methylphenidate it has fewer cardiovascular side effects than has amphetamine, it is well absorbed orally (although slower than methylphenidate or amphetamine), and it has a longer half-life than methylphenidate (seven to eight hours).

Interestingly, the therapeutic efficacy of pemoline is often delayed two to four weeks (see Calsi, Grothe, and Elia, 1990).

The side effects of the CNS stimulants are summarized in Table 9–5, are not severe, and in most cases, are not dramatically different from problems commonly encountered in normal children. It is important to recognize that many of the side effects attributed to CNS stimulants can be observed in normal children. Because their child is on a drug, parents often become more aware of symptoms such as headaches or irritability. Even if these symptoms are normally present in the child, parents tend to attribute them to a drug side effect that leads to concern and potential noncompliance. The more disconcerting side effects such as heart palpitations, minor increases in blood pressure, headaches, decreased appetite, and insomnia that occur in most children in the early phase of treatment will gradually wane once tolerance has developed. Some children may, however, develop severe side effects requiring immediate withdrawal of medication. These problems are less likely to develop if the dosage is slowly increased.

In addition to side effects, other treatment problems should be considered. DA agonists can reduce growth hormone production and if moderate dosages are administered to children chronically, growth potential could theoretically be compromised. Long-term follow-up studies do not

Table 9–5 Mean Severity Ratings by Parents of Side Effects in Children on a Placebo Pill and 0.3 and 0.5 mg/kg Methylphenidate[a]

Side Effect	Placebo	0.3 mg/kg	0.5 mg/kg
Decreased appetite	0.4	1.7	2.6[b]
Insomnia	1.4	2.6	3.1[b]
Stomachaches	0.5	1.0	1.5[b]
Headaches	0.3	0.6	0.8[b]
Prone to crying	1.7	2.2	2.0
Tics/nervous movements	0.7	0.9	1.1
Dizziness	0.1	0.3	0.3
Drowsiness	0.5	0.7	0.7
Nail biting	1.1	1.1	1.3
Talks less	0.4	0.6	0.9
Anxious	2.4	1.8	2.0
Disinterested in others	0.7	0.6	0.6
Euphoria	1.7	1.4	1.8
Irritable	3.2	2.5	2.7
Nightmares	0.6	0.6	0.8
Sadness	1.6	1.9	1.8
Staring	1.3	1.3	1.0

[a]Adapted from Barkley et al. (1990). Scores depict mean values of severity from 0 (no problem) to 9 (severe)

[b] = indicates a statistically significant effect

reveal any significant effects on adult stature, however (Stevenson and Wolraich, 1989). Because central stimulants are used, parents are often concerned about the risk of drug addiction. As will be discussed in Chapter 12, however, the medical prescription of drugs for indicated purposes does not lead to dependence. Finally, children should be withdrawn from medication periodically because of the development of pharmacodynamic and physiologic tolerance and the associated reduction in efficacy. These "drug holidays" are most frequently initiated during the winter and summer school breaks. In addition to their ability to reduce the impact of tolerance, the drug holiday also allows the opportunity for assessment of continued need for medication since many children outgrow their AD/HD.

The effectiveness of the central stimulants has led to the pharmacocentric hypothesis that AD/HD results from reduced DA in the brain. Consistent with this hypothesis are recent PET studies indicating that activation of the orbitofrontal cortex in response to stimuli is partially a DA-mediated phenomenon that is reduced in children with AD/HD. The administration of amphetamine-like drugs reinstates normal activity in this region (see Zametkin et al., 1993). In addition, children with TS often exhibit signs and symptoms of AD/HD when treated with DA antagonists while AD/HD children treated with DA agonists can exhibit signs of TS. These data and the high incidence of obsessive-compulsive disorder in TS provide hints that several disorders associated with inadequate concentration or impulse control could be related to abnormalities in the DA system. The findings suggest that the orbitofrontal cortex is crucially involved in attention and concentration (see Heilmann, Voeller, and Nadeau, 1991; Colby, 1991).

Antipsychotic Drugs

Prototypic Agent: *chlorpromazine* (*Thorazine*)

The psychoses are among the most severe types of psychiatric disorders. The psychotic state, a diagnostic requirement for psychosis, consists of bizarre behavior, an inability to think coherently and comprehend the environment, and most importantly, an inability to recognize the presence of these abnormalities. Mood alterations ranging from severe agitation to total emotional withdrawal are also commonly seen. Psychotic patients often experience abnormal sensations such as hallucinations (mostly auditory) and false beliefs (delusions and paranoid ideation). The psychoses are generally distinguished from cognitive disorders in which psychotic behavior may or may not be present, such as delirium (an acute confusional state) and dementia (characterized by memory disturbance). These cognitive disorders generally have a definable cause such as drug toxicity, metabolic disturbance, or identifiable neuropathology. Psychotic behavior may also accompany other severe forms of psychiatric illness such as depression or bipolar disorder.

Schizophrenia is the most common psychosis, afflicting about 1% of the world's population. It is characterized by recurring episodes of psychotic behavior that usually involve bizarre delusions, prominent hallucinations, thought disorder, or emotional disturbance. These overt components of a psychotic episode are called positive symptoms. In contrast, the patient may also exhibit negative symptoms that include lack of motivation, social isolation, poverty of speech, blunted affect, reduced attention span, and eccentric behavior. The negative symptoms can be part of the psychotic episode and often persist after it, in which case they are referred to as residual symptoms. The negative symptoms of schizophrenia are the most difficult to manage.

The first psychotic episode is preceded by a varying period of schizotypal behavior during which flat affect, odd behaviors, social withdrawal, neglect of personal hygiene, and an inability to integrate appropriately into societal structure are generally seen. As many as 3% of the population may exhibit this syndrome but never have a psychotic break, in which case it is classified as a schizotypal personality disorder and considered a milder form of schizophrenia.

The types of symptoms expressed have long-term prognosticating capability. Schizophrenia dominated primarily by positive symptoms, especially if they are manifested all of a sudden, is quite treatable unless the symptoms are frequent and flagrant. Overall deterioration does not tend to occur and, after ten to 15 years, significant improvement is usually observed, especially with drug therapy. Schizophrenia dominated by negative symptoms, however, has a poor long-term prognosis and although the underlying disease does not seen to worsen, the eventual impact of the negative symptoms on social integration often takes its toll, rendering the patient dysfunctional for life. Overall, about one-fourth of schizophrenic patients (mostly those exhibiting predominantly positive symptoms) improve dramatically with treatment. Another quarter of the patients (mostly those with predominantly negative symptoms) have symptoms for life and usually require institutionalization. The rest show variable or limited improvement.

BIOLOGICAL BASIS OF SCHIZOPHRENIA

Freud and followers of psychoanalytic theory believed that the symptoms of schizophrenia were manifestations of deep-seated psychological trauma in childhood that lay suppressed in the subconscious. This notion held sway in psychiatry for much of this century. The fact that the twin of a schizophrenic patient raised separately is almost 12 times more likely to be schizophrenic than the rest of the population, however, indicates a genetic etiology (see Kendler, 1988). In addition, the high rate of gestational disorders and birth complications involving tissue hypoxia during the sixth and seventh months of pregnancy in mothers of schizophrenics (Lewis and Murray, 1987) suggests a neural substrate. The arrival of new technologies, especially magnetic resonance imaging (MRI) and positron emission tomography (PET), has revealed both structural and functional abnormalities in the brains of many schizophrenics (see Buchanan et al., 1993). Taken together, the weight of these data favors a neurologic basis for schizophrenia, with several lines of evidence pointing to a disturbance in dopamine function.

The Dopamine Theory of Schizophrenia

According to the dopamine theory of schizophrenia, the symptoms of the disease stem from dopamine hyperactivity in the forebrain (Stevens, 1973). This is a pharmacocentric hypothesis based on the observations that (1) all of the current antipsychotic drugs block DA neurotransmission (they are all direct-acting DA antagonists); (2) high doses of DA agonists exacerbate psychotic symptoms in schizophrenics and induce paranoid ideation in normal controls that is remarkably similar to that of schizophrenia (see Carlsson, 1988); and (3) the potency of antipsychotic agents is highly correlated with their ability to bind to the D_2 receptor (see Fig. 10–1; Seeman et al., 1976).

The pharmacologic observations that form the cornerstone of the dopamine theory are supported by evidence of increases in dopamine,

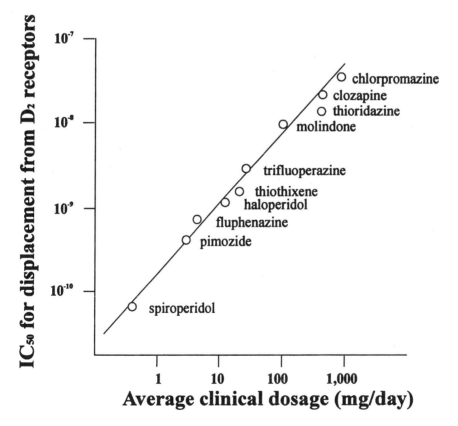

Figure 10–1. The clinically effective daily dosage of several antipsychotic agents is highly correlated with the IC_{50} of these drugs for displacement of spiroperidol from D_2 receptors, implicating a tight correlation between antipsychotic potency and D_2-receptor blockade. (Seeman et al., 1976).

DA-receptor number, and second-messenger production in tissues from schizophrenic patients (Davis et al., 1991). The major problem with this theory is that DA antagonists can block DA receptors within hours of administration yet psychotic symptoms are often not affected for several weeks. In addition, the antipsychotic drugs are most effective against the positive symptoms of schizophrenia and least effective against the negative symptoms (Carpenter and Buchanan, 1994). It is therefore possible that some features of schizophrenia involve dopamine while others do not.

Kraepelin first suggested that frontal lobe pathology was responsible for psychosis. Regional blood flow studies of schizophrenics provide clear evidence of decreased lateral frontal lobe function during tasks that challenge association capacity (Weinberger, Berman, and Zec, 1986). Because of dopamine's important role in regulating frontal lobe function, these data support the involvement of the mesocortical DA system. However, other studies suggest that schizophrenia is associated with increased DA in the amygdala, implicating the mesolimbic system (Reynolds, 1983). The fact that temporal lobe epilepsy is often associated with psychotic symptoms including delusions and hallucinations further suggests the involvement of the amygdala and therefore the mesolimbic system. In addition, many schizophrenics exhibit neurologic signs and symptoms such as defects in stereognosis, balance, proprioception, and visual tracking suggesting impaired integration that can be traced to the temporal lobe. Thus, both frontal and temporal lobe dysfunction are implicated and several postmortem studies have now correlated pathological changes in these brain regions with schizophrenia.

Haug (1962) was the first to demonstrate lateral ventricular enlargement in the brains of schizophrenic patients. This enlargement is associated with neuronal loss in the parahippocampal cortex, other periventricular structures, the hippocampus, the amygdala, and the prefrontal association cortex (see Shelton and Weinberger, 1987, for review). Roberts (1990) proposed that this pathology results from underdevelopment of cortical cells in the parahippocampal region that leads to neurodegenerative changes in the other brain regions to which these cells project. Weinberger (1988) proposed that the negative symptoms are a product of neurodegenerative changes in the parahippocampal region that reduce activity in the frontal lobes. This "hypo-frontality," as Weinberger called it, disinhibits the mesolimbic DA system (primarily the n. accumbens) where excess DA activity is viewed as responsible for the positive symptoms (Fig. 10–2). Although these pathophysiologic hypotheses may provide a mechanism for positive and negative symptoms, they do not reconcile the complexities of the signs and symptoms that can occur in schizophrenia.

Strauss, Carpenter, and Bartko (1974) proposed a three-component model of schizophrenia that has now received considerable support (re-

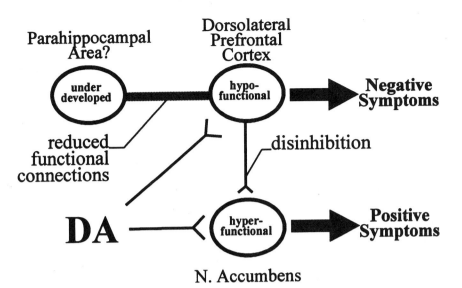

Figure 10–2. The hypofrontality hypothesis of schizophrenia suggests that positive and negative symptoms arise from two distinct areas and pathophysiologies. The negative symptoms are viewed as resulting from reduced activity in the prefrontal cortex secondary to underdevelopment of projection sites in the parahippocampal region. Since the dorsolateral prefrontal region is inhibitory to the n. accumbens, the resulting disinhibition leads to increased activity in this structure and the production of positive symptoms. (Adapted from Weinberger, 1988.)

viewed by Arndt, Allinger, and Andreasen, 1991). This model involves (1) psychotic symptoms (the traditional positive symptoms described above); (2) negative symptoms (restricted affect, limited emotional range, diminished social drive and self-interest, withdrawal, and poverty of speech); and (3) a cognitive and attentional impairment that involves loose association, tangential thinking, and incoherency (formerly classified as positive symptoms). As summarized by Winn (1994), the three types of signs and symptoms have different pathophysiologic processes. The negative symptoms arise from reduced function in the frontal lobes, the positive symptoms result from increased activity in the mesolimbic system, and the cognitive disorder is a consequence of temporal lobe pathology (Table 10–1). Based on this hypothesis, DA antagonists would be most effective against the positive symptoms, partially effective against the thought disorder, and largely ineffective against the negative symptoms. This is the efficacy pattern characteristically seen with most antipsychotic drugs.

Perhaps the key to interpreting the pathological data on schizophrenic brains is that the problem does not necessarily have to occur in the DA system itself but could originate in several target structures sharing projections from or regulating activity in the DA bed nuclei. If this is the

Table 10–1 Symptoms and Structures of Schizophrenia[a]

Psychomotor Poverty Symptoms	Disorganization Symptoms	Reality Distortion Symptoms
Symptoms	**Symptoms**	**Symptoms**
Poverty of speech	Inappropriate affect	Voices speak to the
Decreased spontaneous	Poverty of content of	patient
movements	speech	Delusions of persecution
Unchanging facial	Tangentiality	Delusions of reference
expression	Derailment of speech	Hallucinations
Paucity of expressive	Pressure of speech	
gestures	Distractibility	
Affective nonresponse	Incoherence of speech	
Lack of vocal inflection		
Increased speech latency		
Poor eye contact		
Anatomic associations	**Anatomic associations**	**Anatomic associations**
Dorsolateral-prefrontal	Temporal lobes	Orbitofrontal cortex
cortex		Cingulate cortex
Striatum		

[a]Adapted from Winn (1994)

case, then DA antagonists could still reduce schizophrenic symptoms even if the DA system were intact. This perspective would align with the dopamine theory of schizophrenia and also account for the proposed abnormalities in other neurotransmitter systems as well.

Other Neurotransmitters

Norepinephrine, serotonin, enkephalin, other neuropeptides, and glutamate may be involved in the pathophysiology of schizophrenia (see Ashton, 1992; Ellenbroek, 1993). The similarity between the signs and symptoms of phencyclidine (PCP) toxicity and psychosis are often used to argue for the involvement of glutamate. However, PCP inhibits DA reuptake and stimulates its release both directly and indirectly through NMDA heteroreceptors on the DA terminal. Moreover, antipsychotic drugs block many of the psychotomimetic actions of PCP (see Snell and Johnson, 1985; Chapter 12), suggesting that the dopaminergic actions of PCP may be responsible for the psychotic behavior produced by this drug.

Considerable interest is currently focused on the involvement of serotonin in schizophrenia. Clozapine and risperidone are two antipsychotic drugs that appear to be more effective against the negative symptoms of schizophrenia than other antipsychotic agents. Both block DA and 5HT receptors (see Marder et al., 1993; Marder, 1994). However, selective serotonin antagonists are not effective antipsychotics. This suggests that reducing psychotic symptoms may be more related to balancing the activities of DA and 5HT than simply reducing the activity of dopamine. Regardless of the neurotransmitters involved, it is clear that the antipsychotic drugs are effective at treating psychotic behavior whatever its cause.

THE ANTIPSYCHOTIC AGENTS

Receptor Antagonism

The antipsychotic drugs are a diverse chemical group with the common ability to act directly as competitive antagonists of DA receptors (Fig. 10–3; Table 10–2). The affinity of these drugs for the various DA receptor subtypes varies widely, however. While they all share an affinity for D_2 receptors that correlates with their antipsychotic potency, haloperidol has little affinity for D_1 receptors while clozapine has as much affinity for D_1 as for D_2 receptors. The affinity of antipsychotics for D_3, D_4, and D_5 receptors varies widely as well. The effect of these differences in affinity on the efficacy and side effects of antipsychotic drugs is just now becoming apparent. Affinity for D_4 receptors appears to offer greater efficacy against negative symptoms and a reduced incidence of side effects such as drug-induced parkinsonism.

In addition to their differences in affinity for DA-receptor subtypes, the antipsychotic drugs differ markedly in their affinity for noradrenergic, muscarinic, histaminergic, and serotonergic receptors, where they are also direct-acting competitive antagonists. Their relative differences in affinity for these receptors contribute significantly to their propensity to produce such side affects as sedation, orthostatic hypotension, and parkinsonism, and their relative affinity for $5HT_2$ receptors may influence their relative efficacy against negative symptoms.

The introduction of these drugs in the early 1950s revolutionized the treatment of schizophrenia since it offered the psychotic an alternative to inpatient therapy. Prior to the advent of the antipsychotic drugs in the early 1950s, almost half the hospital beds were occupied by psychotic patients. The percentage dropped to less than 20% after widespread use of these drugs became common. The notion that a drug could reverse many symptoms of what was considered at the time to be a functional disorder brought about by repressed feelings understandably met with considerable skepticism at a time when American psychiatry was dominated by psychoanalysts. Against this skepticism, the need to establish clinical effi-

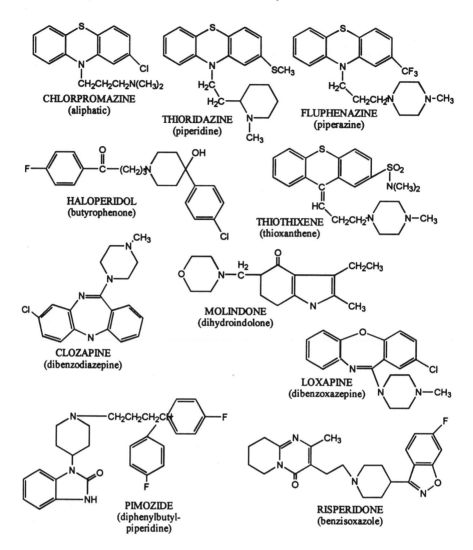

Figure 10–3. Structures and chemical classes (in parentheses) of widely used antipsychotic agents.

cacy in an unbiased fashion led to the development of the double-blind clinical trial. In a double-blind design, neither the patients nor rating physician knows whether the patient is receiving an active drug or a placebo. With this approach, the clinical efficacy of the phenothiazine agents, the first antipsychotics to be used, was quickly established (see Davis et al., 1980). However, not all symptoms responded to medication and it became common to administer huge doses of the drugs in a misguided attempt to alleviate the full spectrum of the disease. Typically, the dose was increased until the patient exhibited immobility and rigidity

Table 10–2 Antipsychotic Drugs

Drug (Trade Name)	EPSE Potential	Potency	Distinguishing Characteristics[a]
Phenothiazines			
Chlorpromazine (Thorazine)	Typical	Low	The industry standard
Thioridazine (Mellaril)	Atypical	Low	The original atypical
Mesoridazine (Serentil)	Atypical	Low	agent
Trifluoperazine (Stelazine)	Typical	High	Active metabolite of
Acetophenazine (Tindal)	Typical	High	thioridazine
Perphenazine (Trilafon)	Typical	High	Very sedating
Fluphenazine (Prolixin)	Typical	High	Depot formulations available
Butyrophenones			
Haloperidol (Haldol)	Typical	High	The first nonpheno-thiazine agent
Thioxanthines			
Chlorprothixene (Taractan)	Typical	High	Sedating and severe autonomic effects
Thiothixene (Navane)	Typical	High	Not strongly sedating
Diphenylbutylpiperidines			
Pimozide (Orap)	Atypical	High	Used mostly in Tourette syndrome
Dibenzoxazepines			
Loxapine (Loxitane)	Typical	High	
Dibenzodiazepines			
Clozapine (Clozaril)	Atypical	Low	No tardive dyskinesia; "wet pillow" Side effect; agranulo-cytosis
Dihydroindolone			
Molindone (Moban)	Typical	High	Least proconvulsive agent
Benzisoxazole			
Risperidone (Risperdal)	Atypical	High	Dose-related EPSEs

[a]EPSE = extrapyramidal side effects

(neurolepsis), and from this strategy arose the term *neuroleptic drug*, which remains a synonym for antipsychotic drug even today (see Haasse and Janssen, 1985). At high doses all antipsychotic drugs also induce a state of detachment from the environment, diminished arousal, and a tendency to sleep that led to their characterization as major tranquilizers. However, with the introduction of newer drugs and the realization that antipsychotic drugs can be effective at dosages that do not tranquilize the patient or induce neurolepsis, these two terms are no longer appropriate.

Antipsychotic Efficacy

Despite their diversity in structure, all the currently used antipsychotic drugs are competitive inhibitors of the D_2 receptor. All of the agents reduce the symptoms of an acute psychotic episode, whatever its cause. Thus, psychotic symptoms resulting from drug overdoses, heavy metal intoxication, and even metabolic disturbances are effectively controlled by this drug class. In most schizophrenics, chronic maintenance therapy significantly reduces the relapse rate and the severity of psychotic episodes as well. While most psychiatrists would agree that the antipsychotic drugs as a class are effective at reducing the positive symptoms seen during a psychotic episode, there are those who would suggest that they are totally ineffective at treating negative symptoms. Although they are clearly less effective at treating negative symptoms (Kay and Singh, 1989), the literature suggests that their relative efficacy in this regard is a matter of degree. Thus, drugs such as clozapine and risperidone appear to be more effective than others in treating negative symptoms.

Unfortunately, many patients are not effectively managed by antipsychotic agents. These treatment failures are generally viewed as falling into two categories. Drug-resistant patients do not appear to respond to any drug no matter how well a drug regimen has been tailored to the patient's needs. Such patients may have more brain pathology than others. The second category is drug intolerance. In these patients, the side effects of the drugs are so pronounced that they outweigh the benefits. New drugs with fewer side effects should reduce the incidence of these treatment failures, and the development of such drugs is a major focus of current research.

It has become common lore that antipsychotic efficacy may require weeks or months to develop, though there is evidence that most patients begin to improve earlier (Ellenbroek, 1993). Whatever its length, the delay makes it difficult to ascribe antipsychotic action to DA-receptor blockade alone when approximately 80% of the brain's DA receptors are occupied within one hour of drug administration. Compensatory processes within the DA system in the continued presence of antipsychotic drugs are therefore thought to be at least partially responsible for the drugs therapeutic benefit.

Several theories have been advanced to explain this efficacy delay. The most popular hypothesis involves the up-regulation of D_2-receptor number (see Chapter 3). This change in response to pharmacologic denervation requires several weeks to develop and thus coincides nicely with the pattern of therapeutic improvement seen in many schizophrenic patients. However, if receptor up-regulation were responsible for antipsychotic efficacy, then one would have to assume that DA hypofunction was present at the time of the psychotic episode. This is simply not consistent with the bulk of the literature.

Bunney (1984) initially proposed that the development of depolarization blockade in the cell bodies of the mesencephalon was responsible for the efficacy delay. (Depolarization blockade occurs when excitable cells are stimulated at a rate that cannot be supported by their refractory period [see Chapter 7].) The antagonism of forebrain DA receptors reduces inhibitory feedback via the striatonigral pathway and other systems, and this increases DA neuron firing rate in the face of a reduced postsynaptic DA signal. Thus, when the receptors are blocked by drug, a feedback circuit increases the activity of the DA neuron. This feedback can become so intense in the presence of a DA antagonist and the dopamine neuron can fire at such a high rate that it cannot support an action potential and a state of depolarization blockade occurs. Once this blockade has developed, afferent DA signals become dramatically depressed. Bunney reported that the time course over which depolarization blockade develops in animals coincides with the delay in antipsychotic efficacy in humans. The fact that depolarization blockade in the mesencephalon would reduce DA activity at all target sites is significant in light of studies suggesting a common action of antipsychotic drugs in the nucleus accumbens.

As discussed in Chapter 3, drugs acting on neurotransmitter systems can alter neuronal phosphorylation status and regulate transcription. Immediate early genes such as c-fos are regulators of transcription. Recently, it has been observed that all antipsychotic drugs share the ability to activate c-fos. What is more important, the margins of the n. accumbens (the so-called shell region, which is an important site of convergence of the prefrontal and limbic cortices that is regulated by DA fibers from the ventral tegmental area) also exhibits c-fos activation in response to antipsychotic drugs (see Deutch et al., 1991). It is intriguing to speculate that the delay in antipsychotic efficacy is a consequence of the slowly evolving alterations in phosphorylation and transcription that would occur in the shell region because of depolarization blockade resulting from chronic antipsychotic drug treatment.

Clearly, we are far from a complete understanding of antipsychotic drug action. However, the mechanism underlying certain side effects of these drugs is becoming clearer. In fact, the propensity of some drugs to produce parkinsonian side effects while other drugs are much less potent in this regard may be a result of depolarization blockade in selected regions of the mesencephalon. Whatever the mechanism, the propensity of some antipsychotic drugs to produce so-called "extrapyramidal" side effects while others do so less frequently led to a widely used classification of antipsychotic drugs as either typical or atypical, respectively.

Acute Extrapyramidal Side Effects

The term extrapyramidal was historically used to describe the basal ganglia and its connections. The corticospinal tract is often called the pyramidal tract and the term extrapyramidal referred to those neuronal projections involved with motor control that were not part of the pyramidal tract. Although the term is no longer in common use, its historical association with certain side effects of antipsychotic drugs remains.

Acute extrapyramidal side effects (EPSEs) fall into three categories: parkinsonian side effects, dystonia, and akathisia (Table 10–3). Although all the antipsychotic drugs can produce EPSEs, certain drugs do so more commonly. If the administration of an antipsychotic normally produces EPSEs, it is called a typical agent. Haloperidol is the most widely known typical agent. If an antipsychotic drug does not normally produce EPSEs, it is called an atypical agent (see Table 10–2). Thioridazine and clozapine are examples.

Drug-induced Parkinsonism

The best-known EPSE is drug-induced parkinsonism. The tremor, rigidity (cogwheel type), bradykinesia, and postural instability that can accompany the use of antipsychotic drugs are the EPSEs that led to their division into typical and atypical categories. The period of maximum risk for their development is one to four weeks following treatment initiation al-

---

Table 10–3 Acute Extrapyramidal Side Effects (EPSEs)

Acute dystonic reactions
  a—midline muscle cramps
  b—opisthotonus
  c—torticollis
  d—oculogyric crises
  e—pharyngeal/lingual spasms
Akathisia
  a—inability to sit still
  b—fidgety or restless
  c—bursts of locomotion which, if associated with a perioral
    tremor, are called the rabbit syndrome
Parkinsonian side effects
  a—rigidity (cogwheel type)
  b—tremor
  c—bradykinesia or akinesia
  d—postural instability and a stooped posture

though they can develop any time during therapy, especially when the dosage is increased to quell a psychotic episode. Parkinsonian side effects occur in 20 to 30% of all treated patients (Marsden et al., 1975) but they are more commonly seen with typical agents, especially in the elderly, than with atypical agents.

White and Wang (1983) proposed that the development of parkinsonian symptoms results from depolarization blockade of DA neurons forming the nigrostriatal pathway following the administration of D_2 antagonists. Figure 10–4 diagrams part of the direct pathway (see Chapter 9) forming the striatonigral feedback system. Independently of the action of DA on the outflow neurons to the globus pallidus, DA activity in the striatum feeds back to the substantia nigra via this system and regulates

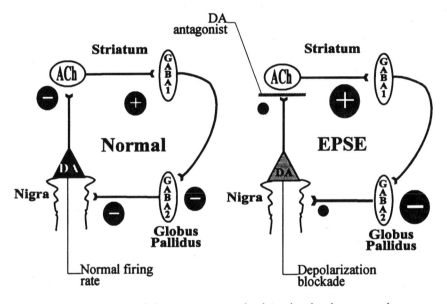

Figure 10–4. Depiction of the circuitry involved in the development of acute extrapyramidal side effects (EPSEs) resulting from depolarization blockade of dopamine (DA) neurons projecting from the substantia nigra pars compacta to the striatum. Normally DA is inhibitory to the cholinergic (ACh) interneurons in the striatum. These cholinergic interneurons excite the GABA-1 cells projecting to the globus pallidus. This GABA projection neuron in turn inhibits the next GABA neuron (GABA-2) which is inhibitory on DA neurons in the compacta. As a result, an increase in DA release leads to inhibition of the DA neurons and feedback inhibition. When a DA antagonist blocks DA in the striatum (left) the disinhibition of the DA neurons in the compacta leads to a dramatic increase in the DA neuron firing rate, leading to depolarization blockade. The depolarization blockade leads to dramatic decreases in DA release and loss of competition between the DA antagonist and DA. This produces a complete loss of DA activity and parkinsonian side effects. (The size of the black circles containing + for excitation and − for inhibition is indicative of the degree of activity across a synapse.)

the firing rate of DA neurons. Reduced activity in nigrostriatal neurons disinhibits the cholinergic interneurons of the striatum. This increases the excitatory drive on the first GABA neuron in this pathway (GABA-1). With GABA-1 hyperactive, the second GABA neuron (GABA-2) is inhibited and its firing rate decreases, thereby disinhibiting the dendritic field of the DA neurons in the substantia nigra. This disinhibition increases the firing of the spontaneously active dopamine neurons and the release of DA in the striatum—a classic long-loop feedback system. This increase in DA neuron activity in the presence of a DA antagonist results in increased DA catabolism and increased homovanillic acid in the CSF, a characteristic consequence of antipsychotic drug treatment.

The striatonigral feedback system was only designed to operate within the confines of physiologically relevant levels of DA, however, and in the presence of a DA antagonist, the disinhibition may be so profound that the DA neuron fires too fast to maintain normal Na^+ channel cycling. Depolarization blockade then occurs. Since depolarization cannot be effectively transmitted to the striatum, DA release in the striatum is blocked.

The development of depolarization blockade has several consequences. First, the inhibition of DA release reduces both D_1 and D_2 actions in the striatum, mimicking the pathophysiological deficit of Parkinson's disease and thus its cardinal features. Second, the inhibition of DA release reduces competition between dopamine and antagonist molecules for access to the D_2 receptor. This loss of competition increases the potency of the DA antagonist, yielding effective blockade in the striatum at lower than anticipated levels of the antipsychotic drug. Third, the depolarization blockade that occurs throughout the mesencephalon reduces DA release in the mesocortical and mesolimbic systems, contributing to antipsychotic efficacy as described above.

The coadministration of an antimuscarinic drug with an antipsychotic drug prevents depolarization blockade. Blocking the muscarinic receptors on GABA-1 neurons reduces GABA-1 activity, disinhibiting GABA-2 and reinstating inhibition of the DA cell bodies in the substantia nigra. By preventing depolarization blockade, antimuscarinic drugs reinstate DA release in the striatum and prevent parkinsonian side effects. However, they do not prevent depolarization blockade in the mesolimbic and mesocortical systems since the fibers that feed back to these cell bodies are not regulated by ACh. Thus, depolarization blockade and the reduction in dopamine release in the striatum is avoided and reduces parkinsonian symptoms without interfering with depolarization blockade in the mesolimbic and mesocortical pathways which maintains antipsychotic efficacy.

Patients who develop EPSEs while receiving antipsychotic therapy are often given antimuscarinic agents. Although benztropine is commonly used and effective, it is a poor choice. Benztropine is a DA reuptake inhibitor besides being a potent antimuscarinic agent (see Chapter 9). The increase in dopamine it produces will enhance the competition for access to the DA receptor between the dopamine that is released and the DA antagonist administered. As a result, the degree of DA-receptor blockade will be reduced. However, this action will also occur in the mesolimbic and mesocortical system, thereby reducing antipsychotic efficacy. A higher dose of antipsychotic might then be needed. Antimuscarinic agents that are more ACh-specific such as trihexyphenidyl and orphenadrine are therefore better choices.

Several antipsychotic drugs possess antimuscarinic actions as well as DA antagonist actions. These are the atypical antipsychotic agents thioridazine, mesoridazine, clozapine, and pimozide. Their antimuscarinic actions reduce the tendency to develop depolarization blockade, thereby decreasing the incidence of EPSEs associated with their use.

The variable ability of the antipsychotic phenothiazines to antagonize ACh muscarinic receptors is a classic example of structure–activity relationships in pharmacology. The first drugs to be widely used in the treatment of psychosis were the phenothiazines. The phenothiazine structure consists of two benzene rings joined by a sulfur and nitrogen atom (see Fig. 10–3). Three different side chains are joined to the nitrogen atom that confer different antipsychotic and antimuscarinic potency. Piperidine phenothiazines such as thioridazine are the least potent antipsychotics and the most potent antimuscarinic drugs. Their antimuscarinic actions make them least likely to produce EPSEs. An aliphatic substitution produces phenothiazines such as chlorpromazine that possess low antipsychotic potency and intermediate antimuscarinic actions. Although the aliphatic phenothiazines have antimuscarinic effects, they are still classified as typical antipsychotics. The piperazine substitution produces phenothiazines such as fluphenazine that are potent antipsychotics with little affinity for muscarinic receptors. The piperazine substitution also reduces alpha-antagonistic effects decreasing the severity of autonomic side effects antipsychotic drugs often produce. Thus, the side-chain substitution on the phenothiazine structure determines the drug's antimuscarinic potency and its atypical or typical classification. The thioxanthene antipsychotics also have aliphatic and piperazine substitutions.

Dystonia

Dystonia is usually the first EPSE to develop after antipsychotic drug therapy begins. When it occurs dystonia appears within five days of starting treatment in 90% of cases. Dystonia is often expressed intermittently for periods of a couple of hours, although longer durations are not uncommon. When all antipsychotic agents are considered, the incidence of dystonia is estimated at 16 to 25% of the treated population. With typical agents such as haloperidol as many as half the patients may be affected (Arana et al., 1988), while atypical agents produce dystonia in only 5%. Patients with a family history of dystonia, younger patients, and patients receiving high doses of typical agents are at increased risk. The severity as well as the incidence of dystonia depends on the type of antipsychotic used and the dose administered. Coadministration of an antimuscarinic agent such as trihexyphenidyl reduces dystonia in most patients.

Akathisia

Akathisia is the most common EPSE. It affects 20 to 40% of patients treated with antipsychotics and develops during the first month of treatment. Again, its incidence is higher when typical agents are used and lower with atypical use. Akathisia has both an objective and a subjective component. The former is apparent motor restlessness that is manifested as continuous shifting of posture (from one foot to another while standing or an inability to sit still). The latter is expressed by the patient as a feeling of tension and a desire to move. When it develops, akathisia is particularly troublesome in paranoid patients with delusions of control by outside forces since they often perceive these subjective feelings as evidence of such control (Van Putten, 1975). Although all of the antipsychotic agents can produce this side effect, the benzamides such as sulpiride, remoxipride, and metoclopramide appear more likely to induce it (see Ellenbroek, 1993). These drugs are not used in the United States except for metoclopramide, which is used solely as an antiemetic. Antimuscarinic drugs are effective at reducing both the objective and subjective components of akathisia. In patients who do not respond to antimuscarinic drugs, $beta_2$-blockers such as propranolol or $alpha_2$ agonists such as clonidine can be used.

Although EPSEs are common side effects of antipsychotic drugs they can be misinterpreted by physicians. Rigidity, akinesia, and dystonia are sometimes confused with catatonia and can lead to an increase in medication that exacerbates the side effects. Similarly, akathisia can be confused with psychotic agitation. If it were assumed that any dramatic change in motor expression during therapy is more likely a drug side effect than a worsening of the disease process, there would be fewer treatment errors.

"Why not just use atypical antipsychotic agents and preclude the incidence of EPSEs in the first place?" First, atypical antipsychotic drugs are not devoid of EPSEs; rather, they exhibit lower incidences. Second, the development of other side effects with atypical agents or the need to administer very large doses to deal with a severe psychotic episode precludes the use of some atypical drugs, especially the low-potency ones. Thus, it is not always possible to use an atypical agent.

Chronic EPSEs

Two EPSEs, tardive dystonia and tardive dyskinesia, may develop late in the course of antipsychotic therapy. (Tardive is derived from the same root as tardy.) Tardive dystonia is similar to acute dystonia. Like acute dystonia, it responds to a reduction in the antipsychotic dosage or to the coadministration of an antimuscarinic drug. In contrast, tardive dyskinesia (TD)—with its bizarre hyperkinetic movements—is often made worse by antipsychotic dosage reduction or antimuscarinic therapy and is the most frequent cause of drug intolerance and noncompliance (Table 10–4).

TD is an extrapyramidal movement disorder that should not be confused, as it often is, with acute EPSEs. In contrast to the paucity of movement associated with drug-induced parkinsonism, TD is a choreiform movement disorder involving excessive movement. The lips may smack, the patient appears to be chewing something very large, and the tongue may protrude intermittently. Although it is most commonly manifested in the lingual-facial-buccal musculature, TD can be expressed in any muscle group and, if the respiratory accessory musculature is affected, it can be life-threatening. Based on the balance hypothesis of striatal function (Chapter 9), this choreic movement disorder is thought to result from excessive DA relative to ACh activity. Thus, unlike EPSEs, TD is usually ex-

Table 10–4 DSM-IV Criteria for Tardive Dyskinesia

A—Involuntary movements of the tongue, jaw, trunk, or extremities have developed in association with the use of an antipsychotic medication
B—The involuntary movements are present over a period of at least four weeks and occur in any of the following patterns:
  1—choreiform movements (i.e., rapid, jerky, nonrepetitive)
  2—athetoid movements (i.e., slow, sinuous, continual)
  3—rhythmic movements (i.e., stereotypies)
C—The signs and symptoms in criteria A and B develop during exposure to a neuroleptic medication or within four weeks of withdrawal from an oral (or within eight weeks of withdrawal from a depot) antipsychotic medication
D—There has been exposure to an antipsychotic medication for at least three months or one month if age 60 or older
E—No other known neurologic or general medical condition can account for the appearance of the symptoms
F—The symptoms are not better accounted for by an antipsychotic-induced acute movement disorder (e.g., antipsychotic-induced acute dystonia or akathisia)

acerbated by reducing the administered dose of antipsychotic or by treatment with an antimuscarinic agent.

The longer patients are treated and the higher the dosage used, the greater the likelihood that they will develop TD. The overall incidence of TD is estimated at 10 to 15% on antipsychotic medication with a range over several studies being 0.5 to 54% (Kane and Smith, 1982). There are various risk factors including advanced age, more pronounced frontal lobe hypofunction, and a history of severe acute EPSEs. In addition, menstruating women are more likely to develop TD, which probably reflects the enhancement of DA-receptor responsiveness by estrogen (see Waddington, 1989, for review). Atypical antipsychotics, especially clozapine and risperidone, are less likely to induce TD than other antipsychotic agents.

There are two broad categories of tardive dyskinesia: breakthrough and withdrawal. In breakthrough TD, the symptoms develop during the course of antipsychotic therapy so that the movement disorder "breaks through" the DA-receptor antagonism. But TD is more often seen during withdrawal from antipsychotic medication in the days and weeks following the discontinuation of therapy as the antagonist clears from the body. Tardive dyskinesia is more likely to be persistent when it develops during treatment, and it leaves the patient with an overt movement disorder that laypersons would regard as crazy behavior. Occasionally, the underlying psychosis resolves but the movement disorder remains.

Klawans (1973) proposed that tardive dyskinesia results from DA receptor up-regulation in the striatum, and this remains the most widely quoted hypothesis. In its current form, chronic D_2-receptor antagonism leads to the proliferation of DA receptors and thus to a hypersensitive DA state in the striatum, producing excessive movement in accord with the balance hypothesis of striatal function. Breakthrough TD develops when the dosage of DA antagonist is inadequate to occupy the increased receptor number brought about by chronic treatment (see Fig. 10–5). Alternatively, antipsychotic dosage reduction during therapy unmasks receptor proliferation or the administration of an antimuscarinic agent during therapy reduces ACh activity, and both tip the DA : ACh balance in favor of dopamine, thereby producing dyskinesias. Conversely, withdrawal of antipsychotic medication unmasks an increased receptor population that becomes progressively more stimulated by released dopamine as drug levels in the brain decrease.

The dopamine-hypersensitivity hypothesis is supported by the fact that DA agonists can induce symptoms very similar to TD and that DA-receptor up-regulation requires time to develop, accounting for the delayed onset of the dyskinesias. However, most animals exhibit receptor proliferation and hypersensitivity with antipsychotic treatment while

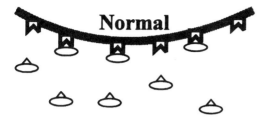

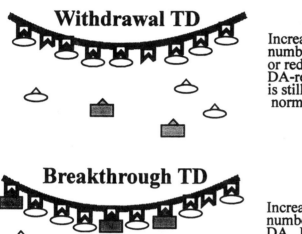

Figure 10–5. Depiction of the DA hypersensitivity model of TD where receptor-site upregulation is proposed to participate in the development of withdrawal and breakthrough dyskinesias. As DA-receptor number increases as a result of chronic antipsychotic treatment, the number of molecules available to block the receptors is decreased. If the receptor proliferation leads to proportionately more receptors than molecules of antipsychotic, breakthrough TD will occur. More commonly, withdrawal of antipsychotic therapy leads to an unmasking of the proliferated receptor population and an associated increase in DA activity, producing the dyskinesias (withdrawal dyskinesias).

most treated patients do not develop TD. Moreover, receptor proliferation requires only a few weeks to develop in animals while TD requires several months. Once developed, D_2-receptor proliferation gradually decreases following antipsychotic drug withdrawal and therefore cannot account for cases of permanent TD. Thus, the dopamine-hypersensitivity hypotheses must be incomplete. I believe that D_2-receptor proliferation is

Table 10–5 Antipsychotic Drug Side Effects

Class	Drug	Receptor	Potency	Acute EPSE	Anti-muscarinic
Phenothiazines, aliphatic	Chloroproma- zine	D_2	+	++	++
Piperidine	Thioridazine	D_2	+	+	+++
Piperazine	Fluphenazine	D_2	++++	++++	+
Thioxanthine	Thiothixene	D_2 & D_2	+++	++	+
Butyrophenone	Haloperidol	D_2	++++	++++	—
Dibenzodiazepine	Clozapine	D_4 $5HT_2$	++	—	+++
Dihydro- indolone	Molindone	D_2	+++	++	—
Dibenzisoxazole derivative	Loxapine	D_2	+++	++	—
Dibenzoxazine	Risperidone	D_2 $5HT_2$	+++	— (Higher dose)	—
Diphenylbutyl- piperidine	Pimozide	D_2	+++	+	+++

permissive for the development of TD and that other factors are also involved (Carvey et al., 1990). Thus, D_2-receptor proliferation must be present for TD to occur, but other factors—including an imbalance between the various DA-receptor populations within the striatum (especially D_1 and D_2), reduced GABA activity in the striatum or substantia nigra, tissue loss in the striatum, and more pronounced neuropathology in the frontal cortex leading to disinhibition of the striatum (see Casey, 1995)—will determine the severity and permanence of the dyskinesias.

Whatever its underlying cause, the medical management of TD is problematic (see Gardos and Cole, 1995). Increasing the administered dose of an antipsychotic drug in breakthrough TD or reinstating therapy for withdrawal TD usually alleviates symptoms. However, this strategy usually only delays the expression of symptoms and, in many cases, makes TD worse. Dopamine-depleting drugs such as tetrabenazine and reserpine can be effective but are associated with significant side effects that complicate their use. $GABA_A$ agonists can be effective and the benzodiazepines are often used, but these drugs may also exacerbate psychotic symptoms. Switching the patient to an antipsychotic drug such as clozapine that does not produce TD does not usually relieve the symptoms but provides antipsychotic action while a reversible dyskinesia wanes.

Table 10–5 (cont'd)

Sedation	Orthostatic Hypotension	TD	Seizure Threshold	Malignant Syndrome	Quinidine-Like Effect	Increase Prolactin
+++	+++	++	++++	+++	+++	+++
+++	+++	+	+++	+++	+++	+++
+	+	+++	+++	+	++	+++
+/++	++	++	+	+	+	+++
+	+	+++	+	+	—	+++
+++	++	—	++	+/−	—	—
++	+	++	—	+/−	—	+++
+	+	++	+	+/−	—	+++
+	+/−	— (Higher dose)	+	—	—	+
+++	++	+	+	+	—	+++

Other Side Effects

Beside being DA antagonists and possessing variable potencies as muscarinic antagonists, the antipsychotic agents have other actions that contribute to the development of side effects (see Table 10–5).

Cardiovascular effects

All of the antipsychotic agents possess some affinity for alpha$_1$ receptors where they act as direct-acting antagonists. The piperazine phenothiazines are among the least potent while the aliphatic phenothiazines such as chlorpromazine are among the most potent. Chlorpromazine's ability to block alpha$_1$ receptors together with its intermediate antimuscarinic actions can produce profound cardiovascular side effects. Orthostatic hypotension (alpha$_1$ blockade) and tachycardia (antimuscarinic effect) are commonly observed early in treatment until tolerance develops. CNS regulation of autonomic function may also be compromised and this too contributes to cardiovascular symptoms. All phenothiazine antipsychotic and chlorpromazine and thioridazine in particular also have direct cardiotoxic effects on the heart: the so-called "quinidine-like" effects. (Quinidine is a class I$_A$ antiarrhythmic agent that inhibits Na$^+$ flux, depresses phase-0 depolarization, and slows conduction through the His-Purkinje system of the heart.) As a result, sinus tachycardia, widening of the QRS interval, and T-wave blunting can develop rapidly in some patients and may be lethal in overdose situations. The mechanism for this quinidine-like effect is unknown. The butyrophenones, thioxanthines, and the diphenylbutylpiperidines are much less potent in this regard. The greater cardiotoxic effects of chlorpromazine and thioridazine may, in part, reflect their low potencies as antipsychotics, which requires higher dosages.

Other autonomic side effects

In addition to their actions on the cardiovascular system, the antipsychotic drugs have several other autonomic effects that are related to their variable potencies as antimuscarinic antagonists. These include dry mouth, paralysis of accommodation leading to the inability to focus vision on near objects, nasal stuffiness, constipation, and urinary retention. Interestingly, clozapine, an atypical agent with significant antimuscarinic potency, produces sialorrhea in many patients. This effect does not exhibit significant tolerance and patients often complain of waking up with a wet pillow.

Effects on the endocrine system

Dopamine, acting at D_2 receptors, is prolactin inhibitory factor. All antipsychotic agents with the exception of clozapine, which has low affinity for D_2 receptors, will elevate prolactin levels. This effect is dose dependent and correlated with antipsychotic efficacy, reflecting the ability of the drugs to enter the CNS and block D_2 receptors. The prolactin increase can lead to gynecomastia and even galactorrhea in males although these effects are more common in females.

Dopamine also plays a role, albeit indirect, in the regulation of growth hormone (GH) secretion. Since GH secretion is highly episodic, however, predicting the effect of these agents is difficult. Antipsychotic drugs also disrupt the regulation of several gonadotrophins and reduce corticotrophin levels. Together with other hypothalamic effects, this contributes to alterations in sexual behavior including decreased libido, inability to achieve erection, and reduced frequency of orgasm. Paradoxically, priapism (prolonged painful erection) is associated with the chronic use of thioridazine. An overall increase in melanoctye-stimulating hormone accompanies the chronic use of phenothiazines. This increase can lead to a darkening of skin color and may contribute to the photosensitivity experienced by some patients, especially those taking chlorpromazine.

Antiemetic effects

As DA antagonists, all of the antipsychotic agents will reduce CTZ-mediated emesis although thioridazine, clozapine, and risperidone are much less potent in this regard. The antipsychotic drugs in general are effective antiemetics, but they are not generally used for this purpose because of their serious side effects. Instead, the DA antagonist metoclopramide is most commonly used. Despite its DA antagonism, it is not an effective antipsychotic, probably because of its limited penetration into the CNS. Therefore, metoclopramide can be administered at dosages that effectively block DA receptors in the chemoreceptor zone without a significant risk of central side effects.

Weight gain and hypothermia

Since many antipsychotic drugs inhibit NE and 5HT receptors that are involved in appetite suppression, their use is often associated with weight gain. The tendency of all members of this drug class to reduce motor activity contributes to weight gain as well. Molindone is exceptional, however, since it is much less likely than other antipsychotic drugs to produce weight gain, offering a treatment alternative for obese psychotics.

As DA antagonists, the antipsychotic agents reduce body temperature. This mild hypothermic action is likely mediated by a direct action of dopamine on the hypothalamus and an indirect effect associated with reduced motor activity.

Neuroleptic malignant syndrome

Occasionally in hypersensitive patients, a potentially fatal condition called neuroleptic malignant syndrome develops. Its symptoms are similar to the malignant hyperthermia resulting from gas anesthetic use (see Chapter 7) and is characterized by excessive muscle rigidity and severe hyperthermia. Muscle rigidity is the likely cause of this hyperthermia although a paradoxic DA-mediated response by the hypothalamus cannot be ruled out. Although dantrolene (a Ca^{2+} channel antagonist that acts specifically on the sarcoplasmic reticulum) can be used to relieve the muscle rigidity and hyperthermia, this drug does not attack the cause of the problem, which is thought to originate centrally, at least in part. Thus, the direct-acting DA agonist bromocriptine or the indirect-acting DA agonist levodopa is usually more effective. These treatments are not generally effective for malignant hyperthermia, however, suggesting that the mechanism involved is different from that of neuroleptic malignant syndrome.

Seizure threshold

Increased dopamine in the CNS raises the seizure threshold (making it harder to have a seizure), perhaps because of dopamine's overall inhibitory effect on the brain (see Chapter 9). The DA antagonists as a class therefore lower seizure thresholds. The aliphatic phenothiazines and clozapine are most potent while molindone appears least potent in this regard. The epileptogenic actions of the antipsychotic drugs become important considerations in the treatment of some emergency room patients since those experiencing temporal lobe seizures can be readily misdiagnosed as psychotics. The epileptogenic actions of the antipsychotics also interfere with their use in patients experiencing hallucinations and delusions during alcohol withdrawal (delirium tremors; see Chapter 12) since they already have a reduced seizure threshold.

Systemic lupus erythematosus

All of the antipsychotic agents increase the production of polyclonal IgM autoantibodies directed against nuclear material and cardiolipin. The production of these antibodies is the hallmark of systemic lupus erythematosus (SLE), which can be difficult to manage and in some cases life-threatening. Although the IgM titer is increased, clinical symptoms of SLE rarely occur. However, chlorpromazine use has been associated with several cases.

Psychological and cognitive effects

Because schizophrenia itself alters association processing, mood, and behavior, separating the effects of the antipsychotic drugs on these processes from those associated with the underlying disease is difficult. In normal, healthy volunteers the antipsychotics depress overall emotional responsiveness, blunting affect. Their effects on memory consolidation and recall are negligible, but they can slow thinking and retard psychomotor function. Some volunteers even experience dysphoria. The benefits antipsychotic drugs provide to the patient, however, far outweigh these relatively subtle effects.

Sedation

The antipsychotics have a calming effect. Since dopamine plays a role in arousal, all the antipsychotic drugs will produce sedation at sufficiently high dosages. However, agents with antihistaminergic properties (like the aliphatic and piperidine phenothiazines) and antimuscarinic actions are more likely to produce sedation at dosages commonly used in antipsychotic therapy. Thioridazine, chlorpromazine, and clozapine are particularly potent in this regard. As with sedative-hypnotic drugs, however, tolerance to this effect develops quickly.

CLOZAPINE

Clozapine is a low-potency, atypical antipsychotic agent. Its potency as an antimuscarinic ranks among the highest of the antipsychotic drugs. Its affinity for the $5HT_2$ receptor is tenfold higher than its affinity for the D_2 receptor. In addition to these characteristics, three aspects of clozapine distinguish it from other members of the antipsychotic drug class (see Meltzer, 1993, for review).

Foremost is its ability to relieve psychotic symptoms in patients refractory to all other forms of antipsychotic therapy. Clozapine is effective not only in reducing negative symptoms in many patients, but also positive and cognitive symptoms in patients who do not respond to other antipsychotic agents. Thus, it is the treatment of choice for drug-resistant patients. Second, not one case of TD has been reported with the use of clozapine. This feature makes clozapine truly atypical with regard to chronic extrapyramidal side effects. Finally, unlike all other current antipsychotics, clozapine has very little D_2-receptor affinity. This property is probably responsible for its reduced acute EPSE profile, its failure to cause TD, its reduced antiemetic properties, and its insignificant effects on serum prolactin levels. Moreover, its greater affinity for the D_4-receptor subtype has forced the scientific community to reconsider the involvement of D_2 receptors in the expression of psychotic symptoms in general and to consider the role of D_4 receptors in negative symptoms in particular. However, its potency as a $5HT_{2A}$- and $5HT_7$-receptor antagonist is similar to risperidone and may be important for its actions against negative symptoms since both drugs appear to be more effective in this regard than other antipsychotics.

Clozapine does have side effects that distinguish it from other atypical antipsychotics. These include a paradoxic tendency to produce sialorrhea despite the drug's potent antimuscarinic action. Transient hyperthermia is commonly observed at the start of therapy and can be confused with the early development of neuroleptic malignant syndrome. The course of hyperthermia is benign in most cases and responds to normal antipyretic medications such as aspirin. Most importantly, clozapine can cause leukopenia and agranulocytosis.

Although all the antipsychotic agents, and in particular the phenothiazines, can reduce white blood cell (leukopenia) and granulocyte (agranulocytosis) counts, these effects are rare and usually not life-threatening. However, the incidence of agranulocytosis associated with clozapine therapy is ten to 20 times higher than with other antipsychotics (Meltzer, 1993). In fact, the incidence was so high that clozapine was withheld from the U.S. market. Because of its unique capacity to improve the symptoms of treatment-resistant and treatment-intolerant patients, however, the drug was introduced to the American market in 1990 with the provision that white blood cell counts be monitored weekly. This provision significantly raises the cost of clozapine therapy. Gershon and Meltzer (1992) have shown that the clozapine metabolite N-desmethylclozapine can dramatically compromise myeloid cell function and mitosis. This raises the interesting possibility that those patients who develop agranulocytosis may biotransform clozapine differently from the rest of the population.

RISPERIDONE

Risperidone is chemically unrelated to any of the current antipsychotics and the newest to be approved for the American market. Like clozapine, it has greater affinity for $5HT_{2A}$ and $5HT_7$ receptors than for D_2 receptors at clinically used doses, but its ability to block D_4 receptors is lower than that of clozapine. It is also antagonistic to alpha and histamine receptors. Although it has little affinity for muscarinic receptors it is not a typical antipsychotic agent. It is classified as atypical because at effective antipsychotic doses it does not produce significant D_2-receptor blockade. If the dosage is increased beyond the therapeutic range (6 to 10 mg/day), however, it will produce EPSEs. Thus, risperidone's dose-response curve is such that it provides antipsychotic efficacy at doses that produce little risk for EPSEs.

PHARMACOKINETICS OF ANTIPSYCHOTIC DRUGS

The pharmacokinetics of the antipsychotic agents have been well studied but the large number of available agents and the complex metabolism some of them undergo often produce confusion. A few important generalizations can be made, however (see Fig. 10–6).

Inter- and intrapatient variability in the absorption of the antipsychotic drugs is common. This can be reduced by delivering drugs in liquid formulations. A contributing factor to the variability in absorption is the coadministration of antimuscarinic drugs or the antimuscarinic activity of the antipsychotic agents themselves, which can reduce gastroduodenal motility, slow drug transit time, and thereby reduce absorption. Once absorbed, the drugs are oxidized primarily by the P-450 system and then conjugated. Several metabolites are active such as the 9-hydroxyrisperidone product of risperidone. Other drug metabolites such as mesoridazine (the product of thioridazine) can be more potent than the parent compound. A significant first-pass effect occurs and parenteral administration is usually associated with increased plasma levels. Microsomal enzyme-inducing drugs such as carbamazepine increase the biotransformation rate of many antipsychotic drugs, as do the tars in cigarette smoke. Chlorpro-

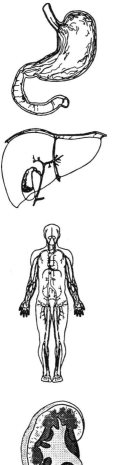

Erratic oral absorbtion with increased bioavailability following parenteral administration. Depot formulations available.

Biotransformation by oxidation followed by glucuronide conjugation. Some metabolites are active.

Highly protein and membrane bound. Concentrates in many tissues and brain concentrations may be higher than in plasma. Some autoinduction of biotransforming enzymes leading to pharmacokinetic tolerance.

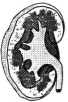

Excreted primarily in urine with some excreted in bile. 20 to 40 hour half-lives enable once-a-day dosing.

Figure 10–6. The general pharmacokinetics of the antipsychotic drug class are summarized in this figure. As a class, they are handled by the body in a similar fashion.

mazine and thioridazine can induce their own metabolism (autoinduction) and this may lead to pharmacokinetic tolerance.

Once the drugs reach the general circulation, they become extensively bound (~85%) to plasma proteins though tenfold differences in the amount of unbound drug have been reported in patients taking the same drug. Since most of the antipsychotics are very lipophilic, they tend to concentrate in lipid-rich structures. Brain concentrations can actually exceed plasma levels. Most of the drugs have half-lives of 20 to 40 hours, allowing once-a-day dosing. The acid metabolites and glucuronic acid conjugates are excreted primarily in the urine, and metabolites have been detected in urine for months after treatment ends.

Plasma Levels and Efficacy

Because of the wide variability in plasma levels and the production of active metabolites, the use of plasma levels to predict therapeutic responsiveness is fraught with problems. Some success has been achieved with the neuroleptic radioreceptor binding assay (NRBA; Creese and Snyder, 1977). This assay measures plasma D_2-receptor inhibitory activity. Patient plasma is tested for its ability to displace radiolabeled spiroperidol from a rat or calf striatal tissue preparation. Since whole plasma is used, parent drug and active metabolites are being assessed for their aggregate capacity to bind to the DA receptor. Variability in plasma binding and the production of active metabolites are therefore readily accommodated by this assay. With the NRBA and more traditional assays such as chromatography, a minimum therapeutic value has been established for several drugs including chlorpromazine, fluphenazine, haloperidol, and thiothixene.

Depot Formulations

In chronic treatment of the psychotic patient, compliance is a critical aspect of therapeutic management. Depot formulations have been developed to address this problem. Most often, they are produced by replacing the hydroxyl group on the drug with a long-chain, fat-soluble ester such as decanoate. This is done with fluphenazine, haloperidol, and flupenthixol. Depot formulations release the drug very slowly following intramuscular injection and are then rapidly de-esterified once they reach the blood, freeing the active drug to act. Depot formulations can yield effective antipsychotic plasma levels for up to a month.

Although depot formulations have reduced many compliance difficulties, their reduced ability to allow quick or subtle changes in drug dosage can be a problem in patients whose symptoms fluctuate frequently or have unexpected psychotic episodes. Oral supplementation can be used, but if severe EPSEs develop, withdrawing the medication is impossible and dialysis is ineffective at removing the drug from the blood. Therefore, the use of depot formulations is often restricted to patients who have had long histories of side-effect-free therapy.

Antidepressant Drugs

Prototypic Agent: *Imipramine (Tofranil)*

S adness is but one of several characteristics that, in various combinations, constitute a major depressive disorder (Table 11–1). Clinically, depressed patients may be apathetic, may fail to derive pleasure from normal life events (anhedonia), may suffer excessive anxiety, or may be inappropriately irritable. Thus, "not all clinically depressed patients are sad, and many sad patients are not clinically depressed" (Agency for Health Care Policy and Research, 1993).

A depressive disorder may be either unipolar or bipolar. Unipolar illness is characterized by one abnormal mood, usually depression, although unipolar mania also occurs. In contrast, bipolar disorder or manic-depressive illness involves mood swings between depression and mania. Clinical depression is much more common in women (20–25% lifetime risk) than in men (7–12%) while the incidence of bipolar disorder is equivalent for both sexes (Agency for Health Care Policy and Research, 1993). The peak age of onset of depression for women is between 35 and 40 while in men the incidence increases gradually with age. A genetic predisposition is thought to exist for mood disorders, especially bipolar disorder.

The treatment of depression involves drugs, psychotherapy, and electroconvulsive therapy. A small but significant proportion of patients fail to respond or experience only mild improvement regardless of the treatment involved. Approximately 15% of depressed patients will require hospitalization. Many patients spontaneously remit within a year but they often relapse, and in such patients the prognosis is poor. Identifying depressed patients and implementing appropriate therapy is critical since

Table 11–1 DSM-IV Criteria for Major Depressive Episode

A—Five (or more) of the following symptoms have been present during a two-week period and represent a change from previous functioning; at least one of the symptoms is either (1) depressed mood or (2) loss of interest or pleasure that is not due to a general medical condition or mood-incongruent delusions or hallucinations.

  1—depressed mood most of the day, nearly every day as indicated by either subjective report (*e.g.*, feels sad or empty) or observation made by others (*e.g.*, appears tearful)
  2—markedly diminished interest or pleasure in all or almost all activities most of the day, nearly every day (as indicated by either subjective account or observation made by other)
  3—significant weight loss when not dieting or weight gain (*e.g.*, a change of more than 5% of body weight in a month), or decrease or increase in appetite nearly every day. In children consider failure to make expected weight gains
  4—insomnia or hypersomnia nearly every day
  5—psychomotor agitation or retardation nearly every day (observable by others, not merely subjective feelings of restlessness or being slowed down)
  6—fatigue or loss of energy nearly every day
  7—feelings of worthlessness or excessive or inappropriate guilt (which may be delusional) nearly every day (not merely self-reproach or guilt about being sick)
  8—diminished ability to think or concentrate, or indecisive, nearly every day (thereby subjective account or as observed by others)
  9—recurrent thoughts of death (not just fear of dying), recurrent suicidal ideation without a specific plan, or suicide attempt or a specific plan for committing suicide.

B—The symptoms are not part of another psychiatric condition

C—The symptoms cause clinically significant distress or impairment in social, occupational, or other important areas of functioning

D—The symptoms are not due to a drug or other physiologic condition (*e.g.*, hypothyroidism)

E—The symptoms are not better accounted for by bereavement, or after the loss of a loved one, the symptoms persist for longer than two months or are characterized by marked functional impairment, morbid preoccupation with worthlessness, suicidal ideation, psychotic symptoms, or psychomotor retardation

60 to 80% of the patients who remain in therapy will improve (Fawcett, 1993). Many clinically depressed individuals, however, receive no medical care for this disorder.

THE BIOGENIC AMINE HYPOTHESIS OF DEPRESSION

In the early 1950s, the antihypertensive drug reserpine was found to produce depression as a side effect, the antituberculosis drug iproniazid was found to improve depression, and amphetamine was known to elevate mood. These observations suggested an organic cause for depression and sparked a debate over the relative contributions of nature and nurture to mood disorders. Although the debate continues to this day, the research that eventually led to our current understanding of the mechanisms by which reserpine, iproniazid, and amphetamine act suggested a central role for both NE and 5HT in depression, fostering the catecholamine and indole amine hypotheses of depression, respectively. Once again, a major advance in our understanding of brain function and dysfunction was made by determining how drugs work.

The Catecholamine Hypothesis

According to the catecholamine hypothesis, the symptoms of depression stem from reduced norepinephrine levels in the CNS (Schildkraut, 1965; Bunney and Davis, 1965). Since reserpine produced depression and amphetamine elevated mood, it was presumed that the pathogenesis of depression could be understood once the mechanisms of action common to both of these drugs were resolved. Reserpine was eventually shown to deplete NE, 5HT, and DA, while amphetamine proved to primarily act by increasing NE and DA. It was further observed that agents elevating dopamine in the CNS produced transient euphoria but did not necessarily relieve the depressed state, which indicated that reductions in the catecholamine NE might be responsible for depression. These findings formed the basis for the catecholamine hypothesis of depression.

Since the mid-1960s, thousands of studies have attempted to validate this hypothesis with surprisingly little success (see Potter and Manji, 1994, for review). The examination of plasma, urine, and CSF levels of vanilla mandelic acid (VMA) and 3-methoxy-4-hydroxyphenylglycol (MHPG), the major catabolic products of norepinephrine, have been inconclusive. Studies on noradrenergic receptors were also inconsistent. The inconsistencies among the studies have engendered strong criticism, but this is often met with the argument that depression is a consequence of altered NE levels only in some patients.

Indole Amine Hypothesis

While many investigators focused their efforts on norepinephrine, others examined the serotonergic system. Reserpine's ability to deplete 5HT, iproniazid's action as a monoamine oxidase inhibitor, and the growing evidence that hallucinogenic drugs produced their mood-altering effects through 5HT suggested a role for this indole amine in depression. The seminal studies of Asberg, Traskman, and Thoren (1976) demonstrating reduced levels of the major oxidation product of serotonin (5-hydroxyindoleacetic acid [5HIAA]) in suicide victims implicated 5HT in depression. Since the mid-1970s, several studies have replicated these findings and have demonstrated reduced brain 5HT in suicide victims as well (see Meltzer and Lowy, 1987, for review). Moreover, parachlorophenylalanine (PCPA), a serotonin depletor, precipitates depression in patients who respond favorably to antidepressant drugs that elevate brain serotonin. In addition, tryptophan, the precursor to serotonin, is reduced in the plasma of many depressed patients and 5HT$_2$ receptors are increased in the frontal cortex of suicide victims, suggesting reduced 5HT release (see Owens and Nemeroff, 1994). Thus, on balance, a large body of evidence favors a serotonin deficiency in depression while the evidence for norepinephrine's role is meager at best.

NE AND 5HT IN NEURONAL PROCESSING

One of the troubling aspects of the thousands of papers that have been written about the roles of norepinephrine and serotonin in depression is that they fail to explain how a deficiency in these neurotransmitters translates into depressive symptoms. A theoretical paper by Foote and Morrison (1987) offers such a mechanism: The locus ceruleus (LC) projects its NE-containing processes to several brain areas including layer VI of the cortex (Fig. 11–1). This projection forms a dense sheet of terminals overlying the white matter beneath the cortical mantle. These fibers branch and innervate all layers of the cortex in an orderly fashion, although there is regional heterogeneity. Thus, primary sensory and motor regions are highly innervated while the temporal cortex is almost devoid of noradrenergic innervation. The functional unit of the cortex is the six-layered cortical column. A single LC fiber can alter the activity of thousands of these columns. Intracellular recordings of the neurons in a cortical column reveal a high level of background activity that reflects the extensive intracortical communication among the columns. Norepinephrine reduces this background activity by inhibiting corticocortical communicating fibers. When environmental sensory stimuli are processed, this information is transferred by thalamocortical afferents to the cortical mantle where it induces an electrical response. In order to be detected, the amplitude of this input must be higher than the background activity. If the amplitude of the incoming sensory volley is not large relative to the amplitude of the normal background, it may not be detected as "non-background" (Fig. 11–2).

Afferent sensory neurons give off collaterals that either directly or indirectly increase activity in the LC. Activation of the LC stimulates the release of NE from the terminals of the LC projection system and this re-

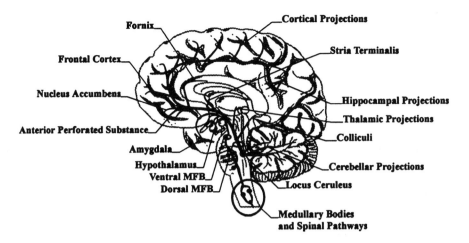

Figure 11–1. The norepinephrine pathways of the brain.

duces corticocortical activity. Incoming sensory activity (which is delayed by thalamic processing) is then transmitted to cortical cells that are more likely to detect or attend to incoming sensory signals. In a sense, the LC induces a generalized alerting response to incoming sensory activity by increasing the signal-to-noise ratio of sensory processing. Consistent with this notion is the fact that during sleep the LC firing rate declines and during dreaming it almost ceases. The sleep-associated reduction in LC activity facilitates corticocortical communication while reducing attention to external sensory processing.

Serotonergic fibers from the raphe nuclear groups perform a similar function. Fibers from the dorsal and medial raphe innervate several layers of the cortex, particularly layer IV (Fig. 11–3). In most regions the 5HT and NE fibers do not overlap, suggesting that each influences the activity of a different set of cells. Alternatively, NE and 5HT may regulate different states of neural processing in a column. Like NE, 5HT modulates the activity of cortical neurons. Whereas NE is thought to regulate sensory processing, 5HT is thought to regulate limbic processing. Thus, the raphe nuclei are activated in response to alterations in the behavioral state of the animal (fight or flight, hunger, sexual arousal, etc.). Once activated, the serotonergic fibers increase the signal-to-noise ratio for processing state-dependent activities by inhibiting corticocortical activity that could potentially interfere with their detection. Messages from afferent limbic fibers carrying behavioral-state activity to the cortex are thus attended to more readily. This facilitated signaling mediated by 5HT enables cortical cells to respond more readily to signals originating in limbic structures such as the septum or amygdala in much the same manner that NE facilitates cortical responsiveness to sensory signals.

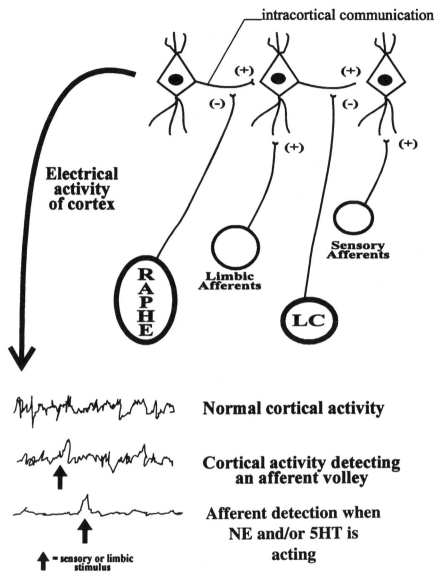

Figure 11–2. The role of NE and 5HT in cortical processing. By inhibiting intracortical communication, NE and 5HT fibers can enhance the signal-to-noise ratio of sensory and limbic processing, respectively.

Foote and Morrison hypothesized that an individual whose brain is deficient in NE would be less attentive to sensory signals and more likely to process then abnormally, leading to psychomotor retardation, withdrawal, hypersomnolence and a reduced appetite, while an individual deficient in 5HT would be less likely to process emotional stimuli ade-

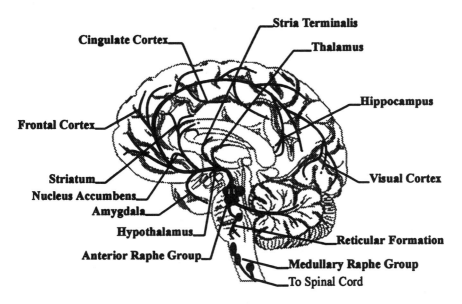

Figure 11–3. The serotonin pathways of the brain.

quately, leading to flat affect or inappropriate emotional responses to environmental events, producing anhedonia. Persons deficient in NE and/or 5HT would also be more likely to misinterpret sensory or behavioral state activity, to integrate them poorly with past experience, and thus to develop a distorted sense of the environment. The administration of antidepressant drugs that increase NE or 5HT activity would thus reinstate normal levels of cortical integration and reduce symptoms of depression.

Although the ideas set forth by Foote and Morrison offer a possible explanation for the consequences of brain NE and 5HT deficiency, they do not address the cause of that deficiency. Interestingly, both neurotransmitters are involved in the production of melatonin, the secretion of which is greatly influenced by the brain's biological clock. This suggests that anomalous biological rhythms may be responsible for disruptions in NE and 5HT and might lead to some forms of depression.

CIRCADIAN PERIODICITY IN DEPRESSED PATIENTS

Whether or not we are aware of it, we are very much influenced by the periodic events occurring in our environment—circadian, lunar, and annual rhythms. Virtually every bodily function studied exhibits entrainment to these external cycles. Dopamine levels in the striatum, beta-adrenergic-receptor numbers in the frontal cortex, and levels of hormones all vary with the light–dark cycle. These rhythmic fluctuations serve an adaptive purpose. Daily patterns in activity reduce predation by nocturnal animals on diurnal species. Lunar cycles synchronize mating behaviors and annual rhythms lead to migratory behavior that maximizes access to food sources. As any one who has experienced jet lag knows, being out of synch with one's environment can have a negative effect on mood. It is not surprising, then, that the normal circadian rhythms of many physiologic processes are disrupted in depressed patients. Although rhythm disturbances are not found in all depressed patients, disrupted periodicity may contribute to the pathogenesis of depression in many of them (see Kupfer, Monk, and Barchas, 1988; Shafii and Shafii, 1990).

The suprachiasmatic nucleus (SCN), located in the rostral hypothalamus just superior to the optic chiasm, is the brain's endogenous clock. It receives a separate afferent projection from the retina whose sole function apparently is to detect the presence or absence of light and convey this information to the SCN. In turn, the SCN projects to a number of different hypothalamic nuclei that regulate activity in the superior cervical ganglion. Efferent sympathetic autonomic nervous system (SANS) fibers from the superior cervical ganglion project to the pineal gland, thereby regulating the release of melatonin (Fig. 11–4). In concert with the pineal gland, the SCN is responsible for synchronizing endogenous rhythms with external light cues. Since neurotransmitter levels, receptor numbers, and probably second-messenger actions wax and wane over the 24-hour period, disruptions in this temporal organization could easily lead to inappropriate interactions among several neurotransmitter systems and thereby contribute to depression (see Wirz-Justice et al., 1996). Melatonin's involvement is supported by studies in which depression developed after melatonin was given during the day when its levels are normally low. Moreover, during the winter months when the photoperiod is short, melatonin levels are high for a longer period of the day. This probably contributes to a seasonal depression that occurs in the winter months and is now called seasonal affective disorder (SAD).

A remarkably consistent body of research (Campbell et al., 1995) indicates that exposing SAD patients to bright light (at least 2,500 lux) activates the SCN and reduces depression (normal room light is 750 lux and sunlight is 10,000 lux). Exposing these patients to a bright light at a specified time of day (usually early in the morning) phase-shifts their circadian rhythms, brings them into synch with the environment, and elevates their mood.

Abnormalities in endogenous circadian rhythms, disruptions in the brain's clock, and the biogenic amine hypotheses of depression may all be interrelated. Serotonin and melatonin share tryptophan as a precursor and their brain levels depend in part on the availability of circulating

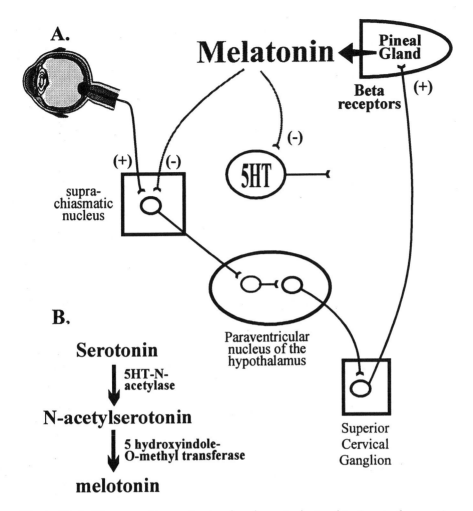

Figure 11–4. The suprachiasmatic-pineal pathway is depicted in A as is the negative effect melatonin has as a feedback inhibitor to the suprachiasmatic nucleus and to serotonergic neurons (+ = excitatory; − = inhibitory). In B the relationship between serotonin and melatonin biosynthesis is depicted.

tryptophan. In addition, melatonin inhibits serotonergic neurons (Fig. 11–4). If melatonin levels were increased because of prolonged exposure to dark or because of a genetic or functional disturbance in the endogenous clock, less tryptophan would be available for 5HT synthesis in serotonergic neurons and serotonergic neuron activity would be decreased by the action of increased melatonin. Excess melatonin therefore can lead to reduced activity of the serotonergic system, which is consistent with the indole amine hypothesis of depression. In addition, norepinephrine released from the terminals of the superior cervical ganglion increases the release of melatonin through a beta-adrenergic mechanism. As will be discussed below, one of the consequences of chronic antidepressant activity is down-regulation of beta-adrenergic receptors. Chronic antidepressant drug treatment would thus lead to reduced melatonin release and a reduction in the depressant actions of melatonin.

Although the theories advanced above offer intriguing hypotheses about the etiology of depression and the role of norepinephrine and serotonin in them, we are far from a complete understanding of this illness. It is likely that depression has several etiologies and results from alterations in neurochemicals in addition to norepinephrine, serotonin, and melatonin. As will be seen in the next section, however, all of the currently used antidepressant drugs increase the activity of norepinephrine and/or serotonin. Since these drugs are effective in two-thirds of depressed patients, it is clear that these two neurotransmitters are involved with depression in the majority of cases. Thus, whether genetic abnormalities in neurotransmission exist, endogenous periodicity is disrupted, or other CNS functions not described in this brief review of depression occur, any model of depression must accommodate the noradrenergic and serotonergic actions of the antidepressant drugs.

THE ANTIDEPRESSANT DRUGS

Several drug classes have antidepressant properties (Fig. 11–5). Some have a three-ring structure and were thus named the tricyclic antidepressants (TCAs). The TCAs are all competitive reuptake inhibitors of norepinephrine and serotonin. Whether or not the side-chain amine is secondary or tertiary (i.e., $-NHCH_3$ or $-N[CH_3]_2$, respectively) determines the affinity of these drugs for other receptors such as muscarinic and alpha$_1$-adrenergic receptors, where they act as competitive antagonists. Other antidepressants do not have a tricyclic structure and have been called atypical, heterocyclic, or second-generation agents. They are also competitive reuptake inhibitors of norepinephrine and serotonin. Within this group are the newest additions to the antidepressant family, called the selective serotonin reuptake inhibitors (SSRIs) which, as the name implies, inhibit the reuptake of serotonin only. A third group of antidepressants is the monoamine oxidase inhibitors (MAOIs), which act as competitive or irreversible inhibitors of the NE and 5HT catabolizing enzyme monoamine oxidase (MAO). The irreversible inhibitors are comprised of two chemical classes best characterized as the hydrazines (e.g., phenelzine) and the nonhydrazine agents (e.g., isocarboxazid). A new class of MAO inhibitors called the reversible inhibitors of monoamine oxidase competitively inhibit MAO.

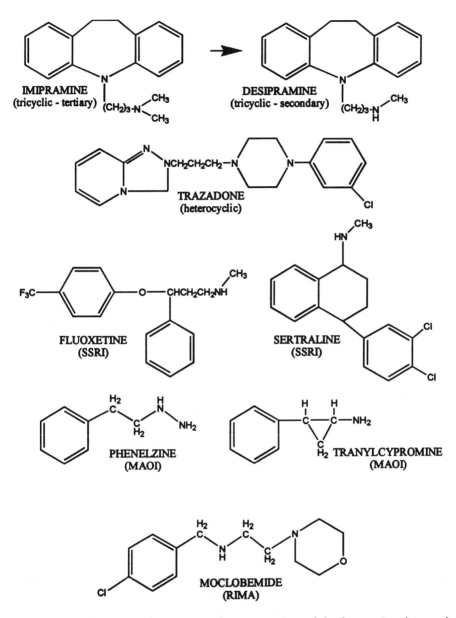

Figure 11–5. The chemical structures of representatives of the four major classes of antidepressants. Imipramine a tertiary amine, is biotransformed into the secondary amine desipramine.

The Reuptake-Inhibiting Antidepressants

The TCAs and heterocyclics are competitive inhibitors of the high-affinity norepinephrine and serotonin transporters. As such, they bind reversibly to the neurotransmitter acceptor site on the transport protein. Unlike levodopa or amphetamine, however, the antidepressants are not substrates for the transport protein, so they are not transported into the cytoplasmic pool of the terminal. Regardless, inhibiting reuptake increases the concentration of the neurotransmitter in the synapse and extends the time it has to bind with its receptors. These drugs are therefore indirect-acting agonists.

The TCAs inhibit the reuptake of NE and 5HT to varying degrees. Desipramine inhibits the reuptake of NE more so than 5HT while clomipramine inhibits the reuptake of 5HT more so than NE. The heterocyclic antidepressants, except for the SSRIs, similarly inhibit the reuptake of NE and 5HT to varying degrees. The consequences of this reuptake inhibition are complex.

Increasing the concentration of NE and/or 5HT in the synaptic cleft increases the number of interactions between these neurotransmitters and their receptors. Acutely, the neurotransmitter levels are raised in a brain where it is hypothesized that NE and 5HT are low. As is the case for the antipsychotic drugs, however, an efficacy delay is associated with the use of reuptake inhibitors. Thus, depressive symptoms do not decrease immediately, but only after several weeks of treatment. The acute action of the reuptake inhibitors to increase NE and 5HT is therefore not consistent with the biogenic amine hypothesis of depression. Compensatory responses by the brain to the drug is therefore likely responsible for the antidepressant effects of these drugs.

Chronic exposure to these antidepressants produces norepinephrine and/or serotonin receptor-site down-regulation. This down-regulation occurs at postsynaptic receptors as well as alpha$_2$-adrenergic autoreceptors and 5HT autoreceptors located on the cell body. It would be expected that postsynaptic alpha$_1$-adrenergic receptor-site down-regulation would occur. This is not a consistent finding, however, because the TCAs and most of the non-SSRI heterocyclics are competitive antagonists for this receptor and can even produce alpha$_1$-adrenergic receptor-site up-regulation. Whether or not postsynaptic alpha$_1$-adrenergic receptors up- or down-regulate, the predominant effect on beta-adrenergic and/or serotonergic postsynaptic receptors is down-regulation, which is inconsistent with the biogenic amine hypothesis. Thus, postsynaptic receptor down-regulation would result in a net decrease in neurotransmitter activity instead of the increase predicted by the biogenic amine hypothesis (Fig. 11–6). What is consistent with this hypothesis, however, is the increase in

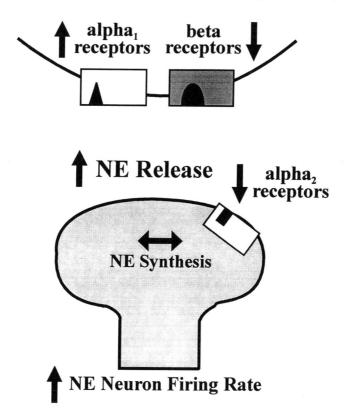

Figure 11–6. Chronic treatment with tricyclic antidepressant (TCAs) produces several changes in the function of the target neurons of norepinephrine (NE) neurons as well as in the NE neuron itself. The net effect of these changes is summarized by the arrows.

NE neuron firing rate that accompanies chronic TCA use first reported by Crews and Smith (1978) and the increase in 5HT neuron firing rate that accompanies chronic use of the SSRIs (Owens and Nemeroff, 1994). These changes occur as a consequence of autoreceptor down-regulation.

Activation of alpha$_2$ autoreceptors located on noradrenergic terminals decreases future NE release by reducing neurotransmitter synthesis and by changing the phosphorylation status of the proteins responsible for neurotransmitter release (see Chapter 3). Activation of this receptor also reduces the neuron firing rate through an unknown mechanism. In serotonergic neurons, analogous autoregulation is thought to result from a postsynaptic action of 5HT released from an axon collateral that inhibits the serotonin cell body (Fig. 11–7). Even though the receptor mediating this effect (5HT$_{1A}$) is technically postsynaptic, it is located on the serotonergic cell body and activated by serotonin and thus is still classified as

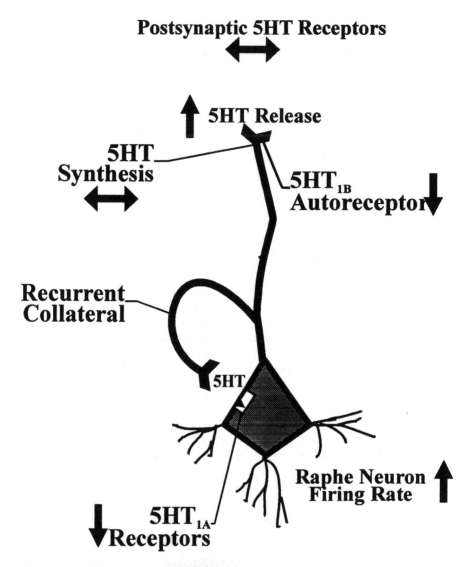

Figure 11–7. Chronic treatment with selective serotonin reuptake inhibitors produces several changes in the function of the target neurons of serotonergic fibers as well as in the serotonin (5HT) neuron itself. The net effect of these changes is summarized by the arrows.

an autoreceptor. With chronic reuptake inhibition, these autoreceptors down-regulate. This has three consequences: (1) Neurotransmitter synthesis that had been formerly decreased by the acute actions of the reuptake inhibitors normalizes or increases slightly; (2) neurotransmitter release similarly returns to normal or is slightly increased; and, most importantly, (3) the neuron fires at a faster rate. The net result of these three effects is an increase in NE and/or 5HT activity as predicted by the biogenic amine hypothesis.

Although the down-regulation of autoreceptors produced by these drugs and the net effect this produces on neurotransmitter activity is consistent with the biogenic amine hypothesis, it may not be the only mechanism through which antidepressant effects can occur. Heninger and Charney (1987) demonstrated that one of the consistent effects of the TCAs is a reduction in NE-mediated cAMP reduction. Findings similar to these in the 5HT system have been observed following SSRI treatment. These data suggest that alterations in receptor numbers and firing rates may not be as important to antidepressant action as the overall alterations in the molecular response of the cell (see Hyman and Nestler, 1993, for an extensive review). This notion is supported by the fact that another antidepressant drug class, the monoamine oxidase inhibitors, similarly increases norepinephrine and serotonin, albeit through a different mechanism.

Monoamine Oxidase Inhibitors

Function of monoamine oxidase (MAO)
MAO is a unique member of the group of mixed-function oxidases that are specific for the biogenic amines. MAO can be found throughout the body, especially in the gastrointestinal tract, liver, and blood. It is also found in neurons and glia. MAO is best viewed as a scavenger enzyme: It prevents the circulation of otherwise-harmful dietary amines (pressor amines) and reduces the nonspecific action of biogenic amines released from the adrenal glands and nervous system.

Two major isoforms of MAO are currently known: MAO-A and MAO-B. They were originally defined pharmacologically through their selective inhibition by clorgiline and selegiline, respectively. They are located in mitochondria and substrate access is facilitated by low-affinity pumps located on the mitochondrial membrane. Compared to MAO-B, MAO-A is found in slightly higher concentrations in the periphery, especially the gut. Although both isoforms are found in the brain in approximately equal quantities, regional heterogeneity suggests system specialization. MAO-A preferentially oxidizes 5HT but will also oxidize NE and DA. MAO-B preferentially oxidizes DA but will also oxidize NE and 5HT. The relative concentration of types A and B in the brain vary by species and even by variety in some cases.

MAO inhibition
MAO inhibitors (MAOIs) falls into two general categories referred to as first- and second-generation agents. All of the first-generation MAOIs

are irreversible inhibitors of MAO. When oxidized by MAO, their metabolites covalently bind to MAO, inactivating it. Once the covalent bond is formed, both the enzyme and drug are destroyed. Because the drug is destroyed, they are referred to as "suicide inhibitors." Pargyline, selegiline, and clorgiline covalently bind to and inactivate the flavin cofactor of MAO. Tranylcypromine and the others inhibit MAO by covalently binding to the enzyme itself. Once the inhibitor has attached to its binding site, the MAO is permanently inactivated and new protein must be synthesized to restore function. This takes time. Even after treatment stops, weeks can pass before adequate numbers of MAO enzymes can be synthesized to reinstate normal oxidative function.

In contrast, the second-generation drugs are reversible inhibitors of MAO-A (RIMAs). Unlike the first-generation agents, RIMAs form a reactive intermediate complex that dissociates from the enzyme, leaving MAO-A again free to oxidize substrate. Thus, even though the absorption, distribution, biotransformation, and excretion of both classes of inhibitors are similar, the RIMAs permit the release of functional MAO after a few hours. The result is a dramatic but transient reduction in MAO activity without the toxicity associated with irreversible inhibition. Whereas the dosages of the first-generation agents must be increased gradually over several weeks because of the risk of toxicity, the RIMAs can be administered at therapeutic dosages immediately and thus can achieve therapeutic plasma levels quickly. Moreover, the dosages of RIMAs can be adjusted subtly to achieve the most appropriate plasma level for an individual. The irreversible MAOIs cannot be manipulated in this fashion and if side effects do develop, the patient must live with them while new enzyme is being synthesized. The RIMAs therefore represent a significant therapeutic advancement in the use of MAOIs. Although these drugs are widely used in other countries, they are not yet available in the United States.

Monoamine oxidase inhibition and the biogenic amine hypothesis
Only MAO-A inhibitors are effective antidepressants. Inhibition of MAO-A increases levels of 5HT within the CNS more so than NE and DA. Since NE and DA can be catabolized by both MAO and COMT, MAO-A inhibition drives their catabolism through the O-methylation pathway. However, 5HT is almost exclusive oxidized and MAO-A inhibition does not leave an alternate pathway. Thus, MAO-A inhibitors will have a more profound effect on 5HT than on NE and DA. The irreversible MAOIs also have affinity, albeit low, for NE and 5HT transporters and are therefore reuptake inhibitors. This combination of MAO and reuptake inhibition classifies the MAOIs as indirect-acting agonists. It is assumed that the mechanism of the antidepressant effects of the

MAOIs is similar to that of the reuptake inhibitors. Thus, as a result of their indirect-agonist effects, 5HT and NE activity is initially increased and eventually leads to a down-regulation of autoreceptors. A net increase in neuronal firing eventually accompanies this down-regulation coincident with a decrease in the severity of symptoms. Like the reuptake inhibitors, an efficacy delay occurs and symptomatic improvement should not be anticipated until after the patient has been on drug for several weeks. These drugs are most likely to have clinical effects once MAO-A activity has been inhibited 70 to 85%. MAO-A activity is conveniently monitored in platelets and is presumed to reflect brain MAO activity.

Antidepressant efficacy and choice of drug

The antidepressant drugs provide significant therapeutic benefit in approximately two-thirds of patients. The advent of the SSRIs brought with it the perception that these drugs were more efficacious than the older agents. This is not true, however, and no antidepressant drug class has been shown to reduce the symptoms of depression more so than another (Fawcett, 1995). Although it is true that SSRI therapy may be more effective in depression, this "effectiveness" is a consequence of increased patient compliance due to the significantly lower incidence of side effects that accompanies the use of these drugs compared with that seen with other antidepressants.

A significant number of patients exhibit dramatic therapeutic benefit from antidepressant drug therapy. All symptoms of the depressive syndrome are influenced in some patients and few would argue with the capability of the antidepressant drugs to as least reduce the severity of depression in most patients. Antidepressant efficacy is, however, sometimes difficult to interpret in many patients and vegetative signs such as improved sleep patterns, reduced autonomic dysfunction, and a normalization of disrupted circadian rhythms have been used to indicate a positive response (see Kupfer, Monk, and Barchas, 1988; Shafii and Shafii, 1990). As seen in Figure 11–8, the relative effects of the antidepressants for NE and 5HT vary from the 1,000-fold-greater selectivity for NE seen with maprotiline to the greater relative selectivity for 5HT seen with fluoxetine. The question, "Which antidepressant drug is most appropriate for a given patient?" therefore becomes important.

Since it is likely that depression is a consequence of several etiologies and may involve NE deficiencies in some, 5HT deficiencies in others, and deficiencies in both neurotransmitters in still others, several strategies have been used to determine which agent is most appropriate for a given patient. The symptoms that predominate the clinical picture may be use-

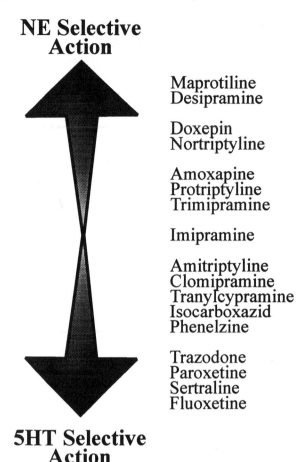

Figure 11–8. The relative specificities of several antidepressants for the norepinephrine (NE) and serotonin (5HT) transporter are schematized in this diagram.

ful in determining drug choice. Thus, for instance, patients who experience difficulty with sleep or have suicide ideation may be more responsive to 5HT-preferring agents. Evaluation of body fluids that show reductions in NE and/or 5HT metabolites may be helpful. Provocative tests such as the dexamethasone suppression test and amphetamine challenge are used as well. The regulation of the pituitary-adrenal axis involves 5HT. Peripherally secreted corticosteroid interacts with serotonergic neurons in the CNS to increase 5HT activity and suppress adrenocorticotropin hormone (ACTH) secretion. The administration of dexamethasone (a synthetic steroid) should depress cortisol secretion by reducing ACTH release. Failure to suppress cortisol with dexamethasone (a negative dexamethasone suppression test) is thought to result from decreased CNS 5HT, implicating the choice of an agent more selective for 5HT.

Amphetamine, on the other hand, increases brain norepinephrine more so than 5HT. Patients exhibiting a transient increase in mood may be more likely to respond favorably to an antidepressant more specific for NE. These tests are only somewhat helpful in identifying the most appropriate drug and the choice of antidepressant therefore remains empiric in most cases; i.e., trial and error dictate which drug will be best. It is also possible that symptoms which do not respond to traditional antidepressants are the result of alterations in other neurotransmitter systems (see Ashton, 1992; Strange, 1992). The involvement of other neurotransmitter systems might suggest that the actions of NE and/or 5HT as well as the choice of which drug to use may not be as important as initially assumed. This makes the choice of drug for a particular patient even more problematic. Moreover, electroconvulsive shock therapy (ECT) is still used and can be very effective in patients suffering from reactive depression or those who do not respond well to traditional drugs. Interestingly, ECT increases NE-stimulated cAMP production and increases 5HT receptor sensitivity, both of which are consistent with the biogenic amine hypothesis of depression (see Heninger and Charney, 1987).

It is likely that the choice of antidepressant and the etiology of depression will remain topics of controversy for some time. From a practical perspective, however, it appears that the most important issue in the choice of antidepressant is the ability of the patient to tolerate the drug's side effects. This is especially true since many patients exhibit patterns of waxing and waning depression that may require prophylactic therapy. These patients are more likely to remain compliant with a drug that produces minimal side effects. Therefore, the side effects of the drugs unfortunately more often dictate the choice of drug than the presumed neurotransmitter deficit.

SIDE EFFECTS OF ANTIDEPRESSANT DRUGS

The TCAs are associated with the greatest morbidity and mortality of all the commonly prescribed centrally acting drugs. In addition to their action as NE and 5HT reuptake inhibitors, these drugs variably block muscarinic, histaminergic, adrenergic, and serotonergic receptors and possess quinidine-like effects, all of which complicate the management of the overdose patient who, in some cases, may have attempted suicide with the antidepressant drug. These additional TCA actions may also produce several bothersome side effects—including orthostatic hypotension, sedation, dry mouth, and constipation—that reduce patient compliance. Because of side effects like these, 75% of treated patients are receiving subtherapeutic doses rendering them susceptible to the underlying morbidity of depression (McCombs et al., 1990). Indeed, the potential for fatal overdose and the numerous side effects associated with TCA use drove the development of the heterocyclic antidepressants. Understanding the side effects of antidepressant drugs is therefore a critical factor in the effective management of the depressed patient. These issues are discussed extensively in several excellent reviews (Hollister and Claghorn, 1993; Lejoyeux et al., 1992; Frenkel, Quitkin, and Rabkin, 1988; Baldessarini, 1989), summarized in Table 11–2 and described as follows.

Cardiovascular Side Effects

The cardiovascular effects of the TCAs are notorious and, in overdose situations, life-threatening. They result from a combination of NE-reuptake inhibition, muscarinic antagonism, quinidine-like effects, and alpha$_1$-adrenergic antagonistic actions. Although the phenothiazines have similar properties, the additional actions of the TCAs as NE-reuptake in-

Table 11–2 Side Effects of the Four Major Classes of Antidepressant Drugs

Effect	TCAs	Atypicals	SSRIs	MAOIs
Orthostatic hypotension	+++	++	− −	+++/− −[a]
Muscarinic-mediated cardiac effects	+++	++	− −	− −
Quinidine-like effects	++	+	− −	− −
Tyramine effect	− −	− −	− −	+++/− −[b]
Antimuscarinic effects (dry mouth, urinary retention, constipation, movement disorders, fatigue, myoclonus, memory impairment, delirium)	+++	++	− −	− −
Switch phenomenon	+++	+/−	− −	− −
Sedation	+++	++	− −[c]	+/− −[c]
Reduced seizure threshold	+	++	− −	− −
Nausea and vomiting	+	+	++	+
Tremor	++	++	++	++
Weight gain	++	+	+	− −
Hepatotoxicity	− −	− −	− −	++[d]/− −

[a]Significantly less so for the RIMAs

[b]Does not apply for RIMAs

[c]Insomnia with SSRIs and RIMAs

[d]Hydrazine MAOIs only

− − = not observed; +/− = rarely observed; + = seldom observed; ++ = often observed; +++ = usually observed

hibitors with beta-adrenergic actions give them a more dramatic cardio-vascular role.

Alpha₁-receptor antagonism

The TCAs, heterocyclics, and MAOIs produce orthostatic hypotension to varying degrees based in part on their peripheral alpha₁-adrenergic antagonistic effects as well as their central actions (see Table 11–2). In general, TCAs having a secondary amine side-chain structure have less affinity for the alpha₁-adrenergic receptor and produce less orthostasis. The non-SSRI heterocyclics and MAOIs have moderate affinity for alpha₁-adrenergic receptors while the SSRIs are virtually devoid of this action. The orthostatic effects of the antidepressants are troublesome and one wonders why agents with significant alpha₁ affinity would be used at all. Excess SANS activity characterizes many depressed patients, however, and in these patients, reducing sympathetic activity with an antidepressant that has significant alpha₁ antagonism can be beneficial.

Antimuscarinic antagonism

The antimuscarinic actions of some antidepressants contribute to their cardiovascular effects. Reducing muscarinic activity increases heart rate and conduction velocity through the His-Purkinje system. The resulting positive chronotropy and dromotropy can lead to heart palpitations that provoke anxiety in depressed patients. In general, the tertiary amine TCAs are most potent in this regard, followed by the secondary amines and the non-SSRI heterocyclics. It is not a problem with the MAOIs and SSRIs. Muscarinic antagonism potentiates the actions of drugs that are also potent NE-reuptake inhibitors. Thus, loss of muscarinic activity combined with increased beta-adrenergic receptor activation can lead to profound tachycardia.

Quinidine-like actions

Quinidine is an antiarrhythmic agent at therapeutic levels that produces arrhythmias at higher doses (see Chapter 10). Like the phenothiazines, the TCAs and to a lesser extent the non-SSRI heterocyclics can have quinidine-like actions. The MAOIs and SSRIs are devoid of this effect. The hydroxylated forms of the parent TCAs are actually responsible for the quinidine effect (see Baldessarini, 1989), so concurrent use of microsomal inducing agents enhances the production of these potentially dangerous metabolites. The quinidine-like actions of the TCAs are potentiated by their alpha-adrenergic and muscarinic effects and are a critical consideration in the overdose patient. Imipramine is clearly the most potent in this regard, followed by amitriptyline, clomipramine, doxepin, and maprotiline.

Hypertensive crisis and MAO-A inhibition

Eating foods that contain large amounts of tyramine and other pressor amines can produce a potentially fatal hypertensive crisis in patients taking irreversible MAO-A inhibitors. (Pressor amines are a group of chemicals in the environment that have indirect-acting adrenergic agonist actions.) This effect is often referred to as the "tyramine effect," the "cheese effect," or the "pickled herring, Chianti wine, and cheese effect." In addition to its ability to oxidize biogenic amines, MAO-A biotransforms pressor amines into inactive metabolites. However, patients on irreversible MAO-A inhibitors cannot biotransform these agents and NE is released via the amphetamine-like actions of tyramine (Fig. 11–9). If tyramine levels are high, the peripheral stores of NE can be released so quickly that blood pressure and heart rate rise sharply. Stroke and arrhythmias can occur in predisposed patients. In otherwise normal patients, this increased SANS tone creates feeling of lightheadedness, headache, nausea, vomiting, and generalized anxiety that are often reasons for noncompliance. Because of this problem, the use of the MAOIs as antidepressants almost ceased, but it is now known that the potential risk of the tyramine effect is generally overstated (see Cooper, 1989, for review).

In addition to the tyramine effect, the irreversible MAOIs produce other cardiovascular effects. Tyramine is converted to octopamine in the periphery by DA-beta-hydroxylase located in noradrenergic terminals. Octopamine is a false neurotransmitter that is sequestered in synaptic vesicles and released like NE although it has very little affinity for adrenergic receptors. Patients on irreversible MAOIs can build up sufficient octopamine levels to produce a NE "depletion effect" that further contributes to orthostatic hypotension. Because of these cardiovascular effects associated with the ingestion of pressor amines, the reversible inhibitors of monoamine oxidase were developed (RIMAs). Because access to the active site on MAO by the reversible inhibitors is competitive, high concentrations of tyramine "outcompete" the inhibitors and are effectively neutralized. Thus, the pressor response to tyramine in the presence of a RIMA is negligible (Amrein et al., 1989; Simpson and de Leon, 1989).

Other Antimuscarinic Effects

The antimuscarinic potency of the antidepressants is highest for the tertiary amines followed by the secondary amines and then the non-SSRI heterocyclics. The MAOIs (both irreversible and the RIMAs) and the SSRIs do not have antimuscarinic action. Antimuscarinic side effects include sedation, dry mouth, constipation, urinary retention, and tachycardia. Higher doses of tertiary TCAs can produce weakness, fatigue, memory loss, delirium, psychosis and movement disorders including akathisia, dyskinesias,

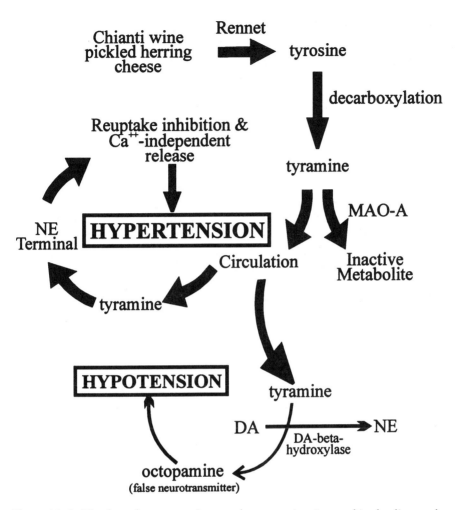

Figure 11–9. The fate of pressor amines, such as tyramine, ingested in the diet are depicted in this schematic. Certain food such as Chianti wine and aged cheeses contain proteins that are converted in high quantities to tyrosine by rennet found in these foods. The high quantities of tyrosine are decarboxylated by the bacteria found in the GI tract to tyramine, which can then be absorbed into the portal circulation. The pressor amine tyramine is normally oxidized by monoamine oxidase type A (MAO-A) to an inactive metabolite. In the presence of a monoamine oxidase inhibitor (MAOI) however, it enters the systemic circulation and eventually norepinephrine (NE) terminals where it acts as a substrate for the transporter protein including Ca^{2+}-independent NE release and as a competitive reuptake inhibitor. Hypertensive crisis can result from the increase in NE activity produced, which is further exacerbated by the MAOI's inhibition of normal NE catabolism. Chronically, tyramine can also be beta-hydroxylated in the NE terminal to the false neurotransmitter octopamine which, as a result of depletion of the vesicular pool of NE, can contribute to hypotension.

and myoclonus. Myoclonus, a purposeless intense contraction of a muscle group, is thought to be a 5HT-mediated phenomenon (Jacobs, 1986) that is probably enhanced by antimuscarinic activity. TCAs that increase 5HT activity through reuptake inhibition and also have antimuscarinic actions (e.g., amitriptyline) are most likely to produce this side effect.

Also potentially related to their antimuscarinic potencies is the so-called "switch phenomenon," which is a highly controversial, presumed effect of the TCAs. Switch characterizes a drug-induced episode of mania resulting from antidepressant therapy. The switch phenomenon may be a consequence of a drug's antimuscarinic potency since tertiary amine TCA use is associated with more manic episodes than other drugs. Studies have shown that prior to the advent of the tricyclic agents, the incidence of manic episodes in depressed patients was 3% and thereafter 9% (see Janowsky and Overstreet, 1995, for discussion). Whether or not this increased incidence represents a group of subclinical bipolar patients or a drug-induced side effect may not be as important as an appreciation for the possibility that the switch might occur in some patients.

Effects on Sleep

Because of their antimuscarinic actions, the TCAs and non-SSRI heterocyclics promote drowsiness and sleep in keeping with their designation as minor tranquilizers. Phenelzine is mildly sedating while the nonhydrazine, irreversible MAOIs and the RIMAs can actually be activating and lead to insomnia, probably because of their lower $alpha_1$-adrenergic antagonist potency. Sedation is not an issue with the SSRIs, and many patients report insomnia with chronic treatment, perhaps as a result of their ability to disrupt 5HT-mediated sleep induction (see Stokes, 1993). As a rule, the more a drug increases NE activity acutely, the less sedating it is, but at higher dosages even desipramine is sedating.

The antidepressants alter sleep architecture in a manner different from the sedative-hypnotic drugs. Thus, the antidepressants and the TCAs in particular increase the amount of time spent in stage II and IV sleep whereas the sedative-hypnotics enhance stages II and III. The antidepressants delay the onset of the first REM episode, which often occurs immediately after sleep onset in many depressed patients. Normalization of REM latency has been used as an index of drug responsiveness and as a confirmation of appropriate drug choice.

Weight Gain

Weight gain is common with antidepressants and is often a cause of noncompliance in depressed patients. Both serotonin and histamine stimulate the satiety center and increased activity at their receptors in the hypothalamus may be responsible for decreasing appetite. Desipramine, the least-potent TCA at blocking histamine and 5HT receptors, has the least effect on weight while flunarazine, a drug that induces 5HT release, has been shown to reduce the craving for carbohydrate that is responsible for obesity in some patients (Rapoport, 1989). These data suggest that antidepressants which block both 5HT and histamine receptors, such as amitriptyline, nortriptyline, and imipramine, are most likely to produce weight gain.

Other Effects

Like the antipsychotics, TCAs and maprotiline in particular reduce the seizure threshold (Jabbari et al., 1985). Seizures become increasingly likely during chronic high-dose therapy following a dramatic increase in dosage or as part of the overdose profile. Although all of the antidepressants can produce nausea and vomiting, the SSRIs are most potent. Indeed, aside from insomnia, nausea and vomiting are the most common side effect of the SSRIs. The nausea and vomiting associated with antidepressant use are probably a result of centrally mediated effects and occur independent of stimulation of the CTZ. All antidepressants and the TCAs in particular increase tremor. Nonspecific beta-adrenergic receptor blockers such as propranolol can be effectively used to reduce the severity of tremor, implicating increased NE as its cause. However, the SSRIs also produce tremor, and since they are highly specific for the 5HT system, the cause of antidepressant-induced tremor remains unknown. The TCAs, heterocyclics, and especially the SSRIs are associated with a delay in orgasm as well as impotence. Finally, the hydrazine MAOIs, such as phenelzine, are associated with hepatotoxicity in a small number of cases (Tollefson, 1983). This hepatotoxicity may manifest itself early on as a peripheral neuropathy secondary to a pyridoxine deficiency.

PHARMACOKINETIC CONSIDERATIONS

TCAs and Non-SSRI Heterocyclics

The pharmacokinetics of the TCAs and non-SSRI heterocyclics are similar. Overall, these compounds are almost totally absorbed following oral administration. Those with significant antimuscarinic activity reduce gastric motility and delay absorption. The high lipid solubility of the TCAs and the non-SSRI heterocyclics yields very high apparent volumes of distribution and they are highly bound to plasma proteins. Unbound drug distributes selectively to tissues (10 : 1 tissue to plasma ratio) and readily enters the CNS. The TCAs and non-SSRI heterocyclics undergo significant first-pass metabolism mainly by oxidation and hydroxylation. Side-chain demethylation also occurs and can convert tertiary amine TCAs to biologically active secondary amines. Thus, the tertiary amines imipramine and amitriptyline are respectively converted into desipramine and nortriptyline. Such biotransformation is always associated with a reduction in affinity for muscarinic and adrenergic receptors. Almost all of the phase I products are glucuronidated and excreted in the urine. Very little enterohepatic recycling takes place and only 3 to 10% of the parent compound is excreted unchanged.

The half-lives of the tricyclic and non-SSRI heterocyclic agents vary from 20 to 80 hours. These are wide interindividual variations. Probably as a result of genetic factors, the relationship between dosage administered and plasma level attained is difficult to predict.

SSRIs

The pharmacokinetics of fluoxetine have been extensively studied and represent an important characteristic of this drug. Fluoxetine is well absorbed orally; its bioavailability is estimated at approximately 72% (see Stokes, 1993). It has a half-life of one to three days and its active metabolite norfluoxetine has a half-life ranging from seven to 15 days. This extended half-life of the parent compound and its metabolite readily allows for once-a-day dosing and reduces the potential rebound effects associated with the use of other short-acting agents. Fluoxetine is not significantly plasma bound and is excreted mostly in urine.

MAOIs

The irreversible MAOIs are well absorbed following oral administration and only moderately protein bound. The elimination half-lives of these agents are generally considered to be around three hours. Since they are suicide inhibitors, however, their metabolites become bound to MAO and their covalently bound forms will remain in the body until the MAO-inhibitor complex is eliminated. The hydrazines (phenelzine and isocarboxazid) are biotransformed by acetylation and since about half the population are slow acetylators genetically, the half-lives of these agents can be extended dramatically. In contrast to the irreversible inhibitors, the RIMAs behave pharmacokinetically more like traditional drugs in that their activity is terminated by the usual routes of biotransformation and excretion. Approximately half of the moclobemide found in plasma is bound to proteins and its half-life is one to three hours.

ANTIDEPRESSANT TOXICITY

TCA *Toxicity*

TCA toxicity is a major concern because these drugs are primarily used in a group of patients who often have suicidal tendencies to begin with. Antidepressants were the leading cause of drug-related deaths in the United States in 1988 (Litovitz et al., 1988). The major signs and symptoms of overdose include cardiovascular toxicity, CNS depression, and such antimuscarinic effects as paralysis of accommodation and urinary retention (Table 11–3). Depending on the agent, cardiac toxicity may be preceded by sinus tachycardia and hypertension due to inhibition of NE reuptake. The tachycardia can last for days if the drug also has significant antimuscarinic activity. The quinidine-like effects can cause conduction block, fibrillation, electromechanical dissociation, asystole, and death. If these

Table 11–3 Signs and Symptoms of Tricyclic Antidepressant Toxicity

Cardiovascular signs
  Tachycardia/bradycardia
  Conduction block
  Fibrillation
  Asystole
  Hypertension/hypotension

CNS signs
  Agitation
  Disorientation
  Delirium
  Hallucinations
  Myoclonus
  Severe dystonia
  Seizures

Antimuscarinic signs
  Paralysis of accommodation
  Inability to sweat
  Warm, flushed skin
  Decreased secretions
  Hyperthermia
  Loss of bowel sounds
  Urinary retention
  Mydriasis/normal pupils

effects predominate, hypotension will result from myocardial depression. Drugs with potent alpha$_1$-adrenergic antagonistic actions tend to produce hypotension. The cardiovascular effects are accompanied by significant CNS signs and symptoms including delirium, agitation, hallucinations, myoclonic jerks, dystonia, and seizures. The seizures are often self-limiting but can develop into status epilepticus. Although coma can be treated with the cholinomimetic agent physostigmine if it occurs, the seizures are often unresponsive, which suggests that they are only partially an antimuscarinic effect of the drugs.

The peripheral signs resulting from the blockade of muscarinic receptors include loss of visual accommodation although narrow-angle glaucoma is rare even in the toxic state; inability to sweat; warm, flushed skin; decreased salivation; increased temperature (especially if dystonia or myoclonus is part of the presentation); reduced gastrointestinal motility; and urinary retention. Mydriasis may occur if antimuscarinic potency is not counteracted by significant NE-reuptake inhibition. This constellation of central and peripheral signs and symptoms largely represents anticholinergic toxicity. It can be recalled with the mnemonic, "Hot as a hare, blind as a stone, mad as a hatter, and dry as a bone."

Because of the potentially lethal consequences of tricyclic antidepressant overdose, precautions must be taken in its management (see Krishel and Jackimczyk, 1991, for review). In general, no assumption should be made about the number of pills consumed as the potential for lethal toxicity always exists due to wide interpatient variability in bioavailability and susceptibility. Pediatric patients are more likely to succumb. Patients should have cardiac monitoring, an open i.v. line, and continuous ventilatory assessment. If their mental status changes, naloxone, thiamine, dextrose, and oxygen may be needed. Treatment of agitation or aggressive behavior should not include the antipsychotics because they can further reduce seizure threshold. Because of gastrointestinal stasis (antimuscarinic actions), lavage should be started immediately. This is most successful in reducing the duration of symptoms if it begins within six hours of ingestion. After lavage, activated charcoal should be given. A catheter should be inserted to maintain urinary secretion.

Sodium bicarbonate is the mainstay in the treatment of cardiovascular toxicity. Alkalinization both circumvents the direct quinidine-like effects of these drugs on Na$^+$ channels and reduces the amount of unbound drug. Because the cardiac toxicity results from quinidine-like effects on Na$^+$ channels, quinidine, procainamide, and disopyramide are all contraindicated. Sodium bicarbonate also helps avoid the tendency toward seizures. If seizures do occur, intravenous diazepam is the treatment of choice. The antimuscarinic signs can be alleviated by administering the cholinomimetic physostigmine. This acetylcholinesterase inhibitor is a tertiary amine that readily penetrates the BBB and is therefore effective at reducing the central as well as the peripheral muscarinic blockade.

Toxicity of Non-TCA Antidepressants

As can be seen, the toxic profile of TCA overdose is a serious matter. The advent of newer antidepressants, especially the SSRIs, has been a great advantage in avoiding potentially fatal overdoses. MAOI toxicity can be associated with significant morbidity and in some cases mortality although the clinical sequelae are not nearly as dangerous as is TCA overdose. The toxic syndrome involves agitation, hyperactivity, hallucinosis, hyperpyrexia, convulsions, and delirium. These are all thought to represent the central manifestations of increased levels of biogenic amines.

Drug Interactions

The antidepressants interact with several other drugs. The classic teaching example is the reduced efficacy of the antihypertensive drug guanethidine (a vesicular pool depletor). As NE-reuptake inhibitors, the TCAs and non-SSRI heterocyclics prevent guanethidine from being taken up into NE terminals, thereby blocking access of the drug to its locus of action. The antidepressants in general will potentiate the effects of any coadministered drug that increases biogenic amine activity. Because of their quinidine-like effects, the TCAs should be used with extreme caution in patients on antiarrhythmic medications. Antimuscarinic-induced gastrointestinal stasis will delay gastrointestinal transit time, thereby affecting the absorption of virtually any other drug administered enterally. Since the TCAs and non-SSRI heterocyclics produce sedation, additive effects with other sedative-hypnotic drugs should be anticipated. Since they are highly protein bound, an increase in the level of unbound drug should be anticipated when other drugs that have affinity for plasma proteins are coadministered (phenytoin, aspirin). Certain steroids (e.g., birth control pills) that are metabolized in the hepatic microsomal enzyme system reduce TCA biotransformation and potentiate toxicity. On the other hand, enzyme inducers such as cigarette smoking and barbiturates reduce plasma levels.

The MAOIs interact with several drugs that act via biogenic amines. Since MAO catalyzes the breakdown of norepinephrine, epinephrine, serotonin, and other biogenic amines, the action of any drug that enhances the activity of these neurotransmitters would be potentiated. This is especially true of the sympathomimetics, and such an interaction can lead to hypertensive crisis. The hepatic biotransformation of the hydrazine MAOIs will interfere with the biotranformation of several other drug classes including the anesthetics, analgesics, antihistamines, alcohol, and some sedatives. Life-threatening hyperpyrexia can follow the administration of meperidine with an MAOI or an SSRI. This effect is thought to be mediated by 5HT release.

The administration of an SSRI and an MAOI can produce the so-called serotonin syndrome, involving hyperthermia, rigidity, myoclonus, extreme fluctuations in vital signs, and dramatic alterations in mental status. Lethality is extremely rare, however. The syndrome is effectively managed with nonspecific 5HT-receptor antagonists such as cyprohepta-dine. The SSRIs are also potent inhibitors of hepatic microsomal oxidases. Any drug that depends on this system for biotransformation, such as codeine, acetaminophen, and diazepam, would exhibit higher than anticipated plasma levels.

Despite the success of antidepressant monotherapy, a significant minority of patients remain refractory to treatment. Some of these patients may benefit from combining an MAOI with a TCA or an SSRI. At one time this strategy was considered extremely dangerous. With the advent of the RIMAs, however, the combination of MAOIs with other antidepressants has become more common. If toxicity develops, it will reverse itself quickly and, after a brief period of drug washout (less than three days), traditional monotherapy can be safely reinstated.

OTHER USES FOR ANTIDEPRESSANTS

Because of the number of neurotransmitter systems they affect, the antidepressant drugs are used in a number of settings that do not include clinical depression. Reference to the use of TCAs in the management of migraine headache and chronic pain has already been made in previous chapters. These drugs are, however, also used in several other disorders.

The antidepressants, especially fluoxetine, are effective in obsessive-compulsive disorders (OCD; Wood, Tollefson, and Birkett, 1993) where depression is often a core symptom. Clinical trials revealed that antidepressants such as clomipramine that are more selective for serotonin were effective in some patients. Fluoxetine also has been shown to reduce OCD symptoms in nondepressed patients, suggesting that 5HT is centrally involved with this disorder. SSRIs also are being tried in eating disorders such as bulimia and anorexia nervosa.

Imipramine, MAOIs, and in particular the SSRIs can be effective in managing panic attacks. The TCAs, especially imipramine, are also useful in treating nighttime enuresis and geriatric incontinence. Their combined antimuscarinic actions, sedative-hypnotic properties and alpha$_1$-adrenergic antagonism are thought to be responsible. Imipramine and desipramine have also been used with some success in AD/HD patients, especially those with coexisting Gilles de la Tourette syndrome or clinical depression. Because of their antihistaminergic actions, amitriptyline, doxepin, and trimipramine are sometimes used for peptic ulcer. If it is assumed that excess gastric acidity aggravates ulcers, the CNS actions of these drugs would also be expected to reduce the perception of stress that can increase gastric acidity. Finally, the TCAs have been used in the treatment of sleep apnea, peripheral diabetic neuropathy, and narcolepsy.

BIPOLAR DISORDER

The focus of this chapter thus far has been on depression alone. The treatment of manic-depressive illness and its behavioral syndrome is, however, different. In their manic phases, bipolar patients may have inflated self-esteem and be prone toward grandiosity. They may be agitated and euphoric. Psychotic features including delusions and even hallucinations may occur. These behaviors are opposite to those characterizing depression. As patients cycle between manic and depressive phases, they often go through periods of normal behavior. It is as though their moods continuously vary along a continuum polarized by elation and depression.

A positive family history is a definite risk factor for bipolar disorder. The risk of manic-depression or severe recurrent unipolar depression is approximately 20% for first-degree relatives and 70% for monozygotic twins, while in the general population, the incidence is only 1–2% (Goodwin and Jamison, 1990). Thus, there is strong evidence of a genetic basis for the disease. Whereas depression is more common in females (2–3 to 1), manic-depression is equally prevalent in both sexes.

In addition to behavioral changes, bipolar patients also exhibit marked alterations in hormonal functions, sleep patterns and circadian rhythms during their mood swings which, together with the genetic evidence, suggests a neurologic substrate for the disorder. It is difficult, however, to envision how a single neurotransmitter system or specific brain locus could be responsible for the disparate cluster of signs and symptoms that characterizes manic-depression. Thus, it is commonly assumed that the neurologic abnormalities associated with manic-depression must encompass dysfunction in a number of systems that participate in the regulation of mood. These systems are likely to involve the biogenic amines, the cholinergic system and possibly the enkephalin system (see Carroll, 1994). This assumption is also based on the observations that: (1) TCAs alleviate depressive symptoms; (2) cholinergic antagonists trigger mood shifts (the switch phenomenon); (3) antipsychotics alleviate some manic symptoms; and (4) changes in biogenic amines and en-kephalins influence mood. Recent evidence suggests that disruption of a second-messenger system common to all of these neurotransmitters might be involved in the pathogenesis of bipolar disorder.

Pharmacotherapy of Bipolar Disorder

Lithium

Lithium is strikingly effective at moderating the mood swings that char-acterize bipolar patients. What is so remarkable about this therapy is that lithium improves both mania and depression. It is clinically effective in an estimated 80% of appropriately diagnosed patients. Lithium thus has greater efficacy than any other drug used in the treatment of psychiatric disorders (Lenox and Watson, 1994). Moreover, it is even capable of pre-venting the occurrence of episodes of recurrent depression in some unipo-lar patients.

As the lightest of the Ia alkali metals, it was originally assumed that lithium substituted for Na^+ in the generation of action potentials. How-ever, in vitro studies did not support this hypothesis since replacement of Na^+ with lithium was only capable of supporting one or two action po-tentials before the neuron would completely shut down. Other hypothe-ses emerged suggesting an action at DA receptors, inhibiting CA^{2+}-depen-dent release of NE and DA or facilitating the reuptake of catecholamines. Lithium may interfere with the ability of neurotransmitters to stimulate cAMP by antagonizing adenylate cyclase (DiPalma, 1987), although this action is now thought to be more responsible for certain side effects such as its potent diuretic actions.

Recent data support the idea that lithium inhibits the regeneration of phosphinositol and thus reduces the production of the second-messengers diacylglycerol (DAG) and inositol triphosphate (IP_3). Interestingly, the neurotransmitters described above share one common feature—the gen-eration of DAG and IP_3. Since these second messengers are involved in intracellular Ca^{2+} mobilization, activation of prostaglandins, and alter-ations in the phosphorylation of key proteins that regulate neurotrans-mitter release and cytoskeletal changes involved in plasticity, many of the initial observations concerning alterations in catecholamine function, Ca^{2+} mobilization, and receptor changes can be explained through this one common mechanism.

Lithium inhibits the enzyme myo-inositol-1 phosphatase (see Ber-ridge, 1989, for review). Since the inositol cascade depends on recycling of precursors from normal cell metabolism and dietary sources, lithium's inhibition of myo-inositol-1 phosphatase would leave a neuron solely dependent upon dietary sources for its precursor pool to maintain adequate levels of the IP_3 precursor PIP_2. The binding of serotonin, for instance, to its receptor would activate the G protein that activates phospholipase C, which in turn mobilizes PIP_2 (see Fig. 11–10), but the restricted pool of PIP_2 after myo-inositol-1 phosphatase inhibition would eventually lead to reduced levels of DAG and IP_3. By reducing DAG, lithium reduces activation of protein kinase C (Blackshear, 1988). Since PKC is responsible for phosphorylating a number of proteins including one called MARKS (myristoylated alanine-rich C-kinase substrate), it has been proposed that alterations in phosphorylation status are responsible for the therapeutic efficacy of lithium. MARKS is thought to regulate cytoskeletal el-

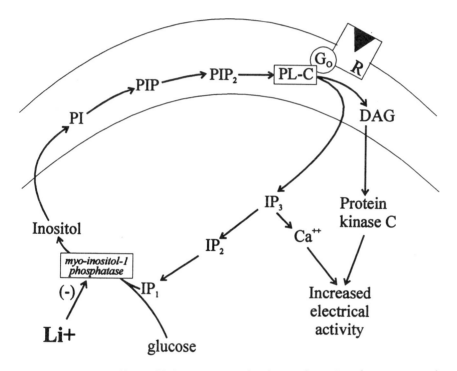

Figure 11–10. The effects of lithium (Li^+) on the electrical activity of a neuron are depicted in this schematic. Normally a neurotransmitter binding to its receptor (R) initiates the production of diacylglycerol (DAG) and inositol triphosphate (IP_3). DAG activates protein kinase C while IP_3 induces CA^{2+} release, both of which lead to increased neuronal activity. IP_3 is subsequently catabolized to IP_2 and IP_1, which then combine with glucose to form inositol via the enzyme myo-inositol-1 phosphatase. The inositol is reincorporated into the membrane, where it is progressively synthesized into the phosphoinositide precursor PIP_2. Lithium, by blocking the activity of myo-inositol-1 phosphatase, depletes the neuron of PIP_2, thereby reducing the ability of the neurotransmitter to increase neuronal activity by its second-messenger systems.

ements involved in neurotransmitter release and plasticity, and altering this protein could have a profound effect on neuronal function (see Lenox and Watson, 1994). More importantly, this effect would depend on the activity of the neuron. If it is assumed that inhibitory and excitatory neurons are most active during the extreme phases of the disease, lithium's blockade of the phosphoinositide cascade would be most effective at those times. Moreover, since the PIP_2 precursor pool could be maintained by the diet, overt drug-induced behavioral alterations such as confusion or dysarthria would not be expected at normal dosages during periods of normal behavior. Indeed, lithium does not normally produce such effects.

Although this hypothesis seems too simple to explain the complex behavioral patterns of bipolar illness, there are several consistencies to it. The concentration at which lithium blocks the phosphoinositide cascade is similar to the concentrations normally achieved in clinical settings. In addition, the time course of the alterations in the phosphorylation of MARKS is consistent with the known clinical effects of lithium. Phosphorylation of MARKS only occurs after seven days of lithium treatment and remains altered for several days after treatment stops. Lithium often requires a week to ten days to attenuate manic episodes and symptom reemergence follows by several days abrupt discontinuation of therapy. The hypothesis that inhibition of the phosphoinositide cascade by lithium is responsible for its therapeutic effects in manic-depressive illness patients has thus acquired significant support.

Lithium Side Effects. Lithium has several side effects (Table 11–4) that are, fortunately, mild at the dosages used clinically. Dysphoria, slowed reaction time, lack of spontaneity, and impaired intellectual function are common early in therapy. These symptoms generally resolve spontaneously or in response to a subtle adjustment of dosage. A fine tremor is frequently associated with lithium treatment although it rarely compromises function. Polyuria and polydipsia are common and probably reflect reduced responsiveness to antidiuretic hormone (ADH) secondary to lithium's inhibition of adenylate cyclase. Inhibition of adenylate cyclase is also thought to be responsible for lithium's well-known inhibition of thyroid function. Conversely, hyperparathyroidism is seen and is exaggerated by the ability of lithium to enhance CA^{2+} reabsorption in the kidney. Nausea and vomiting characterize the initial phase of treatment but are generally transient. Similarly, the competition between lithium and Na^+ in the bowel reduces glucose and water absorption and leads to transient diarrhea and abdominal cramps. Lithium is also associated with a myasthenia-like syndrome, increased intracranial pressure, polyneuropathy, and malignant syndrome although these side effects are rare.

Table 11–4 Side Effects and Toxic Effects of Lithium

Side effects
  Dysphoria
  Slowed reaction time
  Lack of spontaneity
  Impaired intellectual capacity
  Fine tremor
  Polyuria
  Polydipsia
  Compromised thyroid function (goiter)
  Hyperparathyroidism
  Nausea and vomiting
  Diarrhea and abdominal cramps
  Myasthenia-like syndrome
  Increased intracranial pressure
  Polyneuropathy
  Neuroleptic malignant syndrome

Toxic signs and symptoms
  An intensification of normal side effects
  Confusion
  Hyperreflexia
  Gross tremor
  Dysarthria
  Seizures
  Focal neurologic signs
  Cardiac arrhythmias
  Hypotension
  Impaired renal function (rare)

Lithium Pharmacokinetics and Toxicity. Despite the drug's heralded efficacy, management of the patient on lithium can be difficult. Lithium has a very low therapeutic index (2–3) so the therapeutic window, in which plasma levels must be maintained between 0.8 and 1.2 mEq, is narrow. Levels above 1.2 mEq are considered toxic. Lithium toxicity does not necessarily imply a suicide attempt or unintentional overdose. Rather, its mechanism of action coupled with some of its unique pharmacokinetic characteristics occasionally produce an upward spiral of plasma levels that can lead to toxicity even in patients who are followed carefully. The toxicity can develop quickly over a few days.

As in alkali metal, lithium is handled by the body as Na^+ and K^+ are. It is readily absorbed orally and distributed in body water but some tissue binding occurs, giving it an apparent volume of distribution just above body water volume. Although it is a monovalent cation, lithium does not have comparable affinity for monovalent transport proteins and thus does not cross the BBB as readily as Na^+ or K^+. As a result, CSF concentrations of lithium are only half of those of plasma. Disruption of the

BBB, as might occur with heavy alcohol consumption or infection, allows more lithium to enter the brain and quickly leads to CNS toxicity. Distributed in body water, lithium is excreted mostly in urine (95%). Interestingly, lithium is preferentially excreted in sweat. As an alkali metal, it is 80% reabsorbed in the proximal renal tubules with minimal reabsorption in the distal tubules. Conditions that facilitate Na^+ reabsorption, such as dehydration, lead to increased reabsorption of lithium and to toxicity. Thus, even though sweat contains a disproportionate amount of lithium relative to Na^+, the dehydrating effects of exercise increase its reabsorption, producing a net increase in lithium levels and subsequent toxicity. The potential for toxicity is especially prevalent with diuretic agents such as furosemide that, by promoting Na^+ loss, lead to dehydration and increased lithium reabsorption. Extreme caution must therefore be exercised when coadministering diuretics and lithium.

Because of the potential for peak-dose toxicity, lithium is frequently delivered in multiple divided doses or in sustained-release capsules that smooth peak–trough concentration differences. Despite this treatment regimen, plasma levels must still be monitored. Although it is primarily excreted in the urine, some tissue binding occurs, producing a two-phase excretion. Plasma is cleared in six to eight hours and a second, slower excretion phase occurs over a period of a week. For this reason, failure to take a daily dose does not necessarily lead to a severe risk of manic episodes.

Since lithium clearance is similar to that of Na^+, any medical condition that leads to dehydration will increase plasma levels. Slightly elevated levels for even short periods of time lead to intracellular accumulation. Thus, minor elevations of lithium levels increase the inhibition of adenylate cyclase and further reduce ADH sensitivity, contributing to further dehydration and so on. Lithium also reduces aldosterone's ability to stimulate Na^+ reabsorption, which also contributes to dehydration and toxicity. In a sense then, lithium toxicity can be a self-perpetuating process that may occur at the high end of the therapeutic range.

Acutely, plasma levels significantly higher than lithium's therapeutic range are needed to produce signs and symptoms of toxicity whereas after several weeks of treatment the toxicity is more likely to result from intracellular accumulation and can occur at plasma levels as low as the high end of the therapeutic range. In either case, the signs and symptoms of lithium toxicity follow a general pattern of intensified CNS side effects. These are fatal in 10 to 20% of severely intoxicated patients (Table 11–4). Treatment involves symptom-based support and dialysis to reduce the total body burden of lithium. However, reduction of plasma levels does not necessarily resolve the toxic syndrome since its primary cause is intracellular lithium. For this reason, repeated dialysis is generally needed (see Krishel and Jackimczyk, 1991, for review).

Carbamazepine and valproic acid

The antiepileptic agents carbamazepine and valproate have been shown to be effective in some bipolar patients. Their pharmacology was reviewed in Chapter 6. Carbamazepine is structurally related to the TCAs and shares some of their properties. However, the basis for its antidepressant action is unknown and other antiepileptic agents, especially valproate, have been shown to be similarly effective. Carbamazepine and valproate also possess antimanic actions and can be effective in lithium-resistant patients. They may be particularly effective in patients characterized as rapid cyclers.

Drugs of Abuse and Addiction

F or millennia humans have used drugs for nonmedicinal, mind-altering purposes. Now nonmedicinal drug use has reached epidemic proportions in some societies. Although the addictive nature of some drugs contributes to their continued use, they are often taken at first because of their ability to induce euphoria and dreamlike states, or to dissociate users from their surroundings. Many teenagers, however, experiment with drugs because their peers are doing so.

We are beginning to unravel the neurobiology that underlies the actions of "street" drugs. All the drugs considered in this chapter potentially induce dependence, but significant exposure does not necessarily produce dependence in everyone while occasional use can lead to dependence in some people. The ability of a drug to induce dependence thus involves a complex interplay among a neurobiologic predisposition, the unique characteristics of the drug, and the environment in which it is used.

TERMINOLOGY

Confusion surrounds the use of some terms that refer to drug dependence. The following definitions are derived from *The Pharmacological Basis of Therapeutics* (Eighth Edition, Jaffe, Chapter 22, 1990).

Drug abuse can be defined loosely as the use, generally by self-administration, of a drug in a way that deviates from the social norms of a given culture. This is a sociological definition that incorporates the cultural setting in which the pattern of drug use occurs. Coca leaves are chewed by the Peruvian Indians, but this would not be considered abuse because it is socially sanctioned. Most members of a given culture readily recognize an abuse pattern when the consumption of a drug begins to interfere with an individual's ability to conform to social norms. The term drug abuse therefore describes a pattern of use rather than a qualitative or quantitative measure of drug consumption.

Recreational use is the occasional use of a drug for its pleasurable effects. Whether this type of use is accepted by society depends upon the drug and the setting. Recreational use can lead to drug abuse, however. Taking drugs such as marijuana, tobacco, and alcohol is thought to increase the likelihood that other drugs such as cocaine or heroin will be tried (Johnson, 1995) Thus, tobacco, alcohol, and marijuana are often referred to as gateway drugs.

Situational use refers to the consumption of drugs because they are perceived by the user as helpful in a given situation. Coffee and amphetamine consumption by students and truck drivers and self-administration of codeine for a severe ankle strain fall in this category. The gateway notion applies here as well, although situational use is not as likely to lead to drug abuse unless the user begins to consume the drug for recreational purposes.

Drug dependence refers to a pattern of use in which the individual perceives the need to continue usage. This usage occurs without medical need and often despite adverse social and health consequences. It can be characterized as compulsive: When the drug is not available, the individual becomes preoccupied with its acquisition. The term drug dependence can also be applied to the individual taking opioids for chronic pain. All the characteristics of drug dependence are present, but in a medical context. As described in Chapter 4, this type of use rarely leads to addiction. Although chronic pain patients may become dependent on a drug and exhibit compulsive usage, they probably should not be characterized as drug abusers because of the socially unacceptable connotation this term conveys.

Physical dependence is manifested by the overt signs and symptoms of withdrawal from chronic use of a drug. This constellation of signs and symptoms is relatively consistent within a population abusing the same drug class and is called the withdrawal syndrome. Thus, withdrawal from morphine and meperidine produces a similar withdrawal syndrome that is different from the syndrome associated with withdrawal from cocaine and amphetamine. The term physical dependence was originally used to describe physical signs such as diarrhea or vomiting and was distinguished from psychological dependence, the craving for a drug. It is now believed that overt physical signs and craving are all manifestations of "neuroadaptation," albeit in different areas of the nervous system. The term neuroadaptation refers to the alterations in neuronal function brought about by exposure to a drug and encompasses pharmacodynamic, physiologic, and reverse tolerance. Thus, physiologic tolerance to heroin in the myenteric plexus leads to diarrhea upon drug withdrawal and is functionally similar to the tolerance that occurs in the locus ceruleus which is thought to be responsible for the anxiety often seen during withdrawal. The drug craving (psychological dependence) associated with the use of these drugs is now viewed as resulting from reverse tolerance (sensitization) in the nucleus accumbens. The distinction between physical and psychological dependence is therefore artificial and the more encompassing term drug dependence is used.

Addiction is the term used to describe an overall pattern of compulsive drug abuse characterized by consistent preoccupation with drug consumption and procurement and a tendency to relapse after withdrawal. It is the extreme on the continuum of the patterns of abuse described above. The point at which dependence becomes addiction is nebulous. In the past, "addiction" referred to a state of drug dependence in which physical signs of withdrawal occurred when chronic drug use stopped. Since some drugs of abuse, such as amphetamine, do not produce these types of symptoms, they were not considered addictive. This led to confusion, but it is not likely that the terms addict and addiction will leave our vocabulary soon.

Narcotic is technically the term used to describe members of the opioid family. However, it has been generalized by law enforcement agencies and the legal profession to include most commonly abused street drugs.

THE NEUROBIOLOGY OF ADDICTION

Several theories have been advanced to explain drug dependence. These include the redundancy model, in which continued drug exposure activates several different parallel neuronal pathways (Martin, 1986), theories involving the desire to avoid the withdrawal syndrome (see Wise and Bozarth, 1987), and positive reinforcement models where addicts purportedly abuse a drug because it is pleasurable to them (Stewart, de Wit, and Eikelboom, 1984). Unfortunately, these theories are descriptive and derive primarily from studies of the pattern of abuse seen in opioid dependence.

One theory that has been useful is based on the principle of "counteradaptation" (Koob and Bloom, 1988), which incorporates the many changes in the regulation of synaptic physiology that accompany chronic exposure to a drug. In the 1970s and 1980s, these changes were assumed to involve simple alterations in receptor number, neurotransmitter release, and synthesis. Chronic administration of morphine, for instance, led to the down-regulation of enkephalin receptors and to reduced enkephalin synthesis. When the drug was withdrawn, the addict would seek it in order to normalize the enkephalin system. The withdrawal symptoms and drug craving that developed were assumed to be a consequence of the same neuroadaptive processes. From this viewpoint, all aspects of the addiction phenomenon are linked to pharmacodynamic tolerance in the same system. Thus, the reduction in enkephalin activity associated with pharmacodynamic tolerance would produce changes in neuronal function that lead to both the withdrawal syndrome and the craving. For many drugs, however, the development of tolerance and of addiction do not coincide temporally, which suggests that two distinct mechanisms are involved. The theory may account for many aspects of the withdrawal syndrome, but probably not the craving.

Any theory of dependence must explain certain essential features of the addictive process that appear to be common to all drugs of abuse:

1. While different drug groups have different physiologic and behavioral effects, the craving is remarkably similar for all dependence-producing drugs.
2. Environmental factors influence not only the acute effects of drugs but the likelihood of eventual dependence and relapse as well.
3. There are genetic predispositions to drug dependence.
4. With continued exposure to a drug, the desire to consume it increases even though in many cases the ability of the drug to induce euphoria has greatly diminished.
5. For many drugs, the peak of the craving does not occur during abstinence but right at the time of drug's peak effect.

Although the varied acute effects of the different drug classes are easy to understand because each drug class affects different neurotransmitter systems, the similarity of their dependence-invoking effects suggests some action common to all these drugs.

Robinson and Berridge (1993) have advanced an "incentive-sensitization" theory that incorporates the major features of drug dependence and also explains how such a disparate group of drugs can share a similar dependence liability. At the heart of this theory is the development of reverse tolerance or sensitization in the mesolimbic DA pathway. The ability of a drug of abuse to increase dopamine levels in the n. accumbens is viewed as being responsible for establishing "incentive salience," a sense of reward associated with all the salient features of the drug experience including the perception and mental representation of the drug and the events surrounding its consumption. Because of sensitization within this system, the normal desire for the drug (for its pleasurable effects) is transformed into craving. This craving becomes independent of the euphoric properties of the drug and will occur even if consumption is no longer pleasurable. Since sensitization is long-lasting, it can explain why addiction is a relapsing disorder.

The n. accumbens (ventral striatum) lies just anterior and inferior to the caudate and putamen. Although it is structurally similar to the striatum in its internal neuronal architecture, its connections are different (Fig. 12–1). Thus, its primary inputs arise in phylogenetically older regions of the cortex including the entorhinal, temporal, and anterior cingulate cortices. It also receives afferent projections from the amygdala and hippocampus. The n. accumbens projects to the septum, the hypothalamus, and, via the ventral pallidum, to the frontal and cingulate cortices. Based on its connections, it is clearly an important center of limbic function. In addition to its role in the expression of the positive symptoms of schizophrenia (see Chapter 10), the n. accumbens is also an important reward center. Rats will endure significant pain to activate an electrode implanted in this region. Such reward or reinforcement centers are thought to be centrally involved in the associative learning process.

The mesolimbic dopaminergic pathway is an important afferent projection to the n. accumbens. Dopamine is thought to modulate the flow of electrical activity through the n. accumbens and to regulate the "associative" processes that occur there. Increased dopamine activity in the n. accumbens raises the probability that behaviors occurring at the time of increased dopamine will be expressed in the future (e.g., see Phillips, Robbins, and Everitt, 1994).

All drugs that have significant dependence liability are known to increase the release of dopamine in the n. accumbens, including cocaine, amphetamine, opioids, alcohol, caffeine, barbiturates, nicotine, phencyclidine (PCP), and several designer drugs (Fig. 12–1; see also Di Chiara and Imperato, 1988; Robinson and Berridge, 1993; Nestler, 1994). Drugs such as cocaine directly activate the DA system whereas other drugs, such as nicotine, indirectly increase dopamine release. When animal self-administration is used as a model for the craving phenomenon, DA antagonists infused into the n. accumbens prevent self-administration of a drug that would otherwise lead to significant dependence. Drugs that do not affect dopamine or block its activity in the n. accumbens are not self-administered and do not possess abuse potential.

The reverse tolerance (sensitization) phenomenon has been extensively studied in rats self-administering cocaine. In this case, the mechanism of sensitization appears to involve the modulation of second messengers and gene transcription in the n. accumbens as a consequence of

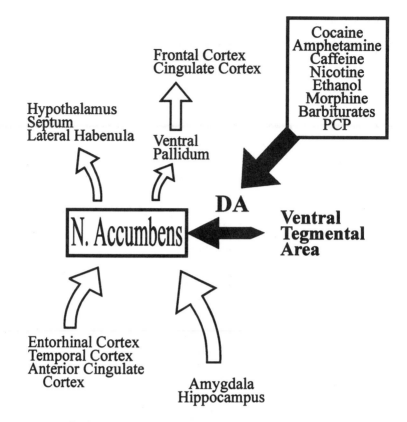

Figure 12–1. All of the currently known drugs that possess dependence liability are known to enhance dopamine (DA) activity in the n. accumbens as depicted in this figure. These drugs increase DA through several different mechanisms as described in the text. Through the afferent and efferent connections of the n. accumbens, this region can readily control the development of contingent reward, leading to "drug craving." This craving is thought to occur independent of the other effects of these drugs such as the withdrawal syndrome, tolerance, and euphoria.

dopamine receptor activation (Fig. 12–2). As reviewed by Nestler (1994), dopamine acts on G proteins to alter the level of cAMP in the n. accumbens. In turn, cAMP activates several protein kinases that regulate transcription factors such as CREB (cAMP response element binding protein). These transcription factors bind to specific promoter regions in the DNA and either increase or decrease the rate at which certain genes are transcribed. A protein product of this cascade is a Fos-related antigen (Fra) protein that is only produced after continued exposure to cocaine.

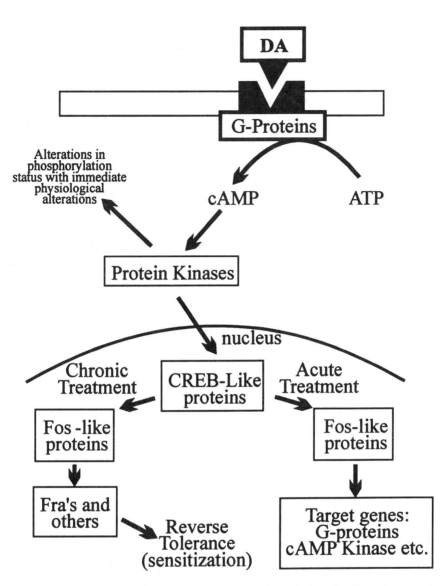

Figure 12–2. As reviewed by Nestler (1994) and described in detail in the text, dependence is thought to be a consequence of reverse tolerance to dopamine (DA) in the n. accumbens. DA activates cAMP which, in turn, activates protein kinases which carry the signal into the nucleus where long-lasting alterations in transcription are thought to occur. Acting through cAMP response element binding protein (CREB), an acute, nuclear response can occur, whereas during chronic treatment, Fos-like proteins have been shown to activate Fra proteins that can lead to reverse tolerance and drug sensitization.

This protein has a half-life of seven to ten days. Its actions therefore continue long after the last cocaine exposure. Fra-mediated changes in neuronal activity, such as receptor sensitivity, the threshold for voltage-gated channels, and neurotransmitter release, could be responsible for reverse tolerance. Through its connections, the sensitized n. accumbens could recruit the activity of other regions of the brain involved in anticipatory need and thereby induce craving. Since stress and other environmental factors increase the release of glucocorticoids that are known to enhance sensitization in the n. accumbens to drugs of abuse (see Kalivas and Stewart, 1991), glucocorticoid-facilitated increases in Fra-like proteins might explain the impact of environmental factors on drug dependence.

Drug-induced changes in the n. accumbens such as the increase in Fra-like proteins or other proteins might also explain the variable susceptibility for dependence within our population. Recent studies have revealed genetic differences in addiction liability and even preferences for a given drug among different strains of rats (see Kosten et al., 1994). These may involve inherited differences in the number of receptors to which the drug of abuse binds, the propensity of the drug to stimulate dopamine release, or the gene loci that regulate the second-messenger cascade of dopamine in the n. accumbens. Addiction susceptibility could therefore be inherited, though still subject to environmental influences. Because of its afferent connections and genetic differences within these pathways, environmental cues or even thinking about past drug experiences would have a variable capacity to activate the n. accumbens once it has been sensitized.

Recent advances in the neurobiology of addiction have provided us with testable hypotheses about he mechanisms underlying the development of drug dependence. Indeed, all of the drugs of abuse described in this chapter (except marijuana, volatile inhalants, and anabolic steroids) have been shown to increase dopamine in the n. accumbens and thus conform to the notion that dopamine sensitization in the n. accumbens is responsible for drug craving. But these drugs differ in several other actions that determine the mood, perceptual, behavioral, and cognitive changes which accompany their abuse. These mechanisms of action also determine the relative safety of the drug, the type of treatment needed by the overdose victim, and the symptoms seen during withdrawal from the drug.

PSYCHOSTIMULANTS

The psychostimulants are a structurally diverse group of drugs (Fig. 12–3) that share the common actions of increasing motor activity and reducing the need for sleep (psychomotor stimulant effects). These drugs also improve concentration and increase reaction time (especially in the

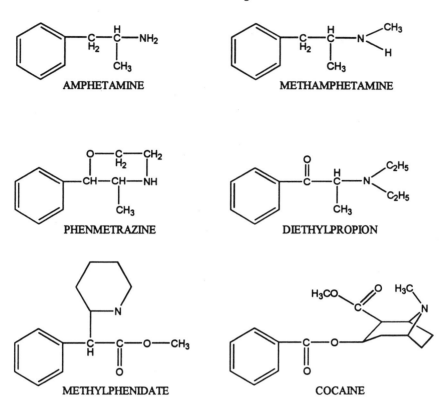

Figure 12–3. The chemical structures of common psychostimulants.

fatigued individual), induce a sense of well-being (euphorogenic effects), and have sympathomimetic effects (increase sympathetic nervous system action). The term central stimulant is also applied to these drugs even though it was formerly reserved for agents that induce seizures such as pentylene tetrazole.

The most commonly used psychostimulants include dextroamphetamine (or simply amphetamine), methamphetamine, phenmetrazine, diethylpropion, and cocaine. These drugs are called by various common names. When amphetamine or methamphetamine is injected intravenously, it is called "speed," but this term is often used to describe the ingestion of amphetamines by any route. Methamphetamine is called "ice" when its free base is extracted into an organic solvent such as ether, pyrolyzed, and smoked. This procedure, applied to cocaine, yields "crack." Drugs used to treat AD/HD such as methylphenidate and pemoline, the pharmacology of which was discussed in Chapter 9, are also classified as psychostimulants. Cathinone (khat), the active substance of the African khat shrub, whose leaves are chewed for their stimulant properties, is also appropriately included in this drug class.

Other drugs have psychostimulant properties but should not be classi-fied as such. These include many antiparkinson drugs such as levodopa and pergolide. Such drugs differ from the psychostimulants in that they all predominantly increase DA activity (Ellinwood, 1975). Caffeine and nicotine share some properties of the stimulant drug class as well but gen-erally do not produce significant euphoria, and at higher dosages they can lead to anxiety and dysphoria.

The anorexiants (appetite suppressors) are often included incorrectly in this category as well. This group of drugs includes phenteramine, benz-phetamine, phendimetrazine, fenfluramine, and phenylpropanolamine. They share many properties with the psychostimulants but are must less potent in this regard. Like the psychostimulants, many anorexiants com-bat drowsiness but they have fewer DA properties, are generally not self-administered by animals, and have negligible addiction liability. Appetite suppression is generally associated with the enhancement of central NE and 5HT activity. Except for fenfluramine, the anorexiants primarily in-crease norepinephrine in the CNS. Fenfluramine is a selective 5HT re-uptake inhibitor and 5HT releasor (see Azmitia and Whitaker-Azmitia, 1995). Its more selective action on the 5HT system and its documented success in reducing carbohydrate consumption have reinforced the no-tion that 5HT is centrally involved in satiety. Fenfluramine has also been used in the treatment of bulimia.

The psychostimulants increase brain DA more than NE levels, and at higher doses they increase 5HT levels. The various effects of these drugs are attributed primarily to the activation of these neurotransmitter sys-tems (Table 12–1) although other neurotransmitters such as glutamate and ACh are probably involved as well, but to a lesser extent. In addition to its effects on NE, DA, and 5HT, cocaine has anesthetic actions ("-caine" properties) that become significant at higher dosages. These anesthetic properties are particularly important considerations in the evaluation and treatment of cocaine overdose victims. Although the psy-chostimulants share many properties, the mechanisms by which the am-phetamine-like drugs and cocaine induce their effects are sufficiently dif-ferent to warrant separate discussion.

Amphetamine, Methamphetamine, Diethylpropion, and Phenmetrazine

The amphetamine-like drugs are all classified as indirect-acting agonists at NE, DA, and 5HT synapses. This action results from their combined actions as reuptake inhibitors, neurotransmitter releasers, and inhibitors of monoamine oxidase (MAO). Methamphetamine differs from amphet-amine by the presence of a methyl group on the amine which appears to confer greater efficacy at the 5HT synapse. Phenmetrazine's actions are

Table 12-1 Psychostimulant Action

Action	Systems Involved
Euphorogenic effect	DA in the frontal cortex and mesolimbic system. NE in the frontal cortex. 5HT in the limbic and frontal cortex
Dependence liability	DA in the mesolimbic system
Sleep antagonism	Cortical NE and inhibition of ACh sleep centers via NE and DA
Anorexic effects	NE and perhaps 5HT in the hypothalamus
Increased concentration and reaction time in the face of fatigue	DA in the orbitofrontal cortex. Reaction time improves because of increased attention
Motor stimulation (locomotion, stereotypies, garrulousness)	DA in the basal ganglia and n. accumbens
Psychotomimetic effects and altered judgment	DA and perhaps 5HT in the frontal cortex, temporal cortex and n. accumbens. Flight of thought impairs judgment
Sympathomimetic effects	Peripheral SANS and central actions in the hypothalamus
Anxiety	Epi release and 5HT in the CNS especially in the amygdala (?)
Respiratory stimulation	DA in the carotid body and NE in the brainstem
Hyperthermia	Primarily as a result of excess locomotor activity and reduced heat loss but also central dysregulation in the hypothalamic temperature regulation center

very similar to amphetamine while diethylpropion is not as potent a releasing agent but inhibits reuptake more so than amphetamine.

In general, the ability of the amphetamines to enhance the effects of NE is thought to be responsible for the more uncomfortable effects of the drugs and to lend a certain degree of anxiety to the high that most users do not like. This jittery, uncomfortable, anxious feeling is, in part, a result of the drug's sympathomimetic actions, which include epinephrine release and central noradrenergic effects. Methamphetamine is less able to increase NE, less associated with peripheral activation at normally ingested doses, and preferred by many users because of this ability to produce a "cleaner" high. Methamphetamine is also more readily pyrolyzed (burned) than amphetamine. The ability to pyrolyze a drug and subsequently inhale it so it passes across the large surface area of the lungs rapidly produces much higher brain levels than other administration routes except for intravenous infusion. As a result, "ice" smokers experience a more intense "rush" followed by more pronounced euphoria than that seen following oral ingestion of methamphetamine or amphetamine.

Amphetamine has a history that dates back to the 1920s. It was used for several purposes, such as appetite suppression, allaying fatigue, and bronchodilation, as well as in the treatment of several ill-defined maladies. Amphetamine inhalers were introduced in 1932 and sold over the counter because of their presumed safety. Amphetamine tablets were also used extensively during World War II to reduce fatigue and enhance endurance. The widespread availability of amphetamines at this time led to an abuse pattern called the *speed run* (see Jaffe, 1990). Users would tape a syringe to their arm and deliver a small quantity of amphetamine every few hours. This might continue for days. During this speed run users were continuously awake, did not eat, were garrulous, and could develop paranoid ideation, psychoses, and movement disorders. At the end of the run they would collapse ("crash") and sleep for days. They would wake up hungry and exhibit signs of clinical depression. Many users would then eat and start taking amphetamines again to allay their depression and reinstate euphoria. By the late 1950s, the abuse potential of the amphetamines was recognized and they were banned from over-the-counter distribution.

Amphetamine abuse, however, has remained stable for years. In addition to its recreational use, it is widely used situationally by truck drivers and others who depend on its sleep-suppressing effects. Recently, methamphetamine abuse has increased with the advent of ice. The intensity of the high achieved by smoking the drug is undoubtedly responsible.

The amphetamines are all indirect-acting agonists of the biogenic amines, especially the catecholamines DA and NE. Their mechanisms of action are as follows: (1) Competitive inhibition of the DA and NE transporter and, at higher doses, they also inhibit the reuptake of 5HT. (2) Ca^{2+}-independent release of DA and NE and to a lesser extent 5HT. This release implies that amphetamines cause the release of a neurotransmitter independent of terminal depolarization. (3) Competitive inhibition of MAO. These three actions are consequences of the structural similarity between amphetamine and the catecholamines DA and NE (Fig. 12–3). Despite these structural similarities, amphetamines are not direct-acting agonists at pre- or postsynaptic receptors. Rather, the structural similarity between the amphetamines and the catecholamines enables them to drive the reuptake cycle; they are all substrates for the reuptake pump.

As depicted in Figure 12–4, Ca^{2+}-dependent release of neurotransmitter floods the synaptic pool (synapse) with catecholamines under normal circumstances. DA that is released will eventually collide with the transporter on the DA neuron terminal. The transporter is a shuttle protein that acts as a facilitated diffusion pump in the presence of Na^+ and K^+ and is responsible for recapturing as much as 85% of released biogenic amine. Once dopamine collides with the binding site on the transporter in the presence of Na^+, the pump tumbles in the membrane and releases its dopamine into the mobile pool (cytoplasm) of the DA terminal. This dopamine can then be resequestered into vesicles (vesicular pool) for rerelease or it may again encounter a free site on the transporter now positioned on the cytoplasmic side of the membrane. If dopamine binds to the pump on the cytoplasmic side of the membrane in the presence of K^+, the transport protein again tumbles and releases its dopamine back into the synapse. Thus, neurotransmitter is recycled between the cytoplasmic and synaptic pools. This recycling increases the time dopamine will be present in the synaptic pool, thereby extending the duration of synaptic activity produced by one terminal depolarization. With each cycle of the transporter, however, more dopamine is resequestered into the vesicular pool. In addition, each cycle exposes dopamine to COMT and MAO in the synapse. These effects combined eventually reduce the extracellular concentration of dopamine and effectively terminate its action. With the loss of dopamine from the synaptic cleft produced by these effects, dopamine is no longer available to shuttle the transporter to the cytoplasmic side of the membrane. Since tyrosine hydroxylase is an extremely active enzyme, however, cytoplasmic dopamine resulting from synthesis is always available to shuttle the pumps to the synaptic side of the membrane. This ensures that the transporters are always trapped on the external surface of the membrane and ready for the next depolarization (see Giros and Caron, 1993 for a review of this process).

Amphetamines disrupt this orderly process. Because of their structural similarities to the catecholamines, they can act as a substrate for the transporter proteins. As a substrate, the amphetamines reversibly compete with the biogenic amines for access to the neurotransmitter binding sites on the transporter protein. The amphetamines are therefore competitive reuptake inhibitors. As substrates for the neurotransmitter binding sites on the transporter protein, they will shuttle the transporter to the cytoplasmic side of the membrane and be released into the cytoplasmic pool. The shuttle protein is now on the cytoplasmic side of the membrane and available to bind molecules of dopamine present there. Once dopamine binds to the now-vacated neurotransmitter binding site, the pump shuttles it back out into the synaptic pool in a Ca^{2+}-independent

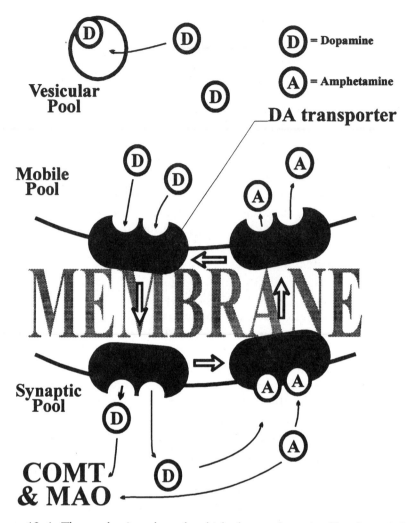

Figure 12–4. The mechanism through which the amphetamine-like drugs induce Ca²⁺-independent release. The DA transporter is a facilitated-transporter "shuttle" protein that carries DA from the synaptic surface to the cytoplasmic surface of the membrane when DA is present in the synaptic cleft. As a shuttle protein, however, it can also carry DA out of the cell and into the synapse if DA binds on the cytoplasmic surface. The structural similarity between DA and amphetamine enables the latter to substitute for DA and carry the transporter to the cytoplasmic side of the membrane. By doing so, the transporter is available for transporting to the synaptic surface of the membrane and thereby induces Ca²⁺-independent release. Amphetamine can also inhibit monoamine oxidase (MAO) although unlike DA, it is not a substrate for catechol-O-methyl transferase (COMT).

fashion. In the presence of the amphetamines, dopamine is therefore transported into the synapse independent of depolarization. Of course, the molecules of amphetamine brought in by the pump could also bind to the neurotransmitter site on the transporter protein after they have been released into the cytoplasmic pool. But since amphetamine has a lower affinity for this site than dopamine and the number of DA molecules far outnumbers those of amphetamine at this time, DA transport predominates. As the amphetamine concentration in the cytoplasmic pool increases, however (when amphetamine has reached high concentrations in the brain and a significant quantity is in the neuron terminals), it will more effectively compete with dopamine in the cytoplasmic pool for access to the reuptake pumps on the cytoplasmic side. As levels increase, amphetamine's ability to stimulate Ca^{2+}-independent release is therefore attenuated. This self-limiting action results in a ceiling effect like that associated with the benzodiazepines. This ceiling effect is probably responsible in part for the low mortality rates associated with amphetamine overdoses. The amphetamines are also MAO inhibitors. Their structural similarity with the biogenic amines allows them to reversibly bind to the neurotransmitter acceptor site on MAO. Although DA was used as the example here, the same mechanisms operate with NE and 5HT. The result is an amphetamine-induced enhancement of DA, NE, and 5HT release independent of normal neuronal activity.

Cocaine

The effects of cocaine depend on its psychostimulant and local anesthetic properties. Although the potency of cocaine in affecting biogenic amines is much higher than its potency as a local anesthetic (10 : 1), recent changes in the pattern of use have made its anesthetic properties more relevant. Cocaine typically has been taken in by insufflation (snorting through the nose), where it is absorbed readily by the vessels in the nasal mucosa and circulated to the body. As a sympathomimetic agent, however, cocaine causes vasoconstriction in nasal arterioles and the associated reduction in vascular flow limits absorption. Achieving plasma levels by this route that approach those seen after intravenous administration is therefore difficult. This changed with the advent of a free-base form of cocaine called "crack" supplied in a compacted, rock form from which an individual dose is "cracked" off. Free-base cocaine is more easily pyrolyzed and aerosolized than cocaine salt and inhalation of the more lipid-soluble free-base form across the enormous surface area of the lungs leads to circulating concentrations comparable to those seen with intravenous administration. The higher plasma levels achieved make the anesthetic properties of cocaine more relevant. These properties are probably responsible for the greater likelihood that cardiac arrest, seizure disorder, and, at very high doses, respiratory depression will occur: actions that are rarely associated with amphetamine overdose and cocaine insufflation. The arrival of crack cocaine has been associated with a marked increase in the number of overdose deaths, not because the potency of the drug has changed, but rather because the pattern of abuse has changed. This abuse pattern is also thought to contribute to the higher dependence liability of crack cocaine.

Cocaine increases dopamine and norepinephrine at normal doses and serotonin at higher doses because it acts as a reuptake inhibitor for these neurotransmitters. There is general consensus on this mechanism of action, but controversy surrounds the issue of whether cocaine acts as a competitive or noncompetitive inhibitor of the transporter proteins. Cocaine's actions have been best studied using the dopamine transporter; several studies suggest that it binds to the protein at a site different from that of dopamine (see Reith et al., 1992). Once bound, cocaine induces a tertiary structural change in the transporter, reducing its capacity to bind neurotransmitter, or it binds so near the neurotransmitter site that it obstructs it. The reuptake pump is thus inactivated (reversibly but not competitively). The alternative hypothesis proposes that cocaine binds to the neurotransmitter acceptor site itself on the transporter protein and thereby acts as a competitive inhibitor. Regardless of the mechanism, the bulky cocaine molecule is not transported across the membrane (as are the amphetamines) and Ca^{2+}-independent biogenic amine release does not occur.

The ability of cocaine to act as an indirect agonist and enhance the action of the biogenic amines is state dependent. Thus, cocaine cannot inhibit the reuptake of a neurotransmitter that is not being released by physiologically relevant processes. Cocaine's ability to induce mood alterations depends on the quantity of DA and NE being released at the time the drug enters the brain. In contrast, the amphetamines that induce the release of neurotransmitter independent of depolarization produce more predictable dose-dependent effects.

Effects of Psychostimulants

The primary effects of the psychostimulants range in intensity from mild to toxic as dose increases (Table 12–1). Barring panic attack resulting from the novelty of these effects in the naive user, the actions of the stimulants are not dramatic and are readily tolerated by the patient at moderate dosages. Many of the effects described exhibit tolerance, however. Although the stimulants are very effective appetite suppressants and sympathomimetics acutely, for instance, tolerance to these effects develop within a few weeks.

The psychostimulants also produce reverse tolerance to some of their effects. Their ability to induce locomotion and stereotypic behaviors increases with continued exposure. Stereotypic behaviors are part of the organism's normal repertoire but they become perseverative to the point of dysfunction. They include compulsions, disassembly and reassembly of mechanical items, inappropriate cataloging of items (license plates, movie stars), and a host of other repetitive behaviors. These behaviors are all part of a toxic psychosis. Thus, an escalating dosing schedule to maintain adequate appetite suppression, for instance, will be increasingly likely to produce behaviors associated with excess dopamine activity or these behaviors will emerge at lower doses because of reverse tolerance. Feelings of elation and a sense of well-being experienced acutely will give way to garrulousness, restlessness, anxiety, akathisia, and auditory and visual hallucinations following extended usage. The picture is one of progressive psychomotor agitation or mania that deteriorates into a psychosis (predominantly paranoid ideation). Because of the risk of dependence, the potential to induce psychotic behavior, and the fact that many effects exhibit tolerance (in particular the appetite-suppressing effects for which these drugs were once widely used), the psychostimulants are all classified by the FDA as schedule II drugs (i.e., high dependence liability, limited clinical use requiring a triplicate prescription form that is registered with the Drug Enforcement Agency).

Cardiovascular effects

The effects of the psychostimulants on cardiovascular regulation are complex and dose dependent. Psychostimulant-induced increases in norepinephrine activity can cause an increase in heart rate, although at lower doses the rate can be decreased slightly due to the baroreceptor reflex. Increased norepinephrine also increases total peripheral resistance, leading to increased blood pressure and a weak pulse. This vasoconstriction reduces the ability to lose heat across the skin and contributes to hyperthermia. In contrast, speed runs may lead to orthostasis as a result of presynaptic norepinephrine depletion. Cocaine can similarly produce orthostasis if plasma levels are high enough to anesthetize postganglionic sympathetic fibers or vascular smooth muscle. In addition, these anesthetic effects interfere with myocardial conduction and lead to arrhythmias.

Respiratory effects

All psychostimulants are respiratory stimulants. Hypoxic drive originating in the carotid body is, in part, a DA-mediated phenomenon that is enhanced by the dopaminergic effects of these drugs (see Chapter 4). Increased norepinephrine levels in the CNS also stimulate the respiratory centers indirectly and increased sympathetic activity produces bronchodilation. Combined, these actions increase minute respiratory volume, and the amphetamines were once used in patients whose respiration was compromised by opioid analgesics. Conversely, the anesthetic properties of cocaine will lead to respiratory depression at higher dosages by depressing the respiratory centers in the brainstem.

Other effects

Mydriasis occurs because of the sympathomimetic effects of these drugs. The effects of the psychostimulants on the bladder sphincter are consistent with their sympathomimetic effects. Increased sphincter tone is typical and amphetamines are used to treat enuresis and incontinence. Psychostimulant effects on the gastrointestinal tract, however, are highly variable and unpredictable. Amphetamine can reduce activity in an active gut but can also stimulate activity in an inactive gut. Headaches occur often. At high levels of cocaine ingestion, its anesthetic actions will counteract its sympathomimetic actions and induce vascular collapse and smooth muscle relaxation.

Toxic Effects of the Central Stimulants

Toxicity from chronic psychostimulant use is serious but not life-threatening. It includes psychomotor agitation, psychotic symptoms, and movement disorders. Patients readily respond to discontinuation of the drug, their symptoms usually resolving within 24 hours. Acute, high-dose ingestion, however, presents a different clinical picture that includes not only neurobehavioral but potentially serious cardiovascular complications. Stimulant overdose victims are seen in the emergency rooms of hospitals throughout the country. Severe, life-threatening toxicity is also encountered in "body packers," individuals who ingest condoms filled with cocaine to smuggle illegal drugs through customs. Because the toxic profiles of the amphetamine-like drugs and of cocaine are different (Hurlbut, 1991), they will be described separately.

Amphetamine

High-dose amphetamine abuse can lead to arrhythmias (usually not fatal), choreoathetoid movement disorders, paranoid ideations, and hyperactivity, leading to myoglobinuria, renal failure, and hyperpyrexia. The vasoconstrictive effects and consequent increase in blood pressure may lead to cranial hemorrhage. Chronic sympathomimetic activity also leads to stimulant vasculitis (necrotizing arteritis), which usually occurs in the gastrointestinal tract or in coronary vessels. The overdose victim is often acidotic from excessive muscle activity, which, together with hyperpyrexia, can lead to convulsions and death. Prevention of the hyperpyrexia in dogs has been shown to prevent amphetamine-induced convulsions and deaths. These convulsions are therefore secondary complications of the acidosis and hyperpyrexia. Excess motor activity, hyperpyrexia, and acidosis may also lead to rhabdomyolitis with tissue destruction and potential renal failure. Patients may experience headache, dizziness, tenseness, irritability, fever, agitation, euphoria, and dyskinesias. They are often garrulous, assaultive, confused, panic stricken, and eventually hallucinatory (auditory and visual). Paranoia and other psychotic symptoms may lead to suicidal or homicidal tendencies. Paranoia is even manifested in the hallucinations, which tend to involve visual distortions of faces that can be gruesome. Patients may also exhibit stereotypic, perseverative behaviors. Most remain aware that their condition is drug induced.

Emergency-room management of these patients is usually best begun with a benzodiazepine although patients exhibiting excessive agitation or paranoid ideation may also require a DA antagonist. Haloperidol is the DA antagonist most commonly used because of its safety, but a phenothiazine such as chlorpromazine that is also a potent alpha antagonist may yield more effective control of the sympathomimetic signs. Patients should be evaluated for cardiac complications and metabolic acidosis. Since most of the ingested amphetamine is excreted unchanged in the urine, acidification of the urine with ammonium chloride will reduce the plasma half-life, which is normally eight to 12 hours, thereby speeding excretion. Acidification can aggravate the acidotic consequences of overdose, especially cardiac arrhythmias and convulsions, however, and this treatment is becoming less popular. Surprisingly, amphetamine overdoses are readily managed and generally not life-threatening, perhaps due to the ceiling effect alluded to above. Several animal studies have shown that amphetamine administered in high doses is neurotoxic (see Ricaurte et al., 1985), but this has not been demonstrated in humans.

Cocaine

The pattern of cocaine toxicity can be very similar to that of amphetamine. Continued intravenous or inhalation abuse can lead to a behavioral pattern like that associated with amphetamine, including paranoid ideations, psychotic symptoms, and choreoathetoid movements. However, toxic doses of cocaine can also produce feelings of anxiety, dysphoria, apathy, and melancholy. This syndrome is called cocaine dysphoria. Olfactory, auditory, and visual hallucinations may be reported. The sensation of bugs crawling under the skin (formication) resulting in the patient picking at and even mutilating the skin is much more common with a cocaine overdose although it has also been reported following high-dose amphetamine use. Formication may be a perceptual distortion of the paresthesias resulting from the anesthetic and vasoconstrictive (sympathomimetic) effects of these drugs.

As with amphetamine, the experienced cocaine user is usually aware of the cause of his condition even at toxic plasma levels. Acute cocaine overdose victims, however, are more often delirious. These patients may become violently aggressive. Their condition can deteriorate rapidly with fatal consequences so cocaine overdose is an important differential diagnosis in any patient presenting with delirium. The management of cocaine overdose is complicated by the drug's anesthetic properties. Consequently, the risk of mortality is significantly greater than with amphetamine.

The pattern of toxicity in the cocaine overdose victim has three phases and is often called the "Casey Jones" reaction (Table 12–2). Early stimulation (phase I) is similar to that of amphetamine with the additional component of cocaine dysphoria. The anesthetic properties of cocaine contribute significantly to the late stimulation and depressive phases. Note that respiratory stimulation switches to depression. Mydriatic pupils may become further dilated. The cardiovascular symptoms observed in these patients must be treated cautiously because some antiarrhythmic agents such as lidocaine are similar to cocaine in their actions and therefore contraindicated.

Cocaine overdose can be treated like amphetamine overdose in the emergency room except that DA antagonists cannot be administered. Due to the greater convulsive properties of cocaine, the administration of the antipsychotic drugs, which reduce seizure thresholds, may exacerbate seizures or even convert intermittent tics and focal convulsions into status epilepticus.

The management of the cocaine overdose victim becomes even more problematic when cocaine is ingested with other drugs. Cocaine intensifies the opioid high and vice versa. Since the half-life of morphine is four hours while that of cocaine is 20–45 minutes, cocaine must be taken intermittently to maintain the intensity of the combined high. This intermittent ingestion can lead to accumulation that produces anesthetic effects. Its respiratory depressant effects combined with those of an opioid can lead to pulmonary edema and fatal respiratory depression at levels of either drug that would otherwise be well tolerated. Treatment with naloxone will reduce the respiratory depressant actions of opioids but not those of cocaine. Administering oxygen before naloxone to such patients will further reduce respiratory drive (see Chapter 4). Potentially fatal respiratory depression can also occur through a different mechanism

Table 12–2 The "Casey Jones" Reaction in the Cocaine Overdose Victim

Phase	CNS Effects	CV Effects[a]	Respiratory Effects
I: Early stimulation	Those effects described in Table 12–1 plus nausea, vomiting, headache, tremor, cold sweats, muscle twitches, tics, and preconvulsive movements	Variable pulse and it is generally elevated 30–50%, skin pallor due to vasoconstriction, and premature ventricular contractions	Increased respiratory rate with possible dyspnea
II: Advanced stimulation	Decreased responsiveness, hyperreflexia, convulsions, status epilepticus, incontinence and possible malignant encephalopathy	Increase in pulse with possible high-output congestive heart failure. CNS hemorrhage is possible but rare. BP begins to fall and pulse becomes rapid, weak, and irregular. Peripheral then central cyanosis develops	Gasping, rapid, and/or irregular respirations (Cheyne-Stokes progressive hypoxia)
III: Depression	Flaccid paralysis, coma, pupils fixed and dilated, areflexia, loss of vital support function, and paralysis of the medullary brain center	Ventricular fibrillations, circulatory failure, with an ashen gray cyanosis. No palpable pulse, followed by cardiac arrest and death	Agonal gasps, respiratory failure, and gross pulmonary edema

[a]BP = blood pressure; CV = cardiovascular effects

when high doses of cocaine and an opioid are taken. The psychostimulant and respiratory stimulant properties of cocaine counteract the sedation and respiratory depressant actions of the opioids, allowing a higher dose of the latter to be ingested. Because of cocaine's shorter half-life, rapid clearance of cocaine may unmask the respiratory depressant effects of the opioid.

Cocaine is also commonly ingested with alcohol. In the body, cocaine and alcohol metabolites conjugate to produce cocaethylene (see Johanson and Schuster, 1995). This chemical is psychoactive and has a much longer half-life than either cocaine or ethanol. As a result, it accumulates in the body and is thought to contribute to organ damage and fatal overdoses at levels of cocaine that are normally not fatal.

The cocaine baby

The number of babies born to mothers who abused cocaine during their pregnancy is staggering (estimated at 150,000/year), as are the health care costs (Agency for Health Care Policy and Research, 1993). Crack babies are born into a withdrawal syndrome consisting of tremors, hyperirritability, altered cries, and cardiovascular and respiratory complications. High-dose abuse during pregnancy may lead to fetal brain ischemia or to low brain weight and altered neurologic signs of all sorts, depending on the location of the lesions in the child's brain. Too few children have reached adulthood to examine the long-term consequences of this pattern of abuse and whether such effects, if any, can be attributed to cocaine will be difficult to determine because of the pattern of polydrug abuse seen in most mothers of cocaine babies.

Caffeine and Nicotine

Caffeine and nicotine are not considered psychostimulants but do produce some of the effects of this drug class. Because both drugs are self-administered by animals and possess dependence liability, their pharmacodynamics will be discussed briefly so that a balanced presentation of the drugs of abuse can be made.

Caffeine

Caffeine is the most widely ingested drug since it is present in a variety of products marketed and sold throughout the world including coffee, cola beverages, teas, maté, and some chocolates. Because of its psychostimulant properties and dependence liability, caffeine is added to some beverages to enhance and maintain consumption in much the same fashion that cocaine was once added to Coca-Cola. The pharmacology of caffeine and its abuse liability were recently reviewed by Griffiths and Mumford (1995).

The effects of caffeine (Table 12–3) are thought to result from its direct-acting, competitive antagonist action at adenosine receptors (Rainnie et al., 1994). Adenosine receptors are found throughout the CNS including the basal ganglia, the n. accumbens, and the bed nuclei of the DA projection systems in the mesencephalon, where adenosine reduces DA release. Acting as an antagonist, caffeine increases dopamine activity, which is probably responsible for its psychomotor stimulant properties and dependence liability (Ferre et al., 1992). Acting through heteroreceptors, adenosine also reduces the release of several neurotransmitters including ACh. By antagonizing these receptors, caffeine increases cholinergic activity in the pedunculopontine-thalamic pathway, which, as discussed in Chapter 6, would combat sedation. Caffeine, like theo-

Table 12–3 Effects of Caffeine

Subjective effects[a]	Increased feeling of well being
	Increased energy
	Increased alertness and concentration
	Increased motivation to work
	Increased desire to talk to others
	Decreased desire to sleep
"Physiologic" effects[b]	Diuresis (as a consequence of increased blood flow)
	Parotid gland salivation
	Increased metabolic rate
	Increased BP and pulse (increased NE and Epi release)
	Increased plasma renin activity
	Smooth muscle relaxation
	Increased secretion of products from many endocrine and exocrine glands (*e.g.*, increased acid, pepsin, gastrin, and parathyroid hormone)
	Antiinflammatory effects (decreased histamine)
Withdrawal syndrome	Headache or cerebral "fullness"
	Drowsiness and yawning
	Increased work difficulty (impaired concentration)
	Anxiety
	Mild depression
	Irritability and decreased contentment
	Decreased sociability
	Flu-like symptoms (muscle aches and heavy feelings in the limbs with nausea)
	Blurred vision

[a] = see Goldstein and Kaizer (1969)
[b] BP = blood pressure

phylline, is also a member of the methylxanthine family of compounds, which are phosphodiesterase inhibitors and which increase the half-life of cAMP. The concentrations needed to produce this inhibition, however, are seldom achieved through dietary sources.

Even though caffeine is known to elevate DA in the n. accumbens, its potency is much lower than the psychostimulants. Although most of the studies report caffeine self-administration in animals, this effect is not observed at all doses. In fact, the self-administration dose-response profile is an inverted U-shaped curve. Thus, at higher administered doses, caffeine possesses aversive effects that reduce consumption and produce dysphoria in humans.

The consumption of high doses of caffeine in the form of over-the-counter tablets is predominated by CNS effects and cardiovascular toxicity. Insomnia, restlessness, and excitement are common and may deteriorate into delirium with convulsions as dosage increases. Caffeine reduces blood flow to the brain, which, at toxic levels, contributes to CNS signs and symptoms. Increased muscle tone with tremors are common. The cardiovascular profile is that of excess sympathetic stimulation, although blocking the autoregulatory effects of adenosine in the heart contribute as well. Nausea and vomiting are commonly seen. Because caffeine produces aversive effects at higher doses, recreational use of caffeine is once tried but seldom repeated.

Nicotine

Nicotine addiction represents the classic argument against the positive reinforcement theory of drug dependence described above. Most smokers recognize the health hazards of smoking and derive little pleasure from their habits. Nearly 20 million smokers attempt to quit each year, yet only 7% of these addicts attain one year of abstinence (Fiore, 1992). Thus, even though much of the enjoyment associated with smoking is gone, the craving remains (Henningfield, Schuh, and Jarvik, 1995).

Nicotine's Mechanism of Action. Nicotine is a direct-acting nicotinic receptor agonist and the drug originally used to distinguish nicotinic from muscarinic cholinergic receptors. Nicotinic activation of autonomic ganglia increases both sympathetic and parasympathetic activity. Nicotine also activates the nicotinic receptors at the neuromuscular junction, increasing muscle tone. In the CNS, nicotine has an alerting effect on the cerebral cortex and induces mild arousal. Nicotine also possesses MAO inhibitory actions which would lead to increased dopamine in the n. accumbens. This action is probably responsible for its dependence liability; its effects on other DA systems—as well as NE and 5HT—that also utilize MAO in their catabolism, contribute to its mild euphorogenic and stimulant properties. In addition to these effects, nicotine has been shown to increase growth hormone, beta-endorphin, vasopressin, and cortisol secretion.

Pharmacokinetics of Nicotine. Nicotine is a tertiary amine that readily crosses membranes. Tobacco contains the more active levorotary racemate of nicotine that is well absorbed across the lungs and mucosal surfaces. Oral ingestion is associated with significant first-pass metabolism yielding the major metabolite cotinine. Pyrolysis at 2,000°F at the tip of a cigarette produces distillation of the nicotine into tar droplets that deliver the drug to the lungs where it is rapidly absorbed into the circulation producing a bolus concentration that is distributed throughout the body within eight seconds. Approximately 50% of nicotine is redistributed from the brain in 20 to 40 minutes with an overall terminal half-life of approximately two hours.

Rapid tolerance develops to the effects of nicotine. This tachyphylaxis is due to pharmacodynamic and physiologic tolerance. As quickly as this rapid tolerance develops, it disappears such that profound effects are experienced after only eight hours of sleep (Srivastava et al., 1991). The tars and other contaminants in cigarette smoke also induce the P-450 system producing pharmacokinetic tolerance to nicotine. This microsomal induction increases the biotransformation rate of several other drugs and is often overlooked in the prescription of medication. Reduced analgesic effects of opioids, decreased sedating effects from several benzodiazepines, and reduced efficacy of several antianginal drugs including atenolol and propranolol should be anticipated in cigarette smokers.

Effects of Nicotine. Overall, the effects of nicotine are similar to those of the psychostimulants including improved concentration and memory as well as appetite suppression (Table 12–4). However, additional effects are related to the carbon monoxide inhaled with cigarette smoke including dizziness, hypoxia, and vascular changes leading to headaches.

Treatment of Nicotine Addiction. The most successful form of treatment for nicotine addiction has been nicotine replacement therapy. Since many health hazards of smoking are a consequence of the smoke in cigarettes, replacing the nicotine with a smokeless delivery system reduces many smoking-related health risks. Nicotine patches and chewing gums reduce the behavioral signs and symptoms of the withdrawal syndrome that contribute significantly to recidivism.

The major deterrents to the success of nicotine patches and chewing gums are the reduced bioavailability of these formulations compared with inhalation and the associated failure of these delivery systems to achieve the plasma nicotine concentrations normally obtained by a single cigarette. Nevertheless, these strategies have been more successful than all other systems and remain established forms of treatment. Nicotine patches and gums are now sold over the counter.

ALCOHOL

Ethanol is a CNS depressant and many of its actions are similar to those discussed in Chapter 6. As with all CNS depressants, ethanol induces dose-dependent depression leading to disinhibition release, ataxia, impaired judgment, sedation, anxiolysis, slurred speech, and eventually stupor, coma, respiratory depression, and death. These effects result from its ability to penetrate membranes where it enhances fluidity and alters the function of embedded proteins (Chin and Goldstein, 1981). It is the re-

Table 12–4 Effects of Nicotine

Subjective effects	Memory facilitation (cortical ACh)
	Improved concentration (frontal lobe DA)
	Euphorogenic effects (frontal lobe DA and increased endorphin release)
	Reinforcing effects (n. accumbens DA)
	Decreased appetite, especially for sweets (increased 5HT)
Physiologic effects[a]	Reduced deep tendon reflexes (ACh action on Renshaw cells)
	Increased metabolic rate (ACh-mediated increase in muscle tone and SANS activation of Epi release)
	Increased heart rate and pulse (SANS)
	Reduced muscle tone in some muscles
	Nausea and vomiting (direct stimulation of the CTZ)
	Reduced taste and smell (ACh effects on sensory trafficking and effects of smoke contaminants upon tongue and nasal receptor systems)
	Tremor (SANS)
Withdrawal syndrome	Craving
	Irritability, impatience, and anxiety
	Lack of concentration
	Insomnia but drowsiness during the day
	Headaches
	Increased appetite and weight gain
	Short-term memory defects
	Decreased heart rate and BP
	Peripheral blood flow increases
	Increased skin temperature

[a]CTZ = chemoreceptor trigger zone (area postrema)

duction in function of these proteins that is responsible in part for the actions of ethanol. At higher concentrations, alcohol can even decrease the function of Na^+-K^+ATPase pumps and the electron transport chain, the effects of which compromise electrical conduction. The net effects of alcohol are slowed neuronal conduction. The resulting impaired sympathetic function along with its smooth-muscle–relaxing effects can reduce vascular tone and decrease total peripheral resistance. This vasodilation is responsible for the red face that is so characteristic of alcoholics who consistently consume high quantities of alcohol.

Although ethanol enters the membrane, its distribution there is not uniform. This suggests that a binding site, perhaps at the protein–lipid interface, could account for the actions of alcohol at moderate doses. Its actions at such doses have been reviewed by Tabakoff and Hoffman (1987) and Gonzales and Hoffman (1991) and are summarized in Table 12–5.

Table 12–5 Effects and Side Effects of Ethanol[a]

Side Effects	Possible Mechanism/Cause
Reduced neuronal conduction	Increased membrane fluidity
Sedation Increased seizure threshold Anterograde amnesia	Benzodiazepine-independent enhancement of GABA function
Euphoria Memory impairment Analgesia Sedation	Delta opioid-like effects Acetylaldehyde conjugation with CAs to produce conjugates with opiate-like effects and neuronal damage
Blood pressure alterations Dependence liability Vasodilation	Acute release of CAs/CNS depression Increased DA in n. accumbens Smooth-muscle relaxation/peripheral neuropathy
Sedation Memory impairment Delirium	Anticholinergic effects
Anxiolysis Sedation Mood alterations	Altered 5HT function; GABA actions
Peripheral neuropathy	Thiamine deficiency (poor diet)
Cirrhosis GI problems	NAD depletion; astringent actions/reduced juices/reduced water-soluble vitamin absorption
Cardiac disease	Alterations in HDL, increased heart work, alcohol-mediated cardiomyopathy
Reduced ADH release	Depression of hypothalamus
Reduced body temperature	Depression of hypothalamus and peripheral vasodilation
Fetal alcohol syndrome	Dietary problems, reduced vitamin absorption, direct effects of alcohol on fetal brain

[a]CA = catecholamines; NAD = nicotine-adenine dinucleotide; ADH = antidiuretic hormone;
HDL = high-density lipoprotein

Effects of Alcohol

GABA effects

Ethanol potentiates the actions of the $GABA_A$ receptor through an unknown mechanism that is independent of the benzodiazepine receptor.
This action likely contributes to its sedative-hypnotic effects, its anticonvulsant properties, its REM-suppressant actions, and its ability to induce
anterograde amnesia. It also explains the additive and perhaps synergistic

depressant effects that occur when ethanol and benzodiazepines are taken together.

Opioid effects

Ethanol has affinity for delta opiate receptors. Moreover, a metabolite of alcohol, acetaldehyde, can condense with catecholamines to form tetra-hydroisoquinolines and salsolinol, which possess opioid-like properties that are reversible by naloxone. These conjugates may also contribute to the neurodegenerative effects of ethanol that, over time, can cause frank loss of neuronal tissue, memory deficits, reduced mental acuity, and permanent motor impairment (see Collins, 1982). The acute opiate-like actions of ethanol probably contribute to its analgesic, euphorogenic, and sedative-hypnotic properties.

Catecholaminergic effects

Although it is a CNS depressant, the acute administration of ethanol releases DA and NE. The release of these catecholamines contributes to ethanol's euphorogenic actions and its ability to induce dependence. In addition, the release of NE in the periphery leads to fluctuations in blood pressure and to the tachycardia some individuals experience after a few drinks. These cardiovascular effects, however, are highly variable. As a CNS depressant, ethanol compromises brainstem function, including that of cardiorespiratory centers. This depressant effect will eventually overcome the catecholaminergic actions of alcohol and depress cardiac function.

Anticholinergic effects

Ethanol markedly reduces ACh release in the reticular formation, perhaps by compromising N-type voltage-gated Ca^{2+} function. This action contributes to the sedation and delirium that often accompany alcoholic intoxication.

Peripheral neuropathy

Demyelination of peripheral nerves is a common finding in alcoholics and is associated with reduced sensory acuity, paresthesias, and reduced conduction velocity. The demyelination is thought to reflect thiamine deficiency because of the alcoholic's poor dietary habits. Together with emotional lability, memory loss, intellectual impairment, ataxia, and paralysis of the external eye muscles, it forms the Wernicke-Korsakoff syndrome, a psychotic disorder that often responds to thiamine therapy.

Liver/GI symptoms

Ethanol biotransformation requires nicotinamide adenine dinucleotide (NAD) and this coenzyme can become depleted in alcoholics. With NAD depletion, several compounds, including glutamate, maleate, and lactate, accumulate in the body and contribute to liver dysfunction (Rogers, Spector, and Trounce, 1981). This can lead to the fatty, cirrhotic liver characteristic of the alcoholic plus impaired gluconeogenesis and hypoglycemia. The resulting impairment in glucose handling contributes to alcohol's mental effects since the brain is an insulin-dependent organ. The effects on membrane fluidity can also disrupt GI function, reducing the absorption of water-soluble vitamins and increasing the secretion of HCl and digestive juices that contribute to gastritis and pancreatitis. Ulcers are exacerbated because alcohol acts as an astringent (dehydrates tissues), further contributing to mucosal irritation. Folate deficiencies resulting from chronic alcohol consumption produces mild anemia while deficiencies in other water-soluble vitamins are associated with the loss of essential antioxidants needed to reduce overall tissue damage.

Cardiac effects

Significant fluctuations in blood pressure are seen with both acute and chronic alcohol intake due to the combined effects of acutely increased NE release, depression of cardioregulatory centers in the brainstem, and the reflex response to peripheral vasodilation. Peripheral neuropathies that accompany chronic use also contribute to autonomic problems and compromise cardiac efficiency even further. The direct effects of alcohol on the heart muscle may eventually lead to cardiomyopathy with associated arrhythmias.

Antidiuretic hormone (ADH)

The generalized CNS depression resulting from ethanol ingestion sharply lowers the release of ADH and induces several poorly characterized hormonal abnormalities. The sudden decrease in ADH along with the increased liquid volume consumption that often accompanies drinking (especially of beer) can produce dramatic diuresis. The astringent properties of alcohol also reduce total body water by drawing water into the blood, further contributing to alcohol's diuretic effect. This effect is probably responsible for the dry mouth ("cotton mouth") experienced the next day.

Body temperature

Contrary to popular opinion, alcohol reduces body temperature. Although the vasodilator effects that accompany acute ingestion lead to a warm feeling because of increased vascular flow to the cutaneous vessels, this preferential shunting of blood to the periphery increases heat loss. At higher doses, hypothalamic depression will compromise the temperature-regulating systems of the body as well. These factors, in combination, can be fatal to alcoholics living on the street or losing consciousness outdoors during cold weather.

Fetal alcohol syndrome

Women who abuse alcohol during pregnancy can give birth to children with a host of medical problems because of the combined effects mentioned above. The increase in membrane fluidity produced by alcohol undoubtedly contributes to abnormal development and teratogenic effects in the fetus as well. The fetal alcohol syndrome includes retarded body weight, microencephaly, underdevelopment, joint abnormalities, facial abnormalities, congenital heart defects, and mental retardation.

Pharmacokinetics of Ethanol

Ethanol is almost completely absorbed from the gastrointestinal tract (primarily the duodenum) and distributed rapidly to the body. Gastric emptying time influences the rate of delivery to the duodenum and, in turn, controls absorption. Straight alcohol reduces gastric emptying time due to its irritant effects. Thus, mixed carbonated drinks containing equivalent quantities of alcohol will intoxicate faster than "straight shots," provided the rate of consumption is the same. Food also delays the emptying of gastric contents and thereby slows delivery of ethanol to the duodenum. In particular, foods high in fat slow ethanol absorption.

Once absorbed, ethanol penetrates tissues readily but is preferentially distributed to the brain because of its disproportionately high perfusion rate. Ethanol is metabolized predominantly by alcohol dehydrogenase in the liver (Fig. 12–5). The activity of this enzyme is limited by its cofactor NAD. Thus, alcohol dehydrogenase saturates quickly and the rate of ethanol metabolism then becomes zero order. Because of its zero-order kinetics, the rate at which ethanol is consumed is more important than the amount consumed. Ethanol is converted to acetaldehyde by aldehyde dehydrogenase, yielding acetate, which is passed to the general metabolism. Genetic polymorphism of alcohol dehydrogenase (see Chapter 2) accounts for the ability of some individuals to "drink like fish" while others get drunk passing a bar on the sidewalk.

Ethanol is also metabolized by the microsomal enzyme system. Although very little alcohol is metabolized by the P-450 system under normal circumstances, the microsomal system becomes proportionately more important as dose increases. Furthermore, the induction of the microsomal system accompanies chronic drinking, leading to pharmacokinetic tolerance. Thus, even though alcohol dehydrogenase does not exhibit induction with chronic ethanol exposure, the microsomal system does and thereby produces tolerance. This induction by alcohol will in-

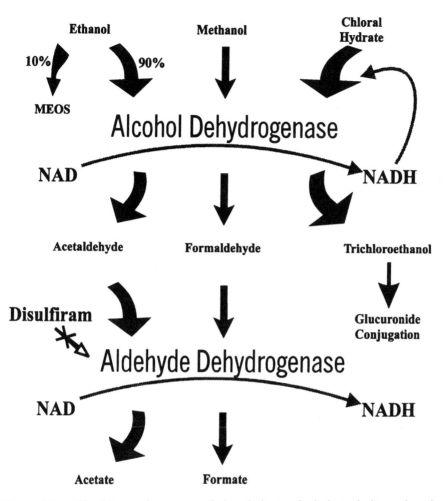

Figure 12–5. The biotransformation of the aliphatic alcohols including ethanol, methanol, and chloral hydrate involves the enzymes alcohol dehydrogenase and aldehyde dehydrogenase. Both enzymes require nicotine-adenine dinucleotide (NAD) as a cofactor, which is reduced to NADH as a result of the oxidation. Ethanol can also be biotransformed by the mixed-function enzyme oxidation system (MEOS) in the liver. The drug disulfiram inhibits the enzyme aldehyde dehydrogenase leading to the buildup of acetaladehyde that contributes to the toxic effects of this drug when ethanol is consumed.

crease the biotransformation rate of other drugs entering this system. Unanticipated alterations in the potency and efficacy of other drugs are therefore common in alcoholics. A small but significant percentage (10%) of alcohol is eliminated through the lungs and other surface body fluids. Dancing and sweating thus speed elimination.

Because ethanol metabolism is zero order, a drug half-life cannot be stated with certainty. The ability to biotransform alcohol depends on body weight and, more importantly, on the liver's weight. On average, it takes about three hours to completely biotransform one ounce of alcohol. Saturation can occur after only a few drinks. One of the more interesting drug interactions associated with ethanol ingestion has to do with its biotransformation and the coadministration of the sedative-hypnotic agent chloral hydrate to yield the Mickey Finn. This drug combination, made famous in many movies, is associated with rapid induction of sleep. Chloral hydrate is actually a prodrug for the active metabolite trichloroethanol (Fig. 12–5). The biotransformation of ethanol drives the metabolism of chloral hydrate by providing NADH for alcohol dehydrogenase. At the same time, the biotransformation of chloral hydrate prevents metabolism of ethanol. The result is increased blood alcohol levels in combination with high trichloroethanol levels and the very rapid induction of sedation.

Ethanol can also be used as an antidote to the ingestion of methanol. The primary concern following methanol ingestion is the production of formaldehyde that can rapidly lead to blindness. By coadministering high dosages of ethanol, methanol biotransformation is inhibited and formaldehyde toxicity reduced.

Tolerance

Pharmacodynamic, physiologic, pharmacokinetic, and behavioral tolerance accompanies chronic high-dose abuse of alcohol (Ashton, 1992). Pharmacodynamic tolerance results from decreased GABA-receptor sensitivity, diminished capacity to depress Ca^{2+} conduction, alterations in the biogenic amine systems, and decreased endogenous opioid concentrations. Taken together, the various forms of tolerance lead to increased consumption and the associated dependency this abuse pattern may produce. Chronic ethanol consumption will also result in cross-tolerance to other sedative-hypnotic agents and to other centrally acting drugs that act through the neurotransmitter systems affected by alcohol.

Withdrawal syndrome

The effects of alcohol withdrawal are a classic example of neuroadaptation, similar to those that follow withdrawal from other CNS depressants. The syndrome includes nausea, weakness, headache, anxiety, and tremor ("the shakes"). If acute consumption is high enough, one drinking binge can produce withdrawal symptoms. Withdrawal from chronic high-dose abuse, however, is more severe and may include all of the above signs and symptoms plus vomiting, abdominal cramps, drug craving, hallucinations, and convulsions. This syndrome peaks 24 to 48 hours after the drug has cleared the body. If it is severe enough, it can enter a phase called delirium tremens (DTs) in which bizarre hallucinations are frequent, tremor is pronounced, and the patient is disoriented, aggressive, and psychotic. Potentially fatal convulsions and cardiovascular collapse can occur. This phase generally lasts five to seven days and is always followed by a protracted withdrawal phase accompanied by severe depression and sleep disturbances.

Disulfiram (antabuse)

Disulfiram is an irreversible inhibitor of aldehyde dehydrogenase. Taking this drug before drinking alcohol prevents the catabolism of acetaldehyde that subsequently accumulates in the body. Acetaldehyde accumulation produces vasodilation, headache, skin flush, hypotension, nausea, vomiting, and eventual circulatory collapse. Disulfiram is also a DA beta-hydroxylase inhibitor. This action (the reduction of DA's anabolic conversion to NE) contributes to the vascular sequelae by reducing the amount of NE available for release. Other drugs with disulfiram-like effects are chlorpropamide, tolbutamide, and metronidazole. Disulfiram is used to treat alcohol abuse. Patients who consent to take this drug will experience severe consequences if they resume drinking. Its use is controversial, however, because the severe interaction of disulfiram and ethanol can have life-threatening cardiovascular effects.

PHENCYCLIDINE (PCP)

Phencyclidine (PCP) was introduced in the 1950s as a dissociative anesthetic. As a dissociative anesthetic similar to ketamine (see Chapter 7), PCP was originally used in surgical procedures. The occurrence of bizarre aftereffects and some reported cases of psychotic-like symptoms lasting for days forced the FDA to withdraw it from the market in 1965. PCP is currently classified as a schedule II drug, but it is also a popular street drug.

PCP is called "angel dust" because it is often sprinkled on marijuana or on tobacco and then smoked. It is also combined with cocaine. Ingested by itself, PCP is well absorbed when taken orally, pyrolyzed and inhaled, or insufflated. It has profound effects on the CNS including psychostimulation, analgesia, anesthesia, depression, hallucinations, and psychotomimetic actions. PCP does not exhibit cross-tolerance with other drugs. Rats trained to recognize the perceptual effects of hallucinogens readily discriminate them from those of PCP. In fact, PCP is readily distinguished from all other drugs of abuse in animal drug-discrimination studies (see Balster, 1991).

Inconsistent absorption and unpredictable effects following oral ingestion kept PCP use low until the late 1970s when pyrolysis and insufflation became popular routes of administration. Its street reputation as a dangerous drug when consumed by these routes led to a decline in use in the 1980s and 1990s. Nevertheless, the low cost and ease with which it is synthesized maintain its availability on the streets despite countermeasures by the federal government to regulate the sale of chemicals used in its synthesis. In contrast to most street drugs, chronic use of PCP produces very little tolerance (only one- to twofold). This contributes to its popularity since the cost of using the drug does not escalate. Moreover, although it induces dependence, there is little evidence of a withdrawal syndrome.

The mechanism of action of PCP

PCP influences CNS function primarily by noncompetitive antagonism of glutamate NMDA receptors (see Johnson and Jones, 1990; Fig. 12–6). These are voltage- and ligand-gated receptors requiring depolarization to displace Mg^{2+} from the ionophore and allow Ca^{2+} and Na^+ to enter the cell (see Chapter 8). PCP binds to a site within the ionophore, preventing cation conductance despite Mg^{2+} displacement. Thus, it is classified as a noncompetitive antagonist of Glu. The site at which PCP binds is called the sigma receptor.

PCP also directly and indirectly influences the activity of several other neurotransmitter systems. It has affinity for the DA transporter although it is not a substrate. It is therefore considered a competitive reuptake in-

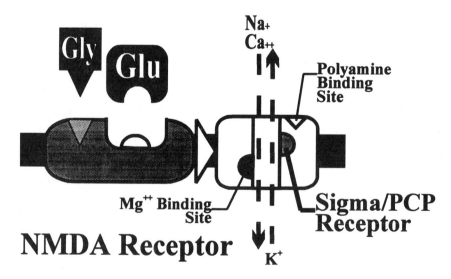

Figure 12–6. The binding site for phencyclidine (PCP) is thought to be located inside the cation channel of the NMDA-receptor complex.

hibitor of dopamine. By blocking NMDA heteroreceptors that normally inhibit DA terminals, PCP also enhances dopamine release. These combined effects produce increased DA activity that contributes significantly to the psychotomimetic effects of this drug. Acting through NMDA receptors, PCP also affects ACh, NE, and 5HT.

Effects of PCP

The many neurotransmitter systems affected by PCP are reflected in its plethora of effects. PCP's ability to influence so many systems also makes it difficult to determine which neurotransmitter system is responsible for a particular effect. Nonetheless, the effects including toxicity are generally dose-dependent. Although PCP is biotransformed in the liver to several metabolites, some of which are active, their potency is reduced and they are not likely to contribute significantly to the actions of PCP.

At low to moderate doses, the behavioral syndrome starts to appear within five minutes when insufflated or an hour when taken orally. The syndrome may last up to 15 hours, which is consistent with PCP's half-life of 16 to 24 hours. The user may experience euphoria or dysphoria and a feeling of numbness. Perception of time may slow. Anxiety and paranoia may develop as the dose increases. Users have reported a variety of experiences: paresthesias, perceptual changes in body size, difficulty in thinking, depersonalization, marked loss of concentration, sensory illusions, increased energy, marked impairment of short-term memory, ataxia, dysarthria, nystagmus, bursts of uncontrolled aggression (almost exclusively in males), delirium, and psychotic symptoms (see Hurlbut, 1991; Brust, 1993). Hallucinations may be combined with feelings of power and invulnerability. With such a diverse set of unpredictable effects, many of which are unpleasant, one has to wonder why the drug remains popular.

The toxic profile of PCP is legendary. Of all overdose victims, PCP patients are the most difficult to manage. The behavioral syndrome seen at higher dosages, especially in males, reportedly includes belligerence, impaired judgment, agitation, and violent, combative behavior. Coupled with PCP's analgesic effects, the perception exists that such patients are not easily restrained. This syndrome has never been systematically studied and may differ little from the behavioral toxicity of other street drugs (Gorelick and Balster, 1995).

The toxic syndrome begins with delirium, increased respirations, laryngeal and pharyngeal hyperactivity, hypertension and tachycardia, hyperpyrexia, increased secretions, muscular rigidity, increased deep tendon reflexes, clonus upon stimulation, stereotypies, rapid horizontal and vertical nystagmus, variable pupil size, and often a blank stare. Loss of pinprick sensations, dysarthria, and ataxia also occur. As toxicity increases, the throat signs diminish and hiccoughing and sustained vomiting may develop. Spasticity, generalized myoclonus, and seizures may also occur and are often associated with a disconjugate gaze. The patient is now stuporous but still somewhat responsive to pain. Eventually, the patient becomes comatose. Aspiration pneumonitis is a major risk because of increased secretions and absent throat reflexes. Stroke, high-output heart failure, and dramatic swings in blood pressure may occur. Seizures are common and may even convert to status epilepticus. Kidney failure is probable if significant rhabdomyolysis had occurred as a result of excessive motor activity. Though patients often have their eyes open ("Eyes open coma"), they die of respiratory or cardiac complications (Hurlbut, 1991). High-dose, chronic administration of PCP produces degenerative changes in neurons and astrocytes including vacuolization, inhibition of microtubule function, reduced neuronal growth, and cell death (Olney, Labruyere, and Price, 1989).

Diazepam is the drug treatment of choice for these patients since it has a calming effect and increases seizure threshold. The patient should be placed in a safe environment where they can be observed and kept away from objects with which they might hurt themselves or others. Restraints should be avoided as they often provoke combative behavior further exacerbating rhabdomyolysis. The antipsychotic drugs should be avoided since they reduce seizure threshold. Continuous gastric suction is indicated since PCP exhibits significant enterogastric recycling due to ion trapping. As discussed in Chapter 2, PCP diffuses into the stomach, where it becomes trapped by ionization. The stomach acts as a sink for PCP, effectively drawing it from the circulation. As a result, the patient may come out of coma temporarily. As coma wanes and gastrointestinal motility returns, the once-trapped PCP is passed into the intestines, where it is again absorbed and recirculated back to the brain to produce coma. This pattern of cyclic comas is considered pathognomonic of PCP overdose.

Patients on PCP arrive in the emergency room with traumatic injuries more often than users of other drugs. The cerebellar effects of PCP (ataxia and nystagmus), its analgesic properties, its cognitive interference, and its ability to produce sensory illusions and a sense of invulnerability all combine to make PCP abusers highly accident prone.

MARIJUANA

Marijuana is the dried female flower of the wild plant *Cannabis sativa.* Pyrolysis of the material releases over 100 substances that are subsequently inhaled in the smoke from a marijuana cigarette. Delta-9 tetrahy-drocannabinol (THC) is thought to be the ingredient most responsible for the mental effects of marijuana and most of the discussion that follows is based on this assumption (Fig. 12–7). But marijuana contains several cannabinoids, such as delta-8 tetrahydrocannabinol, connabidiol, and cannabinol, that have not been systematically evaluated. Thus, it is possible that the combined effects of THC and the other cannabinoids that are potentially synergistic with or antagonistic to it may be responsible for the effects of marijuana.

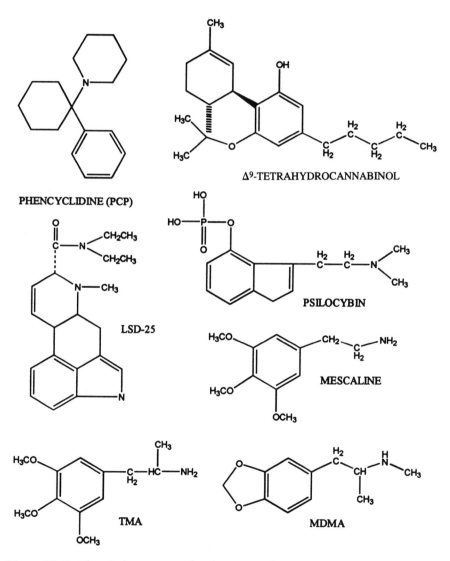

Figure 12–7. Chemical structures of various street drugs.

The normal amount of THC in the cannabis flower is between 2 and 5 mg%. Over the years, the quantity of THC found in confiscated street marijuana has risen to 8 to 10 mg%, suggesting that the plant is being selectively bred for its euphorogenic potency. The THC of hashish (resin-soaked buds of the flower) can approach 15 to 20 mg% while the THC content of hash oil may be as high as 30 mg%. Normal smoking delivers about 18% of the drug to the circulation whereas conditioned smokers who better tolerate the irritant effects of the smoke can take in up to 23% of the drug available in the smoke. In contrast, the bioavailability of THC ingested orally in marijuana cookies, brownies, and teas is only around 6%.

The Mechanism of Action of Marijuana

The effects of THC have been extensively studied in humans and several animal models (Hollister, 1986; Martin, 1986, 1995; Dewey, 1986; Hurlbut, 1991; Brust, 1993). Variable effects are the norm given the differences in dosing schedules, delivery techniques, and brain systems studied.

As an extremely lipophilic substance, THC readily dissolves in membranes and disrupts fluidity in much the same way that gas anesthetics and alcohol do. Like anesthetic gases and alcohol, THC does not disrupt Na^+conductance and therefore does not interfere with depolarization or the speed at which action potentials are conducted. However, its lipophilic properties enable it to enter membranes where specific binding sites (receptors?) have been identified. Thus, as was demonstrated with the anesthetic gases, THC binds stereospecifically to a protein in the membrane (Devane et al., 1988) and it is this action that is thought to be responsible for its psychoactive effects.

THC binding sites are heterogeneously distributed in the brain. Their density is highest in the basal ganglia and cerebellum and moderately dense in the hippocampus and layers I and VI of the cortex. Discrete regions of the brainstem, thalamus, and hypothalamus have a low binding density. These binding sites are linked with G_i. THC taken in with marijuana smoke would thus inhibit the activation of adenylate cyclase by neurotransmitters that work through other G proteins. THC has also been shown to stimulate phospholipase A_2. This would increase the production of arachidonic acid, DAG, and IP_3. It is perhaps this system that is responsible for THC's demonstrated ability to inhibit the voltage-gated Ca^{2+} channel (N channel) that regulates neurotransmitter release. THC is thus best described as a neuromodulatory substance that acts through a specific binding site embedded in the membrane to alter the production of second messengers regulated by other neurotransmitters. Interestingly, a substance called amandamide that binds with high affinity to the THC binding site has been isolated from brain (Devane et al., 1992).

When administered to animals, THC induces a triphasic pattern of change in dopamine and serotonin. Initially dopamine is decreased and serotonin is increased. This pattern is reversed during a second sustained phase followed by a return to normal during the so-called depressive phase. In contrast to the temporal pattern of change seen in dopamine and serotonin, THC consistently reduces acetylcholine, especially in the hippocampus. This decrease appears to be the result of THC's ability to reduce choline uptake.

Psychic Effects of Marijuana

Although marijuana is historically grouped with the hallucinogens, it does not share most of the properties of this drug class and will only produce hallucinations at very high plasma levels. It also has CNS depressant actions, but grouping marijuana with this drug class does not allow for the early phase of stimulation associated with its use. Like PCP, its effects are unique and it is best classified simply as a psychoactive drug.

Marijuana generally produces biphasic psychic changes of euphoria (stimulant phase) and sedation (depressive phase). During the initial stimulant phase, the user describes a "dreamlike" state where time sense is distorted, hearing is less discriminant, and visual distortions can occur (Table 12–6). Concentration can be so compromised that users readily lose their train of thought. Memory consolidation is impaired and appetite is usually suppressed, reflecting THC's effects on ACh and 5HT, respectively. Following the stimulant phase, drowsiness and lethargy are common. As with drugs of the sedative-hypnotic class, sleep latency is reduced, REM latency is increased, and REM suppression occurs. But there is no REM rebound. During the depressive phase, appetite is often increased. At extremely high doses, marijuana can produce a state of memory impairment, confusion, and disorientation bordering on delirium. This type of reaction is rarely seen in the United States, is self-limited when it does occur, and does not require medical intervention.

The psychic effects of marijuana are use and context dependent. First-time users often describe feelings of anxiety that may approximate panic. Such reactions include the characteristic signs and symptoms of sympathetic activation but do not usually require medical intervention other than reassurance. Panic is a common problem in naive users of most street drugs, not just marijuana. However, habitual users sometimes experience feelings of paranoia that can lead to anxiety. The severity of this reaction depends on the environment such that it would be mild at a rock

Table 12–6 Effects of Marijuana

Stimulant/euphoric phase	Dream-like euphoric state Slowed time sense Increased visual acuity (visual distortions can occur) Decreased auditory discrimination Difficulty concentrating (lost train of thought) Reduced appetite Short-term-memory impairment
Depressive/sedative phase	Drowsiness, lethargy, and anergy Increased appetite
Other psychic changes	Reduced aggressiveness Panic attacks Paranoia Hallucinations (very rare) Depersonalization Amotivational syndrome Rare cases of toxic delirium
Other effects[a]	Analgesia (mild) Orthostatic hypotension Tachycardia and heart palpitations Bronchodilation and mild smooth-muscle relaxation Conjunctival reddening and reduced intraocular pressure Slightly reduced testosterone, FSH and LH production Slightly reduced sperm production and possible gynecomastia Reduced muscle strength Potent antiemetic effects Hypothermia Dry mouth and "dry eyes" Moderate antiseizure effects

[a]FSH = follicle-stimulating hormone; LH = luteinizing hormone

concert but intense when alone or in a police station. Contrary to the belief of some, studies in humans consistently demonstrate that marijuana reduces aggressive behavior even though animals injected with THC consistently show aggression.

Amotivational syndrome describes a pattern of behavior that emerges in some habitual drug users after many years and is characterized by the lack of desire to work or excel at any aspect of life. If it occurs, it is most commonly seen in individuals who, as adolescents or teens, consumed large quantities of marijuana for long periods of time. Whether amotivational syndrome is a unique consequence of an interaction between THC and the maturing brain or a personality characteristic of an individual who would have developed this behavior regardless of prior drug exposure is unknown. Nonetheless, it is generally attributed to marijuana use.

Other Effects

THC and marijuana produce several effects that are consistent with its mechanism of action. As described previously, drugs which increase membrane fluidity have analgesic effects and THC falls into this category. Its mild analgesic properties may also result from THC's aspirin-like effect (cyclooxygenase inhibition).

Marijuana induces dose-dependent tachycardia and orthostatic hypotension during the initial stimulant phase of the behavioral syndrome. Tachycardia results from the vagolytic effects associated with THC's inhibition of choline uptake as well as a centrally mediated reduction of activity in the cardiovascular center of the medulla. The basis for the orthostasis is less well understood but probably involves reduced sympathetic outflow mediated by a central effect of the drug—THC's ability to reduce smooth-muscle tone slightly—and its inhibition of choline uptake, which would reduce the activity of preganglionic cholinergic neurons. These combined effects on vascular tone as well as its anticholinergic properties probably contribute to conjunctival reddening that is an invariable characteristic of this drug. Its inhibitory effects on the autonomic nervous system may also be responsible for THC's ability to produce dry mouth and dry eyes and reduce intraocular pressure in a dose-dependent fashion.

Marijuana and THC are famous for their antiemetic effects. Their capacity to reduce the intensity and frequency of nausea and vomiting associated with chemotherapy led to the development of the direct-acting THC agonists dronabinol and nabilone. These drugs are currently available but seldom prescribed due to their psychic effects.

Additional effects associated with THC ingestion include moderate muscle relaxation, increased seizure threshold, hypothermia, and bronchodilation. Although THC is a potent bronchodilator, the resins and particulates in marijuana smoke decrease ciliary motility and irritate the mucosal lining, producing an overall compromise in respiratory function. Marijuana use in humans and THC studies in animals have revealed numerous alterations in hormone levels, and such changes as decreased testosterone levels have been popular subjects for the lay press. The scientific data, however, are inconsistent, and when changes are shown, they are minor and reversible.

The effects of marijuana, including its analgesic and antiemetic properties, its bronchodilatory effects, and its ability to reduce intraocular pressure have often been used as arguments for the legalization of marijuana. It is important to note, however, that in all clinical situations where marijuana could provide therapeutic benefit, other drugs that are generally more potent, more specific, and devoid of psychic properties are available.

Pharmacokinetics of Marijuana

Following inhalation of marijuana smoke, the plasma levels of THC peak within several minutes, fall rapidly within an hour (alpha phase), and decline very slowly thereafter (beta phase). The alpha phase of decline is undoubtedly due to redistribution of the drug from the brain to muscle and then into fat, whereas the much slower beta phase is the result of THC slowly leaving fat tissue. Because of its exceptional lipophilicity, THC and its metabolites can be detected in the body for weeks.

Marijuana is metabolized almost exclusively in the liver, so there is a significant first-pass effect and low bioavailability following oral delivery. Microsomal enzyme induction occurs as a consequence of the tars consumed with the smoke. THC and the other cannabinoids by themselves do not induce the P-450 system. A significant amount of THC is excreted unchanged in the feces (as with most highly lipophilic agents) and enterohepatic recirculation is known to occur. Urinary metabolites are oxidative products and also conjugates.

Some have suggested that THC can accumulate in the body. If this were to occur, it would explain why naive users often fail to perceive a "high" during their first few encounters with marijuana. However, only inactive metabolites of THC accumulate. The failure of naive users to experience euphoria may simply reflect their inability to tolerate the high amounts of inhaled smoke necessary to yield adequate absorption. Experienced users know that the yield is higher if the smoke is inhaled deeply and then held. In support of this argument, THC administered to animals induces consistent cardiovascular changes whether or not the animal has been pre-exposed to the drug. Alternatively, the initiation of the euphorogenic actions of marijuana may require priming (see Chapter 3). Thus, THC might have to act at its endogenous binding sites at least once before initiating the sequence of events hypothesized to be responsible for the euphorogenic actions of the drug.

Tolerance and Dependence

Tolerance to all of marijuana's effects has been demonstrated in both animals and man and it is surprisingly long-lived. According to the counteradaptation theory, such tolerance should be associated with a withdrawal syndrome. Occasional use and even continuous low-dose abuse is not, however, associated with a discernible withdrawal syndrome. In contrast, subjects given high doses of marijuana several times a day for a few weeks, do exhibit withdrawal reactions consisting of irritability, sleep disturbances, nausea, vomiting, diarrhea, tremors, and sweating. These symptoms are generally, though not always, associated with drug craving. Mild cross-tolerance to some effects of marijuana will occur in individuals tolerant to CNS depressants including alcohol and the opiates. Marijuana does not significantly increase dopamine levels in the CNS, and based on current addiction theory, possesses very little dependence liability.

THE HALLUCINOGENS

The hallucinogenic or "psychedelic" drugs are unique in their ability to produce hallucinations without delirium. Thus, unlike the anticholinergic agents, PCP, marijuana, toxic chemicals such as mercury or bromides and, to some extent, the central stimulants, the hallucinogens can give rise to hallucinations in the presence of intact cognitive function and orientation to the environment. Memory is generally not impaired although the internal focus of attention on the subject's own thoughts often disrupts performance on memory tests. Time sense is commonly disrupted and can be either accelerated or slowed (see Table 12–7). In addition to hallucinations, the hallucinogens may affect mood; these usually represent an exaggeration of the predrug mind set and are highly context dependent. They are typically pleasurable but can also be terrifying ("the bad trip"). Somatic signs reflecting sympathetic arousal include increased pulse rate and blood pressure, hyperreflexia, dilated pupils, piloerection, and slight pyrexia. Nausea and vomiting may occur and are particularly prevalent with certain hallucinogens, such as mescaline. Hallucinogenic drugs are commonly used by middle- and upper-class white males, and in this group, abuse has increased over the past two decades despite a decline in the use of many other drugs (Abraham and Aldridge, 1993): 7.6% of the population over the age of 12 have used these drugs at least once.

Chemically, the hallucinogens fall into three major classes (Fig. 12–7):

1. Lysergic acid derivatives (LSD)
2. Phenylalkylamines (mescaline)
3. Indolealkylamines (psilocybin)

In addition to these chemical groups, many designer drugs with hallucinogen-like effects have been developed. These are often referred to as

Table 12–7 The Effects of LSD

Somatic signs	Dizziness
	Weakness
	Tremors
	Nausea
	Mydriasis
	Mild pyrexia
	Piloerection
	Hyperreflexia
	Generalized SANS activation
Perceptual signs	Kaleidoscopic alterations in colors, shapes, and sizes
	Hallucinations in all senses are possible
	Afterimages on moving objects ("trails")
	Synesthesias
	Enhanced auditory sense
Psychic symptoms	Dream-like state
	Coexistence of thoughts
	Alterations in mood (generally pleasant)
	Distorted time sense
	Feelings of estrangement or depersonalization
	Panic attacks in naive users
	Psychotic symptoms in susceptible individuals
	Hallucinogen persisting perceptual disorder (HPPD)

substituted amphetamines or phenylethylamine derivatives (Table 12–8). Most of these drugs do not produce hallucinations until plasma levels are extremely high.

Hallucinations

LSD was first synthesized by Hoffman in 1943. Recognition of its ability to alter mood, induce hallucinations, and generate signs and symptoms resembling psychoses led to the widespread study of its effects soon thereafter. Most of the early work was performed in human volunteers in the early 1950s and is fascinating reading (see Bercel et al., 1956, for instance). The fact that a drug could produce a hallucination offered a strategy for determining the neurobiology underlying this phenomenon. Although some advances have been made, we are still unable to explain the complex neurobiology that leads to the hallucinogenic event.

A hallucination is a visual, auditory, tactile, olfactory, gustatory, or kinesthetic perception in the absence of an external stimulus. It is a conscious experience of sight, sound, taste, smell, or touch in the absence of environmental input. Hallucination differs from an illusion in that the latter is a distortion of an external stimulus. Illusions commonly occur with PCP and anticholinergic intoxication. A hallucination also differs from a delusion in that the latter implies an inappropriate cognitive interpretation of an external event. Hallucinations are "brain-centered" activities that result from the disruption of CNS systems normally responsible for the perception and interpretation of external events. The types of hallucination experienced seem to reflect the normal processing of sensory information as it moves from primary pattern detection to associational integration. The disruption of higher associational areas might also explain the experience of synesthesia that sometimes occurs during the use of hallucinogenic drugs. In a synesthetic hallucination, sensory modalities are mixed up, i.e., colors are heard or sounds are seen. Many of the types of hallucinations experienced with hallucinogenic drugs are seen in patients with specific brain lesions and temporal lobe epilepsy, and it is assumed that the actions of these drugs somehow interfere with neuronal function in these areas (see Cummings, 1985; Asaad and Shapiro, 1986, for discussion).

LSD-induced hallucinations often occur initially as unformed bursts of light, then as geometric forms followed by complex images involving faces, scenes, and even movement within those scenes (Asaad and Shapiro, 1986). This temporal sequence is similar to the pattern of hallucinations that arise from lesions of the primary, secondary, and higher visual association areas and suggests that the hallucinogenic drugs reduce the thresholds for activation sequentially along sensory pathways. Once these thresholds have been reduced, neurons may fire in response to background activity in the absence of an external event, thus producing the hallucination.

The Pharmacodynamics of LSD and Other Hallucinogens

It is generally assumed that, with minor differences, LSD and the other hallucinogens share similar properties which are consistent with their virtually indistinguishable hallucinogenic effects. Our understanding of the mechanisms of LSD evolved in three phases: (1) serotonin antagonism, (2) reduction in the activity of the raphe system, and (3) postsynaptic serotonin agonism (see Jacobs, 1986).

LSD as a 5HT-receptor antagonist

After LSD's hallucinogenic properties were discovered and the structural similarities between 5HT and LSD were characterized, LSD was evaluated for its ability to affect 5HT activity in a bioassay. Since LSD acted as a serotonin antagonist, its hallucinogenicity was thought to be a consequence of reducing 5HT activity in the CNS. But it was soon found that brom-LSD (a brominated form of LSD) also had similar antagonistic actions yet was devoid of hallucinogenic activity.

LSD as a collateral Raphe agonist

Several studies showed that serotonin was the only neurotransmitter to be consistently affected by LSD and that it elevated brain 5HT while reducing its metabolite 5HIAA. Serotonin levels in nerve terminals increased and its metabolite decreased when neuronal firing rate was reduced. A seminal study by Aghajanian and his colleagues (1968) revealed that LSD reduced the normally slow pulsatile firing rate of neurons in the raphe nucleus. Their findings suggested that LSD, acting as an agonist at the receptors mediating collateral inhibition in the raphe system, inhibited the cell bodies and thereby reduced forebrain 5HT activity. Since serotonergic fibers are known to densely innervate the visual and temporal cortices where they are inhibitory, it was assumed that the hallucinogenic experience resulted from disinhibition of these structures. Other studies demonstrating LSD's ability to enhance the stimulus-generalization properties of sensory processing led to the further assumption that internally generated stimuli would be inappropriately generalized to other perceptions and, together with the cortical disinhibition, would produce a hallucination.

This hypothesis was challenged by several observations. First, the behavioral actions of the hallucinogens in animals extend beyond the depression of raphe firing. Second, the hallucinogenic potency of LSD decreases rapidly with consecutive dosing, but LSD-induced inhibition of raphe firing does not. Third, several other hallucinogenic drugs failed to depress raphe firing. Finally, 5HT depletion should block the actions of hallucinogens since it would maximally depress serotonin activity. But destruction of raphe neurons actually enhances the effects of LSD, presumably through receptor-site up-regulation.

LSD as a selective postsynaptic agonist

The data discussed above are consistent with the hypothesis that LSD acts as a selective postsynaptic 5HT agonist. Serotonin receptors mediate both excitation and inhibition in their postsynaptic target structures. The immediate precursor to 5HT, 5-hydroxytryptophan, does not produce hallucinations. Since it increases serotonin release at all serotonergic terminals but does not produce hallucinations, they must arise only when selected 5HT receptors are activated. The receptor originally proposed to mediate this effect was the $5HT_2$ receptor. However, our understanding of the 5HT-receptor system is in continuous flux. Currently, we recognize seven 5HT-receptor families with 18 different subtypes (Glennon and Dukat, 1995). Three different $5HT_2$ receptors have been identified. Until the substrate specificity of LSD for these newer receptors has been systematically studied, the exact mechanism by which LSD acts and the target structures it affects will remain unclear. At present, it is safe to say that LSD exerts its postsynaptic actions in the neocortex, limbic structures, and brainstem, where $5HT_2$ receptors are more dense (see Fig. 12–8).

Dopamine and hallucinogenic drugs
In addition to their actions as 5HT agonists, some hallucinogens (LSD, mescaline, and many substituted amphetamines) are also direct-acting

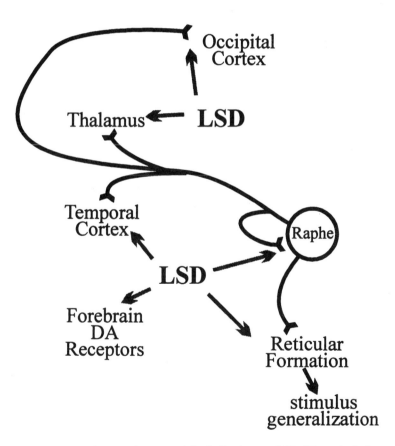

Figure 12–8. Potential sites of action of the hallucinogen LSD. These include postsynaptic targets in the cortex and thalamus as well as autoinhibition through its actions on the receptors activated by the axon collateral. 5HT may also enhance stimulus generalization in the reticular formation.

DA agonists. The ability of levodopa, amantadine (Harper and Knothe, 1973), and many substituted amphetamines to induce hallucinations suggests the involvement of dopamine in the hallucinogenic process. However, DA antagonists can block hallucinations induced by DA without affecting hallucinations induced by LSD. Thus, DA may be involved in the overall actions of the hallucinogens, but it is probably not responsible for the hallucinations they produce.

Effects of Hallucinogens and the Toxic Profile

The effects of hallucinogenic drugs are listed in Table 12–7. These signs and symptoms are induced by as little as 50 μg of LSD, which is generally considered the threshold dose. This means that LSD is one of the most potent drugs known, so handling and administering the synthesized powder can become tricky. Liquid LSD is therefore often added to blotter paper ("microdot"), sugar cubes, or another liquid and then ingested orally. Intravenous injection or insufflation of the hallucinogens is rare and they are unstable during pyrolysis, which prevents ingestion through the lungs. As the administered dose increases, the signs and symptoms intensify, and at very high doses (1 mg) all individuals will experience hallucinations. Although higher dosages are often ingested by experienced users to intensify the hallucinations, their content is not dramatically altered.

Hallucinations are most widely experienced in a dim room or with the eyes closed. Users, even those on "bad trips," are generally aware that the hallucination is drug-related. Experienced users can perform complicated, skilled tasks (depending on size of dose) if requested, although they would rather not be bothered. The user's awareness of the drug-induced nature of the experience and the fact that cognitive function is intact distinguish this drug class from all other drugs that induce hallucinations within the context of a toxic or delirious state.

The psilocybins and the mescaline-like drugs are much less potent than LSD. Psilocybin is most often consumed by eating "magic mushrooms" that are indigenous to parts of the Pacific Northwest, Hawaii, Texas, Florida, and Mexico. Ten to 100 mushrooms must be eaten raw or dry, brewed in tea, or eaten in a stew to obtain a hallucinogenic experience. Psilocybin often induces a characteristic flushing of the face and neck and can induce ataxia. One must always be careful to ensure that a potential overdose victim has not mistakenly consumed mushrooms containing anticholinergic contaminants that would contribute to the hallucination but also possibly induce toxic delirium and death. Mescaline, the least potent of the hallucinogens, comes from the peyote cactus found in arid regions of North and South America. The sun-dried crowns of these cacti (peyote buttons) are consumed dry or in various recipes. Each button contains about 45 mg of mescaline. The threshold for hallucinations is generally considered to be 5 mg/kg. Nausea and vomiting usually herald the onset of the hallucinogenic experience, reflecting the more potent direct-acting DA agonist properties of mescaline relative to the other hallucinogens. Nystagmus, respiratory distress, and hyporeflexia can also occur.

The hallucinogens are absorbed well following oral ingestion and, in each case, the hallucinogenic event begins within an hour. The duration of effect is usually about 12 hours for LSD, six to 12 hours for psilocybin, and six hours for mescaline. Hallucinogenic overdoses are very rare, and when they do occur, drug therapy is not indicated because the potential for fatality is minimal. As with most street drugs, panic attacks in inexperienced users are not uncommon. Victims can become unpredictably violent and belligerent. Segregation in a quiet room with someone present for reassurance is usually all that is required to treat these patients although diazepam may be needed in some cases. Serious medical consequences from a hallucinogen overdose are the exception and invariably involve trauma secondary to activities performed while on drugs. Cardiovascular or other serious medical problems suggest that the patient consumed a substance adulterated with a nonhallucinogenic compound such as PCP or a designer drug (see Hurlbut, 1991; Brust, 1993).

Hallucinogen-induced psychoses
Significant media attention has focused on the fact that the hallucinogenic drugs can induce psychotic behavior and even permanent psychoses in some patients. It is generally assumed, and in some cases established, that these patients were predisposed to psychosis. Evaluation of various Indian tribes who have used mescaline for centuries reveals no elevation in the incidence of psychoses. Moreover, unlike the amphetamines, LSD has variable effects in confirmed psychotics: The amphetamines invariably exacerbate psychotic symptoms while LSD will worsen symptoms in some and have no apparent effect in others. The alterations in symptoms that do occur in these patients reverse with clearance of the drug.

Although early studies suggest that LSD induced a model psychosis, this notion has been abandoned because of the intact cognitive processing that accompanies the LSD-induced hallucination. In addition, the hallucinations in LSD users are primarily visual while those in psychotics are primarily auditory. Although both groups can have any form of hallucination, the hallucinations experienced by psychotics usually occur when their eyes are open whereas the effects of hallucinogenic drugs are most pronounced when the eyes are closed or when the user is in a darkened room.

Hallucinogen persisting perceptual disorder (HPPD)

It is well documented that as many as 35% of users experience a condition called hallucinogen persisting perceptual disorder (HPPD) in *DSM-IV* and more commonly known as "flashbacks." Even one-time users can experience this phenomenon. A flashback is a reinitiation of any aspect of the hallucinogenic experience, including an emotion that occurs without drug ingestion. Flashbacks are most often experienced in the weeks following hallucinogen use, although there have been reports of this disorder occurring five years later. The event is usually short-lived (a matter of seconds) but has lasted for a month in rare cases. Flashbacks in LSD users can be precipitated by DA antagonists or stressful events that are either perceived or real. Their intensity and incidence wane with time.

Studies of hallucinogen users experiencing flashbacks reveal perceptual alterations, including dramatically slower dark adaptation and decreased critical flicker fusion thresholds, particularly in the peripheral visual field (see Abraham and Aldridge, 1993, for review). These studies suggest that the visual systems of flashback patients have a reduced capacity to inhibit afterimages. Neuroscientists generally assume that any sensory system must "inhibit" the impulse activity of previous sensations so that the sensation currently entering the system can be processed appropriately. If this inhibition does not occur, current sensations entering the system will be co-interpreted with those that occurred just moments ago. Such disinhibition is thought to be responsible for the afterimages or trails seen behind moving objects while under the influence of a hallucinogenic drug. The objective measurement of decreased critical flicker fusion thresholds in patients with HPPD suggests that the same disinhibition which occurred during the original hallucinogenic episode is again at work during the flashback. Interestingly, it has been shown that even acute exposure to hallucinogens can induce a long-lasting down-regulation of $5HT_2$ receptors which may be involved in this phenomenon.

Tolerance, Cross-Tolerance, and Dependence

The perceptual and psychic signs and symptoms of the hallucinogenic drugs exhibit rapid tolerance (tachyphylaxis) that usually develops within 24 hours. Because the rate of tolerance is so fast, a daily pattern of use needed for the development of dependence is virtually impossible to achieve, resulting in a very low dependence liability. In addition, there is cross-tolerance among all members of this drug class, so once tolerance develops to one hallucinogen, the potency of all the other hallucinogens is similarly reduced—thus, cross-tolerance (see Carvey et al., 1989). The mechanism of this tolerance is unknown, but because of the speed of its development, it cannot be pharmacokinetic.

Designer Drugs

Many designer drugs are substituted amphetamines, although others share structural similarities with all the hallucinogens. The designer drugs produce neither clear-cut psychostimulant effects nor true hallucinations. Many have been shown to deplete serotonin as well as dopamine and norepinephrine. The mechanism of these effects is unknown.

The most frequently encountered designer drugs are listed in Table 12–8. As a group, they are thought to produce the psychic symptoms of hallucinogens without hallucinations, except at higher doses. Compared to the hallucinogens, they produce more sympathomimetic effects, which complicate the emergency management of overdose victims. Most designer drugs enhance self-esteem and this leads to increased use. During the late 1980s, drugs such as MDA, MDMA ("Ecstasy"), and MDEA

Table 12–8 Designer Drugs

Drug	Distinguishing Characteristics
2,4,5-Trimethoxyamphetamine (TMA)	Structurally resembles both mescaline and amphetamine. Effects are similar to those of mescaline
4-Methyl-2,5-dimethoxyamphetamine (DOM)	Also known as Serenity, Tranquility, and Peace (STP). Hallucinations occur with significant SANS activation
Paramethoxyamphetamine (PMA)	Very potent hallucinogen associated with excessive SANS stimulation and fatalities. Most frequently used as a contaminant to enhance psychic effects of other drugs
Brom-DOM	The most potent phenylethylamine compound, distributed in a microdot formulation. Effects last for ten hours. Overdose is rarely fatal
3,4-Methylenedioxyamphetamine (MDA)	Mild intoxication without hallucinations. Produces feelings of empathy and euphoria. Higher doses produce hallucinations with delirium
3-4-Methylenedioxymethamphetamine (MDMA)	Also known as Ecstasy, Adam, and M & M. Initially synthesized as an appetite suppressant. Used in conjunction with group therapy because of its ability to produce empathy. Known to have induced several deaths secondary to cardiac arrhythmias
3-4-Methylenedioxyethamphetamine (MDEA)	Also known as Eve, with effects similar to those of MDMA

("Eve") were used in group counseling sessions to enhance interpersonal communication and empathy. Under the influence of the drug, patients reported reliving past life events and could discuss these often traumatic experiences openly. A significant grassroots campaign was organized to legalize their use after they were banned by the FDA. Subsequently, the recreational use of these drugs became popular in the 1990s, and many users have felt that their personalities changed dramatically for the better because of the experience. Unfortunately, designer drugs have much lower therapeutic indices than LSD and overdoses can be associated with significant morbidity and even mortality.

Chronic toxic effects include exhaustion, fatigue, depression, nausea, numbness, and flashbacks. Patients exhibiting significant signs and symptoms of sympathetic activation are in a severe state of toxicity and require immediate and aggressive symptomatic treatment. Their signs and symptoms resemble those of amphetamine toxicity and should be managed in a similar way.

ANTICHOLINERGICS

Anticholinergic toxicity has been referred to several times throughout this text in connection with the side effects of many prescription drugs including the antiparkinson agents, tricyclic antidepressants, and antipsychotics (see Table 12–9). The toxic profile is predominantly antimuscarinic. The constellation of symptoms observed in the emergency room that suggests anticholinergic toxicity is generally recalled by the mnemonic, "hot as a hare, blind as a stone, mad as a hatter, and dry to the bone." Because of the risk of death, overdose victims should be treated immediately. GI stasis resulting from reduced cholinergic activity often renders gastric lavage very effective. Lavage should be followed by the administration of activated charcoal. The patient should be cooled and catheterized. Anticonvulsants may be required but antipsychotics should be avoided. Physostigmine, a centrally acting acetylcholinesterase inhibitor, is a direct antidote and will overcome the blockade produced by most of the agents responsible for the anticholinergic syndrome. It must be used cautiously because of the potential for cholinergic toxicity which can produce depolarization blockade of muscles used in respiration (see Chapter 7). Bradycardia and especially excessive bronchial secretions, bronchospasms, and laryngospasms should be monitored carefully in patients treated with this antidote.

Individuals will intentionally ingest substances with anticholinergic effects because at lower doses they produce hallucinogen-like effects as part of the early stages of delirium. Several plants found in the United

Table 12–9 The Anticholinergic Syndrome

Psychic effects	Euphoria
	Anxiety
	Excitement
	Delirium
	Hallucinations (usually visual, formed, and frightening, with loss of insight)
Somatic effects	Mydriasis
	Loss of pupillary light reflexes
	Blurred vision (loss of accommodation)
	Dry, flushed skin
	Vasodilation
	Reduced secretions (saliva, bronchi, and nasal)
	Decreased GI motility
	Hyperpyrexia
	Tachycardia with hyper- or hypotension
	Urinary retention
Toxic effects	Myoclonus
	Extensor posturing
	Seizures
	Coma
	Respiratory depression
	Circulatory collapse
	Death

States (in particular jimson weed, *Datura stramonium*) can produce this syndrome. Adolescents will eat the seeds, chew the roots, or make teas from this plant to experience its effects. Several mushrooms and many over-the-counter medications with antimuscarinic actions act similarly and are used recreationally. Intentional consumption of anticholinergics is therefore common.

VOLATILE INHALANTS

The volatile inhalants are a diverse set of compounds that include glues, aerosols, refrigerants, cleaning fluids, cements, lighter fluid, marker pens, gasoline, volatile anesthetics, fire-extinguisher agents, fingernail polish, bottled-fuel gas, typewriter correction fluid, paint, paint remover, and room deodorizers. These agents are generally sniffed or "huffed" orally either from a bag or directly from the container. It is children who typically abuse these substances.

The inhalant's effects are similar to those of ethanol and other sedative-hypnotics. Despite their structural diversity, they produce similar signs and symptoms. The mood alterations produced are thought to be a consequence of disinhibition release and include a relaxed feeling, light-headedness, and mild euphoria. As dosage is increased, ataxia, diplopia, and slurred speech develop. At higher doses psychotic behaviors, hallucinations, and even seizures may occur. The effects usually last about 30 minutes but are often sustained by repeated administration. As with the sedative-hypnotics, anterograde amnesia may occur. A hangover is rare.

Very little research has been done on the mechanisms of action of this diverse group of drugs. They appear to disrupt the fluidity of membranes. At higher doses, they may uncouple oxidative phosphorylation, leading to effects resembling hypoxia and ischemia in the brain. Although tolerance to their acute effects develops, the presence of a consistent withdrawal syndrome has not been documented.

Some volatile inhalants, especially the halogenated hydrocarbons, can cause cardiac arrhythmias that may require immediate medical attention. Without cardiac complications, however, emergency medical treatment is usually not required because of the short half-lives of volatile inhalants. Sustained chronic use, however, can lead to pathology. This includes kidney, liver, and bone marrow suppression following benzene and chlorinated hydrocarbon exposure; lead encephalopathies in gasoline sniffers; neurodegenerative changes in toluene abusers, and peripheral neuropathies in hexane sniffers. Death is a rare occurrence (Brust, 1993).

ANABOLIC STEROIDS

Since it was first described in the early 1980s, anabolic steroid abuse has risen dramatically, weaving its way into the fabric of many of our school systems. Among high school males, the estimated prevalence was 6.7% in 1988 (Buckley et al., 1988). Most young men who use steroids do so to enhance their athletic performance; others simply want to improve their physical appearance. Unlike other drugs of abuse, the anabolic steroids are not usually ingested for their acute euphoric effects but rather for their long-term effects on muscle mass.

Like the volatile inhalants, anabolic steroids are a diverse group of compounds, but they are all derivatives of the hormone androgen. They include testosterone cypionate, nandrolone decanoate, methandrostenolone, and boldenone undecylenate. Their structures involve a modification of that of testosterone which prevents rapid clearance from the body. The drugs are purchased illicitly from other students, at health spas and gyms, and even through bodybuilding magazines. These same sources also provide anecdotal information about dosage and administration routes. The drugs are commonly administered either orally or intramuscularly in amounts far above those used clinically for any purpose. Many drugs are administered continuously at low or moderate doses. Alternatively, very high doses are used for several weeks followed by a period of abstinence, a pattern called stacking. Because of the high dosages, the clinical literature is not helpful in determining the acute and long-term effects of androgen abuse. What we do know is largely anecdotal and arises from case reports and emergency room experiences.

The acute CNS effects of these drugs, even at high doses, are mild if perceptible at all. Continued high-dose abuse may produce mild euphoria and increased aggressiveness. In some patients, high-dose, continuous use can produce euphoria that often alternates with depression and irritability. Nervousness, hyperactivity, sleep disorders, increased libidos, delusions of reference, psychomotor retardation or acceleration, paranoid ideations, auditory and visual hallucinations, and manic-hypomanic disorders have been reported. Rarely, a psychotic-like state with loose associations and formal thought disorder may occur. The characteristic changes of masculinization are commonly observed: increased performance during heavy work, hirsutism, pronounced brow ridges, increased muscle mass, etc. The toxic effects of these agents rarely constitute a medical emergency except in cases of acute psychotic reactions that are effectively managed with DA antagonists such as haloperidol (Hickson, Ball, and Falduto, 1989). A withdrawal syndrome has been reported and involves depression, chills, nausea, and vomiting.

The mechanism by which anabolic steroids produce their CNS effects is unknown or poorly characterized at best. At the doses commonly taken, they can profoundly influence several hormonal feedback loops and thereby depress pituitary release of LH, FSH, glucocorticoids (e.g., corticosteroid), and TSH. The large circulating levels of steroids and their subsequent metabolic conversion to estradiols are probably responsible for feminizing effects including gynecomastia and reduced sperm production that can be seen in some users. The disruption of these hormonal systems and the neurotransmitter systems they affect is likely involved in their CNS effects.

Appendix: Drug Lists

Chapter 4: Opioid Analgesics and Pain

Prototypical Agent: Morphine

Full Agonists
codeine
heroin
hydromorphone (Dilaudid)
oxymorphone (Numorphan)
hydrocodone (Hycodan)
levorphanol (Levo-Dromoran)
meperidine (Demerol)
fentanyl (Sublimaze)
methadone (Dolophine)
propoxyphene (Darvon)

Partial Agonists/Antagonists
pentazocine (Talwin)
nalbuphine (Nubain)
butorphanol (Stadol)
buprenorphine (Buprenex)

Antagonists
naloxone (Narcan)
naltrexone (Trexan)

Other Agents
dextromethorphan
diphenoxylate with atropine (Lomotil)
loperamide (Imodium)

Chapter 5: Pharmacology of Headache

Prototypical Agents: Aspirin, Ergotamine (Wigraine, Ergostat, Ergomar), and Methysergide (Sansert)

Nonsteroidal antiinflammatory drugs (NSAIDs): acetaminophen, ibuprofen, naproxen
Ergot alkaloids: ergotamine, dihydroergotamine
Serotonin agonists: sumatriptan (Imitrex)
Ca^{2+} channel antagonists: verapamil (Calan), nifedipine (Procardia), nimodipine (Nimotop)

Other Agents
propranolol (Inderal), amitriptyline (Elavil)

Prokinetics/Antiemetics
metoclopramide (Reglan), ondansetron (Zofran), prochlorperazine (Compazine)

Chapter 6: Sedative-Hypnotics and Anxiolytics

Prototypical Agent: Diazepam (Valium)

Benzodiazepines
chlordiazepoxide (Librium)
triazolam (Halcion)
alprazolam (Xanax)
clorazepate (Tranxene)
temazepam (Restoril)
oxazepam (Serax)
halazepam (Praxipam)
lorazepam (Ativan)
flurazepam (Dalmane)
midazolam (Versed)
quazepam (Doral)
estazolam (Prosom)

Benzodiazepine Antagonist
flumazenil (Romazicon)

Barbiturates
amobarbital (Amytal)
secobarbital (Seconal)
pentobarbital (Nembutal)
phenobarbital (Luminal)
methohexital (Brevital)

Others
zolpidem (Ambien)
meprobramate (Miltown)
chloral hydrate (Noctec)
paraldehyde
ethchlorvynol (Placidyl)
glutethimide (Doriden)
methyprylon (Noludar)
ethinamate (Valmid)

Selective Anxiolytic Agents
buspirone (Buspar)
propranolol (Inderal)

Chapter 7: General Anesthetics, Local Anesthetics, and Muscle Relaxers

Prototypical Agent: Halothane (Fluothane)

Gases
enflurane (Ethrane)
isoflurane (Forane)
methoxyflurane (Penthrane)
desflurane (Suprane)
sevoflurane
nitrous oxide
ether
chloroform

Intravenous Agents
thiopental (Pentothal)
methohexital (Brevital)
etomidate (Amidate)
propofol (Diprivan)
ketamine (Ketalar)

Intravenous Opioids
fentanyl (Sublimaze)
sufentanil (Sufenta)
alfentyl (Alfenta)

Combinations
fentanyl/droperidol (Innovar; neurolept-analgesia)
droperidol/nitrous oxide (neurolept-anesthesia)

Neuromuscular Blockers
nicotinic antagonists: tubocurarine, pancuronium (Pavulon), rocuronium
    (Zemuron), gallamine (Flaxedil)

cholinesterase inhibitors: neostigmine (Prostigmin), physostigmine,
    ambenonium (Mytelase), edrophonium (Tensilon)
direct-acting agonists: succinylcholine (Anectine), decamethonium

Local Anesthetics
procaine (Novocaine)
lidocaine (Xylocaine)
cocaine
mepivacaine (Carbocaine)
tetracaine (Pontocaine)
etidocaine (Duranest)
benzocaine
bupivacaine (Marcaine)
chlorprocaine (Nesacaine)
prilocaine (Citanest)
pramoxine (Tronothane)
dyclonine (Dyclone)
proparacaine (Alcaine)

Chapter 8: Antiepileptic Drugs

Prototypical Agent: Phenytoin (Dilantin)

Other Drugs to Consider
phenobarbital (Luminal)
mephobarbital (Mebaral)
primidone (Mysoline)
carbamazepine (Tegretol)
valproate (Depakote)
clonazepam (Klonopin)
ethosuximide (Zarontin)

Adjunctive Drugs
lamotrigine (Lamictal)
MK-801
gamma-vinyl-GABA (Vigabatrin)
gabapentin (Neurontin)

Drugs Used for Status Epilepticus
diazepam (Valium)
lorazepam (Ativan)
phenobarbital (Luminal)
pentobarbital (Nembutal)

Chapter 9: Treatment of Movement Disorders

Prototypical Agent: *Carbidopa/Levodopa* (*Sinemet*)

Antiparkinsonian Drugs
Indirect-acting DA agonists: amantadine (Symmetrel), benztropine
    (Cogentin), selegiline (Eldepryl)
Antimuscarinic agents; trihexyphenidyl (Artane), benztropine
    (Cogentin), biperiden (Akineton), procyclidine (Kemadrin)
Direct-Acting DA agonists; bromocriptine (Parlodel), pergolide
    (Permax), pramipexole (Mirapex), ropinirole (Requip)

Huntington's Disease and Gilles de la Tourette Syndrome Drugs
haloperidol (Haldol)
pimozide (Orap)
thioridazine (Mellaril)
clonidine (Catapres)

Antitremor Drugs
propranolol (Inderal)

Drugs Used for Dystonia
antimuscarinic drugs
benzodiazepines
botulinum toxin (Botox)

Chelators for Wilson's disease
penicillamine (Cuprimine)
trientine (Cuprid)

Drugs for Attention Deficit/Hyperactivity Disorder
d-amphetamine (Dexedrine)
methylphenidate (Ritalin)
pemoline (Cylert)

Chapter 10: Antipsychotic Drugs

Prototypical Agent: *Chlorpromazine* (*Thorazine; an Aliphatic Phenothiazine*)

Other Direct-Acting DA Antagonists
Phenothiazines: thioridazine (Mellaril), mesoridazine (Serentil),
    trifluoperazine (Stelazine), acetophenazine (Tindal), perphenazine
    (Trilafon), fluphenazine (Prolixin)
Butyrophenones: haloperidol (Haldol)
Thioxanthines: chlorprothixene (Taractan), thiothixene (Navane)
Diphenylbutylpiperidines: pimozide (Orap)
Dibenzoxazepines: loxapine (Loxitane)

Dibenzodiazepines: clozapine (Clozaril)
Dihydroindolone: molindone (Moban)
Benzisoxazole: risperidone (Risperdal)

Chapter 11: The Antidepressant Drugs

Prototypical Agent: Imipramine (Tofranil)

Other Tricyclic Antidepressants: amitriptyline (Elavil), clomipramine
    (Anafranil), desipramine (Norpramin), doxepin (Sinequan),
    nortriptyline (Aventyl), protriptyline (Vivactil), trimipramine
    (Surmontil)
Heterocyclic Agents: amoxapine (Ascendin), maprotiline (Ludiomil),
    trazodone (Desyrel)
Selective Serotonin Reuptake Inhibitors (SSRIs): fluoxetine (Prozac),
    paroxetine (Paxil), sertraline (Zoloft), fluvoxamine (Luvox),
    venlafaxine (Effexor)
Monoamine Oxidase Inhibitors (MAOIs): isocarboxazid (Marplan),
    phenelzine (Nardil), tranylcypromine (Parnate)
Antimanic Drugs: lithium carbonate (Eskalith), carbamazepine
    (Tegretol), valproate (Depakote)

Chapter 12: Drugs of Abuse and Addiction

Psychostimulants: amphetamine (Dexedrine), methamphetamine,
    cocaine, methylphenidate (Ritalin), pemoline (Cylert), cathionine
Anorexients: phenteramine, benzphetamine, phendimetrazine,
    fenfluramine, phenylpropanolamine
CNS Stimulants: caffeine, nicotine
CNS Depressants: ethanol
Dissociative anesthetic: phencyclidine (PCP)
marijuana
Hallucinogens: lysergic acid diethylamide (LSD), mescaline, psilocybin
Designer drugs: 2,4,5-Trimethoxyamphetamine (TMA), 4-Methyl-2,5-
    dimethoxyamphetamine (DOM), Para-methoxyamphetamine (PMA),
    Brom-DOM, 3,4-Methylenedioxyamphetamine (MDA), 3,4-
    Methylenedioxymethamphetamine (MDMA),
    3,4-Methylenedioxyethamphetamine (MDEA)
anticholinergics
volatile inhalants
anabolic steroids

References

Abraham, H.D., & Aldridge, A.M. (1993). Adverse consequence of lysergic acid di-ethylamide. *Addiction, 88,* 1327–1334.

Adler, E.M., Yaari, Y., David, G., & Selzer, M. (1986). Frequency-dependent action of phenytoin on lamprey spinal axons. *Brain Research, 362,* 271–280.

Agency for Health Care Policy and Research. Anonymous. Depression in primary care: Vol. I. Detection and diagnosis. Clinical practice guideline, No. 5. U.S. Department of Health and Human Services, Public Health Services. (1993). AHCPR Publ. 93-0550.

Aghajanian, G.K., Foote, W.E., & Sheard, M.H. (1968). Lysergic acid diethylamide: sensitive neuronal units in the midbrain raphe. *Science, 161,* 706–708.

Amrein, R., Allen, S.R., Guentert, T.W., Hartmann, D., Lorscheid, T., Schoerlin, M.P., & Vranesic, D. (1989). The pharmacology of reversible monoamine oxidase inhibitors. *British Journal of Psychiatry Supplement,* 66–71.

Anderson, D.M. (1994). Red tides [published erratum appears in Sci Am 1994 Oct;271(4): 10]. *Scientific American, 271,* 62–68.

Andrade, R., Malenka, R.C., & Nicoll, R.A. (1986). A G-protein couples serotonin and GABA$_B$ receptors to the same channels in the hippocampus. *Science, 234,* 1261–1265.

Angel, A. (1993). Central neuronal pathways and the process of anaesthesia. *British Journal of Anesthesia, 71,* 141–163.

Arana, G.W., Goff, D.C., Baldessarini, R.J., & Keepers, G.A. (1988). Efficacy of anticholinergic prophylaxis for neuroleptic-induced acute dystonia. *American Journal of Psychiatry, 145,* 993–996.

Arndt, S., Alliger, R.J., & Andreasen, N.C. (1991). The distinction of positive and negative symptoms. The failure of a two-dimensional model. *British Journal of Psychiatry, 158,* 317–322.

Asaad, G., & Shapiro, B. (1986). Hallucinations: theoretical and clinical overview. *American Journal of Psychiatry, 143,* 1088–1097.

Asberg, M., Traskman, L., & Thoren, P. (1976). 5-HIAA in the cerebrospinal fluid. A biochemical suicide predictor? *Archives in General Psychiatry, 33,* 1193–1197.

Ashton, H. (1984). Benzodiazepine withdrawal: an unfinished story. *British Medicine Journal, 288,* 1135–1140.

Ashton, H. (1992). *Brain function and psychotropic drugs.* New York: Oxford University Press.

Azmitia, E.C., & Whitaker-Azmita, P.M. (1995). Anatomy, cell biology, and plasticity of the serotonergic system: neuropsychopharmacological implications for the actions of psychotropic drugs. In F.E. Bloom & D.J. Kupfer (Eds), *Psychopharmacology: the fourth generation of progress.* New York: Raven Press.

Bailey, P.L. (1994). Clinical pharmacology and applications of opioid agonists. In T.A. Bowdle, A. Horita, & E.D. Kharasch (Eds), *The pharmacologic basis of anesthesiology.* (p. 83). New York: Churchill Livingstone.

Baldessarini, R.J. (1989). Current status of antidepressants: clinical pharmacology and therapy. *Journal of Clinical Psychiatry, 50,* 117–126.

Balster, R.L. (1991). Discriminative stimulus properties of phencyclidine and other NMDA antagonists. In R.A. Glennon, T.U.C. Jarbe, & J. Frankenheim (Eds), *Drug discrimination: applications to drug abuse research* (pp. 163–180). Washington, D.C., U.S. Gov. Printing Office.

Barkley, R.A., McMurray, M.B., Edelbrock, C.S., & Robbins, K. (1990). Side effects of methylphenidate in children with attention deficit hyperactivity disorder: a systemic, placebo-controlled evaluation. *Pediatrics, 86,* 184–192.

Bartoszyk, G.D., Meyerson, N., Reimann, W., Satzinger, G., & vonHodenberg, A. (1986). Gabapentin. In B.S. Meldrum & R.J. Porter (Eds), *New anticonvulsant drugs.* (pp. 147–163). London: John Libbey.

Basbaum, A.I. (1984). Anatomical substrates of pain and pain modulation and their relationship to analgesic drug action. In M.J. Kuhar & G.W. Pasternak (Eds.), *Analgesics: neurochemical, behavioral and clinical perspectives.* (pp. 97–124). New York: Raven Press.

Beecher, H.K. (1946). Pain in men wounded in battle. *Annals of Surgery, 123,* 96–105.

Bercel, N.A., Travis, L.E., Olinger, L.B., & Dreikurs, E. (1956). Model psychoses induced by LSD-25 in normals. *Archives of Neurology and Psychiatry, 588–611.*

Berridge, M.J. (1989). The Albert Lasker Medical Awards. Inositol trisphosphate, calcium, lithium, and cell signaling. *JAMA, 262,* 1834–1841.

Bianchine, J.R., & Shaw, G.M. (1976). Clinical pharmacokinetics of levodopa in parkinson's disease. *Clinical Pharmacokinetics, 1,* 313–338.

Bjorklund, A., & Lindvall, O. (1984). Dopamine-containing systems in the CNS. In A. Bjorklund & T. Hokfelt (Eds), *Handbook of chemical neuroanatomy.* (pp. 55–122). Amsterdam: Elsevier Science.

Blackshear, P.J. (1988). Approaches to the study of protein kinase C involvement in signal transduction. *American Journal of Medical Sciences, 296,* 231–240.

Bliss, T.V.P., & Lomo, T. (1973). Long-lasting potentiation of synaptic transmission in the dentate area of the anesthetized rabbit following stimulation of the perforant path. *Journal of Physiology, 232,* 331–356.

Bloom, F.E., & Lazerson, A. (1988). *Brain, mind and behavior.* New York: W.H. Freeman.

Bochner, F., Hooper, W.D., Tyrer, J.H., & Eadie, M.J. (1972). Factors involved in an outbreak of phenytoin intoxication. *Journal of Neurological Science, 16,* 481–487.

Bodnar, R.J., Williams, C.L., Lee, S.J., & Pasternak, G.W. (1988). Role of mu_1 opiate receptor in supraspinal opiates analgesia. *Brain Research, 447,* 25–37.

Bourgeois, B.F.D. (1989). Biotransformation and mechanisms of action. In R. Levy, R. Mattson, B. Meldrum, J.K. Penry, & F.E. Dreifuss (Eds.), *Antiepileptic drugs.* New York: Raven Press.

Bowman, W.C., Rodger, I.W., Houston, J., Marshall, R.J., & McIndewar, I. (1988). Structure:action relationships among some desacetoxy analogues of pancuronium and vecuronium in the anesthetized cat. *Anesthesiology, 69,* 57–62.

Braestrup, C., Nielsen, M., Jenson, L.H., Honore, T., & Peterson, E.N. (1983). Benziodiazepine receptor ligands and positive and negative efficacy. *Neuropharmacology, 22,* 1481–1488.

Braun, A.R., & Chase, T.N. (1986). Obligatory D-1/D-2 receptor interaction in the generation of dopamine agonist related behaviors. *European Journal of Physiology, 131,* 301–306.

Bromm, B., Forth, W., Richter, E., & Scharein, E. (1992). Effects of acetaminophen and antipyrine on non-inflammatory pain and EEG activity. *Pain, 50,* 213–221.

Brown, R. (1995). Muramyl peptides and the functions of sleep. *Behavioral Brain Research, 69,* 85–90.

Brust, J.C. (1993). Clinical, radiological, and pathological aspects of cerebrovascular disease associated with drug abuse. *Stroke, 24,* I129–I133.

Buchanan, R.W., Breier, A., Kirkpatrick, B., Elkashef, A., Munson, R.C., Gellad, F., & Carpenter, W.T.J. (1993). Structural abnormalities in deficit and nondeficit schizophrenia. *American Journal of Psychiatry, 150,* 59–65.

Buckley, W.E., Yesalis, C.E.I, Friedl, K.E., Anderson, W.A., Streit, A.L., & Wright, J.E. (1988). Estimated prevalence of anabolic steroid use among male high school seniors. *JAMA, 260,* 3441–3445.

Bunney, B.S. (1984). Antipsychotic drug effects on the electrical activity of dopaminergic neurones. *Trends in Neuroscience, 7,* 212–215.

Bunney, W.E.J., & Davis, J.M. (1965). Norepinephrine in depressive reactions. *Archives in General Psychiatry, 13,* 483–494.

Cabeza, R.J., Zoltoski, R.K., & Gillin, J.C. (1994). Biochemical pharmacology of sleep. In S. Chokrovery (Ed), *Sleep disorders medicine: basic science, technical considerations and clinical aspects.* Boston: Butterworth-Heinemann.

Calsi, K.A., Grothe, D.R., & Elia, J. (1990). Attention-deficit hyperactivity disorder. *Clinical Pharmacy, 9,* 632–642.

Campbell, S.S., Eastman, C.I., Terman, M., Lewy, A.J. Boulos, Z., & Dijk, D.J. (1995). Light treatment for sleep disorders: consensus report. I. Chronology of seminal studies in humans. *Journal of Biological Rhythms, 10,* 105–109.

Carlsson, A. (1988). The current status of the dopamine hypothesis of schizophrenia. *Neuropsychopharmacology, 1,* 179–186.

Carpenter, W.T.J., & Buchanan, R.W. (1994). Schizophrenia. *New England Journal of Medicine, 330,* 681–690.

Carroll, B.J. (1994). Brain mechanisms in manic depression. *Clinical Chemistry, 40,* 303–308.

Carvey, P. (1989). LSD and other related hallucinogens elicit myoclonic jumping behavior in the guinea pig. *Progressive Neuro-Psychopharmacology and Biological Psychiatry, 13,* 199–210.

Carvey, P.M., Kao, L.C., Zhang, T.J., Amdur, R.L., Lin, D.H., Singh, R., & Klawans, H.L. (1990). Dopaminergic alterations in cotreatments attenuating haloperidol-induced hypersensitivity. *Pharmacology, Biochemistry and Behavior, 35,* 291–300.

Casey, D.E. (1995). Tardive dyskinesia: pathophysiology. In F.E. Bloom & D.J. Kupfer (Eds), *Psychopharmacology: the fourth generation of progress.* (pp. 1497–1502). New York: Raven Press.

Catterall, W.A. (1992). Cellular and molecular biology of voltage-gated sodium channels. *Physiological Review, 72,* S15–48.

Cedarbaum, J.M. (1987). Clinical pharmacokinetics of anti-parkinsonian drugs. *Clinical Pharmacokinetics, 13,* 141–178.

Chapman, A., Keane, P.E., Meldrum, B.S., Simiand, J., & Vernieres, J.C. (1982). Mechanisms of anticonvulsant action of valproate. *Progressive Neurobiology, 19,* 315–359.

Charney, D.S., Heninger, G.R., & Kleber, H.D. (1986). The combined use of clonidine and naltrexone as a rapid, safe, and effective treatment of abrupt withdrawal from methadone. *American Journal of Psychiatry, 143,* 831–837.

Charney, D.S., Woods, S.W., Nagy, L.M., Southwick, S.M., Krystal, J.H., & Heninger, G.R. (1990). Noradrenergic function in panic disorder. *Journal of Clinical Psychiatry, 51 Supplement A,* 5–11.

Chase, M.H., Soja, P.J., & Morales, F.R. (1989). Evidence that glycine mediates the postsynaptic potentials that inhibit lumbar motoneurons during the atonia of active sleep. *Journal of Neuroscience, 9,* 743–751.

Chase, T.N., Engber, T.M., & Mouradin, M.M. (1996). Contribution of dopaminergic and glutamatergic mechanisms to the pathogenesis of motor response complications in Parkinson's disease. *Advances in Neurology, 69,* 497–501.

Chin, J.H., & Goldstein, D.B. (1981). Membrane-disordering action of ethanol: variation with membrane cholesterol content and depth of the spin label probe. *Molecular Pharmacology 19,* 425–431.

Clark, D.L., & Rosner, B.S. (1973). Neurophysiologic effects of general anesthetics. I. The electroencephalogram and sensory evoked responses in man. *Anesthesiology, 38,* 564–582.

Clemens, J.A., & Fuller, R.W. (1979). Differences in the effects of amphetamines and methylphenidate on brain dopamine turnover and serum prolactin concentration in reserpine-treated rats. *Life Sciences, 24,* 2077–2081.

Colby, C.L. (1991). The neuroanatomy and neurophysiology of attention. *Journal of Child Neurology, 6,* 90–118.

Collin, E., & Cesselin, F. (1991). Neurobiological mechanisms of opioid tolerance and dependence. In Anonymous, *Clinical neuropharmacology.* (pp. 465–488). New York, NY: Raven Press.

Collins, M.A. (1982). A possible neurochemical mechanism for brain and nerve damage associated with chronic alcoholism. *Trends in Pharmacological Sciences, 3,* 373–375.

Cooper, A.J. (1989). Tyramine and irreversible monoamine oxidase inhibitors in clinical practice. *British Journal of Psychiatry Supplement,* 38–45.

Cooper, J.R., Bloom, F.E., & Roth, R.H. (1996). *The biological basis of neuropharmacology.* New York: Oxford University Press.

Costa, E., Corda, M.G., & Guidotti, A. (1996). On a brain polypeptide functioning as a putative effector for the recognition sites of benzodiazepine and beta-carboline derivatives. *Neuropharmacology, 22,* 1481–1492.

Couch, J.R., Ziegler, D.K., & Hassanein, R. (1976). Amitriptyline in the prophylaxis of migraine: effectiveness and relationship of antimigraine and antidepressant effects. *Neurology, 26,* 121–127.

Coulter, D.A., Huguenard, J.R., & Prince, D.A. (1989). Characterization of ethosuximide reduction of low-threshold calcium current in thalamic neurons. *Annals of Neurology, 25,* 582–593.

Courtney, K.R., & Etter, E.F. (1983). Modulated anticonvulsant block of sodium channels in nerve and muscle. *European Journal of Pharmacology, 88,* 1–9.

Creese, I., & Snyder, S.H. (1977). A simple and sensitive radioreceptor assay for antischizophrenic drugs in blood. *Nature, 270,* 180–182.

Crews, F.T., & Smith, C.B. (1978). Presynaptic alpha-receptor subsensitivity after long-term antidepressant treatment. *Science, 202,* 322–324.

Cummings, J.L. (1985). Organic delusions: phenomenology, anatomical correlations, and review. *British Journal of Psychiatry, 146,* 184–197.

Curran, H.V. (1986). Tranquillising memories: a review of the effects of benzodiazepines on human memory. *Biological Psychology, 23,* 179–213.

Dahlstrom, A., & Fuxe, K. (1964). Evidence for the existence of monoamine-containing neurons in the central nervous system. Demonstration of monoamines in the cell bodies of brain stem neurons. *Acta Psychiatrica Scandinavica, 62,* 1–55.

Dallas, F.A.A., Dixon, C.M., McCulloch, R.J., & Saynor, D.A. (1989). The kinetics of [14]-GR43175 in rat and dog. *Cephalagia, 9, (Supplement 9)* 53–56.

Daval, J.L., Deckert, J., Weiss, S.R.B., Post, R.M., & Marangos, P.J. (1989). Upregulation of adenosine A1 receptor and forskolin binding sites following chronic treatment with caffeine or carbamazepine: a quantitative autoradiographic study. *Epilepsia, 30,* 26–33.

Davis, J.M., Schaffer, C.B., Killian, G.A., Kinard, C., & Chan, C. (1980). Important issues in the drug treatment of schizophrenia. *Schizophrenia Bulletin, 6,* 70–87.

Davis, K.L., Kahn, R.S., Ko, G., & Davidson, M. (1991). Dopamine in schizophrenia: a review and reconceptualization. *American Journal of Psychiatry, 148,* 1474–1486.

Davis, M. (1992). The role of the amygdala in fear and anxiety. *Annual Review in Neuroscience, 15,* 353–375.

Dawson, V.L., Dawson, T.M., Bartley, D.A., Uhl, G.R., & Snyder, S.H. (1993). Mechanisms of nitric oxide-mediated neurotoxicity in primary brain cultures. *Journal of Neuroscience, 13,* 2651–2661.

Deliganis, A.V., & Peroutka, S.J. (1991). 5-Hydroxytryptamine$_{1D}$ receptor agonism predicts antimigraine efficacy. *Headache, 31,* 228–231.

Deutch, A.Y., Lee, M.C., Gillham, M.H., Cameron, D.A., Goldstein, M., & Iadarola, M.J. (1991). Stress selectively increases fos protein in dopamine neurons innervating the prefrontal cortex. *Cerebral Cortex, 1,* 273–292.

Devane, W.A., Dysarz, II, F.A., Johnson, M.R., Melvin, L.S., & Howlett, A.C. (1988). Determination and characterization of a cannabinoid receptor in rat brain. *Molecular Pharmacology, 34,* 605–613.

Devane, W.A., Hanus, L., Breuer, A., Pertwee, R.G., Stevenson, L.A., Griffin, G., Gibson, D., Mandelbaum, A., Etinger, A., & Mechoulam, R. (1992). Isolation and structure of a brain constituent that binds to the cannabinoid receptor [see comments]. *Science, 258,* 1946–1949.

Dewey, W.L. (1986). Cannabinoid pharmacology. *Pharmacological Reviews, 38,* 151–178.

Di Chiara, G., & Imperato, A. (1988). Drugs abused by humans preferentially increase synaptic dopamine concentrations in the mesolimbic system of freely moving rats. *Proceedings of the National Academy of Sciences of the United States of America, 85,* 5274–5278.

Diago, M.P., Sebastian, J.V., & Vera-Sempere, F. (1990). Diphenylhydantoin-induced gingival overgrowth in man: a clinico-pathological study. *Journal of Periodontology, 61,* 571–574.

Dimitriadou, V., Buzzi, M.G., Theoharides, T.C., & Moskowitz, M.A. (1992). Ultrastructural evidence for neurogenically mediated changes in blood vessels of the rat dura mater and tongue following antidromic trigeminal stimulation. *Neuroscience, 48,* 187–203.

Dingledine, R. (1983). N-methyl aspartate activates voltage-dependent calcium conductance in rat hippocampal pyrimidal cells. *Journal of Physiology (London), 343,* 385–405.

DiPalma, J.R. (1987). Lithium toxicity. *American Family Physician, 36,* 225–228.

Dreifuss, F.E., Santilli, N., Langer, D.H., Sweeney, K.P., Moline, K.A., & Menander, K.B. (1987). Valproic acid hepatic fatalities: a retrospective review. *Neurology, 37,* 379–385.

Earnest, M.P., Marx, J.A., & Drury, L.R. (1983). Complications of intravenous phenytoin for acute treatment of seizures. Recommendations for usage. *JAMA, 249,* 762–765.

Eger, E.I.I. (1974). *Anesthetic uptake and action.* Baltimore: Williams and Wilkins.

Ellenbroek, B.A. (1993). Treatment of schizophrenia: a clinical and preclinical evaluation of neuroleptic drugs. *Pharmacology and Therapeutics, 57,* 1–78.

Ellinwood, E.H.J. (1975). Treatment of reactions to amphetamine-type stimulants. *Current Psychiatric Therapies, 15,* 163–169.

Engel, J.I. (1989). *Seizures and epilepsy.* Philadelphia: F.A. Davis.

Evans, C.J., Hammond, D.L., & Frederickson, R.C.A. (1988). The opioid peptides. In G.W. Pasternak (Ed.), *The opiate receptors.* (pp. 23–71). Clifton Park, NJ: Humana Press.

Fadda, F., Gessa, G.L., Marcou, E., & Rossetti, Z. (1984). Evidence for dopamine autoreceptors in mesocortical dopamine neurons. *Brain Research, 293,* 67–72.

Farnebo, L.O., Fuxe, K., Hamberger, B., & Ljungdahl, H. (1970). Effect of some antiparkinsonian drugs on catecholamine neurons. *Journal of Pharmacy and Pharmacology, 22,* 733–737.

Fawcett, J. (1993). The morbidity and mortality of clinical depression. *International Clinical Psychopharmacology, 8,* 217–220.

Fawcett, J. (1995). Compliance definitions and key issues. *Journal of Clinical Psychiatry, 56,* 4–8.

Ferre, S., Fuxe, K., Von Euler, G., Johansson, B., & Fredholm, B.B. (1992). Adenosine-dopamine interactions in the brain. *Neuroscience, 51,* 501–512.

Fiore, M.C. (1992). Trends in cigarette smoking in the United States. The epidemiology of tobacco use. *Medical Clinics of North America, 76,* 289–303.

Fisher, C., Byrne, J., Edwards, A., & Kahn, E. (1971). [Psychophysiologic study of nightmares]Etude psycho-physiologique des cauchemars. *Revue de Medecine Psychosomtique et de Psychologie Medicale, 13,* 7–29.

Foley, K.M. (1985). The treatment of cancer pain. *New England Journal of Medicine, 313,* 84–95.

Foote, S.L., & Morrison, J.H. (1987). Development of the noradrenergic, serotonergic, and dopaminergic innervation of neocortex. *Current Topics in Developmental Biology, 21,* 391–423.

Fozard, J.R. (1982). Basic mechanisms of antimigraine drugs. *Advances in Neurology, 33,* 295–307.

Franks, N.P., & Lieb, W.R. (1981). Is membrane expansion relevant to anaesthesia? *Nature, 292,* 248–251.

Franks, N.P., & Lieb, W.R. (1994). Molecular and cellular mechanisms of general anaesthesia. *Nature, 367,* 607–614.

Frazier, D.T., Narahashi, T., & Yamada, M. (1970). The site of action and active form of local anesthetics. II. Experiments with quaternary compounds. *Journal of Pharmacological Experimental Therapy, 171,* 45–51.

Frenkel, A.R., Quitkin, F.M., & Rabkin, J.G. (1988). Behavioral side effects associated with antidepressants and lithium. In Anonymous, *Behavior and antidepressants and lithium.* (pp. 111–127). New York: Oxford University Press.

Gage, P.W., & McKinnon, D., & Robertson, B. (1986). The influence of anesthetics on postsynaptic ion channels. In S.H. Roth & K.W. Miller (Eds.), *Molecular and cellular mechanisms of anesthetics.* (pp. 139–153). New York: Plenum Press.

Gardos, G., & Cole, J. (1995). The treatment of tardive dyskinesias. In F.E. Bloom & D.J. Kupfer (Eds.), *Psychopharmacology: the fourth generation of progress.* (pp. 1503–1511). New York: Raven Press.

Garratt, J.C., Gent, J.P., Feely, M., & Haigh, J.R. (1988). Can benzodiazepines be classified by characterizing their anticonvulsant tolerance-inducing potential? *European Journal of Pharmacology, 145,* 75–80.

Gerlak, R.P., Clark, P., Stump, J.M., & Vernier, V.G. (1970). Amantadine-dopamine interaction. *Science, 169,* 203–204.

Gershon, S., & Meltzer, H. (1992). Mechanisms of clozapine-induced agranulocytosis. *Drug Safety, 7,* 17–25.

Giros, B., & Caron, M.G. (1993). Molecular characterization of the dopamine transporter. *Trends in Pharmacological Sciences, 14,* 43–49.

Glennon, R.A., & Dukat, M. (1995). Serotonin receptor subtypes. In F.E. Bloom & D.J. Kupfer (Eds.), *Psychopharmacology: the fourth generation of progress.* New York: Raven Press.

Goadsby, P.J., & Edvinsson, L. (1993). The trigeminovascular system and migraine: studies characterizing cerebrovascular and neuropeptide changes seen in humans and cats. *Annals of Neurology, 33,* 48–56.

Goldstein, A., & Kaizer, S. (1969). Psychotropic effects of caffeine in man. 3. A questionnaire survey of coffee drinking and its effects in a group of housewives. *Clinical Pharmacology and Therapeutics, 10,* 477–488.

Gonzalez, R.A., & Hoffman, P.L. (1991). Receptor gated channels may be selective CNS targets for ethanol. *Trends in Pharmacological Sciences, 12,* 1–3.

Goodwin, F.K., & Jamison, K.R. (1990). Course and outcome. In Anonymous, *Manic depressive illness.* (pp. 127–156). New York: Oxford University Press.

Gorelick, D.A., & Balster, R.L. (1995). Phencyclidine (PCP). In F.E. Bloom & D.J. Kupfer (Eds.), *Psychopharmacology: the fourth generation of progress.* (pp. 1767–1776). New York: Raven Press.

Gram, L. (1989). Potential antiepileptic drugs lamotrigine. In R. Levy, B. Meldrum, J.K. Penry, & F.E. Dreifuss (Eds.), *Antiepileptic drugs.* (p. 947). New York: Raven Press.

Graves, D.A., Foster, T.S., Batenhorst, R.L., Bennett, R.L., & Baumann, T.J. (1983). Patient-controlled analgesia. *Annals of International Medicine, 99,* 360–366.

Greenberg, D.A. (1986). Calcium channel antagonists and the treatment of migraine. *Clinical Neuropharmacology, 9,* 311–328.

Greene, P., Shale, H., & Fahn, S. (1988). Experience with high dosages of anticholinergic and other drugs in the treatment of torsion dystonia. *Advances in Neurology, 50,* 547–556.

Griffiths, R.K., & Mumford, G.K. (1995). Caffeine- A drug of abuse? In F.E. Bloom & D.J. Kupfer (Eds.), *Psychopharmacology: the fourth generation of progress.* (pp. 1699–1713). New York: Raven Press.

Griffiths, R.R., & Sannerud, C.A. (1987). Abuse of and dependence on benzodiazepines and other anxiolytic/sedative drugs. In H.Y. Meltzer (Ed.), *Psychopharmacology: the third generation of progress.* (pp. 1535–1541). New York: Raven Press.

Gusella, J.F., Wexler, N.S., Conneally, P.M., Naylor, S.L., Anderson, M.A., Tanzi, R.E., Watkins, P.C., Ottina, K., Wallace, M.R., Sakaguchi, A.Y., Young, A.B., Shoulson, I., Bonilla, E., & Martin, J.B. (1983). A polymorphic DNA marker genetically linked to Huntington's disease. *Nature, 306,* 234–238.

Haasse, H., & Janssen, P. (1985). *The action of neuroleptic drugs.* Amsterdam: Elsevier.

Haefely, W. (1989). Neurochemistry of benzodiazepines, barbiturates and alcohol (conference).

Hales, T.G., & Lambert, J.J. (1991). The actions of propofol on inhibitory amino acid receptors of bovine adrenomedullary chromaffin cells and rodent central neurones. *British Journal of Pharmacology, 104,* 619–628.

Hall, L.W., Woolf, N., Bradley, J.W., & Jolly, D.W. (1966). Unusual reaction to suxamethonium chloride. *British Medical Journal, 2,* 1305.

Hannallah, R.S., Baker, S.B., Casey, W., McGill, W.A., Broadman, L.M., & Norden, J.M. (1991). Propofol: effective dose and induction characteristics in unpremedicated children. *Anesthesiology, 74,* 217–219.

Harper, R.W., & Knothe, B.U. (1973). Coloured Lilliputian hallucinations with amantadine. *Medical Journal of Australia, 1,* 444–445.

Harrison, N.L., Majewska, M.D., Harrington, J.W., & Barker, J.L. (1987). Structure-activity relationships for steroid interaction with gamma-aminobutyric acid: a receptor complex. *Journal of Pharmacological Experimental Therapy, 241,* 346–353.

Hartig, P.R., Branchek, T.A., & Weinshank, R.L. (1992). A subfamily of a 5-HT$_{1D}$ receptor genes. *Trends in Pharmacological Sciences, 13,* 152–159.

Harvery, S.C. (1985). Hypnotics and sedatives. In A.G. Gilman, L.S. Goodman, T.W. Rall, & F. Murad (Eds.), *The pharmacological basis of therapeutics.* (pp. 339–371). New York: Macmillan.

Haug, J.O. (1962). Pneumoencephalographic studies in mental disease. *Acta Psychiatrica Scandinavica, 165,* 1–114.

Heikkila, R.E., Manzino, L., Cabbat, F.S., & Duvoisin, R.C. (1984). Protection against the dopaminergic neurotoxicity of 1-methyl-4-phenyl-1,2,5,6,-tetrahydropyridine by monoamine oxidase inhibitors. *Nature, 311,* 467–469.

Heilmann, K.M., Voeller, K.K.S., & Nadeau, S.E. (1991). A possible pathophysiologic substrate of attention deficit hyperactivity disorder. *Journal of Child Neurology, 6,* 76–81.

Heitkamp, H.C., Huber, W., & Schieb, K. (1996). β-Endorphin and adrenocorticotrophin after incremental exercise and marathon running-female responses. *European Journal of Applied Physiology and Occupational Physiology, 72,* 417–424.

Heninger, G.R., & Charney, D.S. (1987). Mechanism of action of antidepressant treatment: implications for the etiology and treatment of depressive disorders. In H.Y. Meltzer (Ed), *Psychopharmacology: the third generation of progress.* (pp. 535–544). New York: Raven Press.

Henningfield, J.E., Schuh, L.M., & Jarvik, M.E. (1995). Pathophysiology of tobacco dependence. In F.E. Bloom & D.J. Kupfer (Eds.), *Psychopharmacology: the fourth generation of progress.* (pp. 1715–1729). New York: Raven Press.

Herz, A. (1993). *Handbook of experimental pharmacology: opioids I.* Berlin: Springer-Verlag.

Hickson, R.C., Ball, K.L., & Falduto, M.T. (1989). Adverse effects of anabolic steroids. *Medical Toxicology and Adverse Drug Experience, 4,* 254–271.

Higgins, G.A., Nguyen, P., & Sellers, E.M. (1992). The NMDA antagonist dizocilpine (MK801) attenuates motivational as well as somatic aspects of naloxine precipitated opioid withdrawal. *Life Science, 50,* PL 167–172.

Hillis, W.S., & MacIntyre, P.D. (1993). Sumatriptan and chest pain. *Lancet, 341,* 1564–1565.

Hollister, L.E. (1986). Health aspects of cannabis. *Pharmacological Review, 38,* 1–20.

Hollister, L.E., & Claghorn, J.L. (1993). New antidepressants. *Annual Review of Pharmacology and Toxicology, 33,* 165–177.

Hubbard, A.K., Roth, T.P., Gandolfi, A.J., Brown, B.R., Webster, N.R., & Nunn, J.F. (1988). Halothane hepatitis patients generate an antibody response toward a covalently bound metabolite of halothane. *Anesthesiology, 68,* 791–796.

Hurlbut, K.M. (1991). Drug-induced psychoses. *Emergency Medicine Clinics of North America, 9,* 31–52.

Hyman, S.E., & Nestler, E.J. (1993). *The molecular foundations of psychiatry.* Washington, DC: American Psychiatric Press.

Hyman, S.E., & Nestler, E.J. (1996). Initiation and adaptation: a paradigm for understanding psychotropic drug action. *American Journal of Psychiatry, 153,* 151–162.

Insel, T.R., Zohar, J., Benkelfat, C., & Murphy, D.L. (1990). Serotonin in obsessions, compulsions and the control of aggressive impulses. In P.M. Whitaker-Azmitia & S.J. Peroutka (Eds.), *The neuropharmacology of serotonin.* (pp. 574–586). New York: New York Academy of Sciences.

Jabbari, B., Bryan, G.E., Marsh, E.E., & Gunderson, C.H. (1985). Incidence of seizures with tricyclic and tetracyclic antidepressants. *Archives in Neurology, 42,* 480–481.

Jacobs, B.L. (1986). Single unit activity of brain monoamine-containing neurons in freely moving animals. *Annals of the New York Academy of Sciences, 473,* 70–77.

Jaffe, J.H. (1990). Drug addiction and drug abuse. In A.G. Gilman, T.W. Rall, A.S. Nies, & P. Taylor (Eds.), *Goodman and Gilman's the pharmacological basis of therapeutics.* (pp. 522–573). New York: Pergamon Press.

Jaffe, J.H., & Martin, W.R. (1990). Opioid analgesics and antagonists. In A.G. Gilman, T.W. Rall, A.S. Nies, & P. Taylor (Eds.). *Goodman and Gilman's: The pharmacological basis of therapeutics.* (pp. 485–521). New York: Pergamon Press.

Jankovic, J., & Fahn, S. (1993). Dystonic disorders. In D. Retford (Ed.), *Parkinson's disease and movement disorders.* (pp. 337). Baltimore: Williams and Wilkins.

Janowsky, D.S., & Overstreet, D.H. (1995). The role of acetylcholine mechanisms in mood disorders. In F.E. Bloom & D.J. Kupfer (Eds.), *Psychopharmacology: the fourth generation of progress.* (pp. 945–956). New York: Raven Press.

Joels, M., Yool, A.J., & Gruol, D.L. (1989). Unique properties of non-N-methyl-D-aspartate excitatory responses in cultured purkinje neurons. *Proc Natl Acad Sci U S A, 86,* 3404–3408.

Johanson, C.E., & Schuster, C.R. (1995). Cocaine. In F.E. Bloom & D.J. Kupfer (Eds.), *Psychopharmacology: the fourth generation of progress.* (pp. 1685–1697). New York: Raven Press.

Johnson, K.M., & Jones, S.M. (1990). Neuropharmacology of phencyclidine: basic mechanisms and therapeutic potential. *Annual Review of Pharmacology and Toxicology, 30,* 707–750.

Johnson, R.L. (1995). Drug abuse. *Pediatrics in Review, 16,* 197–199.

Jones, B.E. (1993). The organization of central cholinergic systems and their functional importance in sleep-waking states. *Progressive Brain Research, 98,* 61–71.

Jouvet, M. (1978). [Is paradoxical sleep responsible for a genetic programming of the brain?]Le sommeil paradoxal est-il responsable d'une programmation genetique du cerveau? *Comptes Rendus des Seances de la Societe de Biologie et de Ses-filiales, 172,* 9–32.

Kalivas, P.W., & Stewart, J. (1991). Dopamine transmission in the initiation and expression of drug- and stress-induced sensitization of motor activity. *Brain Research, Brain Research Reviews, 16*, 223–244.

Kandel, E.R., Schwart, J.H., & Jessell, T.M. (1991). *Principles of neural science*. New York: Elsevier.

Kane, J.M., & Smith, J.M. (1982). Tardive dyskinesia: prevalence and risk factors, 1959–1979. *Archives in General Psychiatry, 39*, 437–481.

Karacan, I., Thornby, J.I., & Anch, A.M. (1976). Dose-related sleep disturbances induced by coffee and caffeine. *Clinical Pharmacology and Therapeutics, 20*, 682–689.

Kay, S.R., & Singh, M.M. (1989). The positive-negative distinction in drug-free schizophrenic patients. Stability, response to neuroleptics, and prognostic significance. *Archives of General Psychiatry, 46*, 711–718.

Kebebian, J.W., & Calne, D.B. (1979). Multiple receptors for dopamine. *Nature, 227*, 93–96.

Kendler, K.S. (1988). Familial aggregation of schizophrenia and schizophrenia spectrum disorders. Evaluation of conflicting results. *Archives of General Psychiatry, 45*, 377–383.

Kerr, I.G., Sone, M., Deangelis, C., Iscoe, N., MacKenzie, R., & Schueller, T. (1988). Continuous narcotic infusion with patient-controlled analgesia for chronic cancer pain in outpatients. *Annals of Internal Medicine, 108*, 554–557.

Klawans, H.L.J. (1973). The pharmacology of tardive dyskinesias. *American Journal of Psychiatry, 130*, 82–86.

Kolesnikov, Y.A., Pick, C.G., Ciszewska, G., & Pasternak, G.W. (1993). Blockade of tolerance to morphine but not to kappa opioids by a nitric oxide synthase inhibitor. *Proceedings of the National Academy of Sciences of the United States of America, 90*, 5162–5166.

Koller, W.C. (1992). *Handbook of Parkinson's Disease*. New York: Marcel Dekker.

Koob, G.F., & Bloom, F.E. (1988). Cellular and molecular mechanisms of drug dependence. *Science, 242*, 715–723.

Kosten, T.A., Miserendino, M.J., Chi, S., & Nestler, E.J. (1994). Fischer and Lewis rat strains show differential cocaine effects in conditioned place preference and behavioral sensitization but not in locomotor activity or conditioned taste aversion. *Journal of Pharmacology and Experimental Therapeutics, 269*, 137–144.

Krishel, S., & Jackimczyk, K. (1991). Cyclic antidepressants, lithium, and neuroleptic agents. Pharmacology and toxicology. *Emergency Medicine Clinics in North America, 9*, 53–86.

Kroin, J.S., Kao, L.C., Zhang, T.J., Penn, R.D., Klawans, H.L., & Carvey, P.M. (1991). Dopamine distribution and behavioral alterations resulting from dopamine infusion into the brain of the lesioned rat. *Journal of Neurosurgery, 74*, 105–111.

Kuhar, M.J. (1986). Neuroanatomical substrates of anxiety: a brief survey. *Trends in Neuroscience, 9*, 307–311.

Kupfer, D.J., Monk, T.H., & Barchas, J.D. (1988). *Biological rhythms and mental disorders*. New York: The Guilford Press.

Kurtzke, J.F., Bennett, D.R., Berg, B.O., Beringer, G.B., Goldstein, D.O., & Vates, T.S. (1986). On national needs for neurologists in the United States. *Neurology, 36*, 383–388.

Lader, M.H., & Petursson, H. (1981). Benzodiazepine derivatives—side effects and dangers. *Biological Psychiatry, 16*, 1195–1201.

Lance, J.W. (1981). Headache. *Annals of Neurology, 10*, 1–10.

Lance, J.W., & Anthony, M. (1966). Some clinical aspects of migraine. *Archives in Neurology, 15*, 356–361.

Lance, J.W., Lambert, G.A., Goadsby, P.J., & Zagami, A.S. (1989). 5-Hydroxytrypta-
mine and its putative aetiological involvement in migraine. *Cephalalgia, Supplement 9*, 7–13.

Lasagna, L., & Beecher, H.K. (1954). Analgesic effectiveness of nalorphine and nalor-
phine-morphine combinations in man. *Journal of Experimental Therapy, 112*,
356–363.

Lauritzen, M. (1994). Pathophysiology of the migraine aura. The spreading depression theory [see comments]. *Brain, 117*, 199–210.

Leao, A.A.P. (1944). Spreading depression of activity in cerebral cortex. *Journal of
Neurophysiology, 7*, 359–390.

LeDoux, J.E., Iwata, J., Cicchetti, P., & Reis, D.J. (1988). Different projections of the
central amygdaloid nucleus mediate autonomic and behavioral correlates of conditioned fear. *Journal of Neuroscience, 8*, 2517–2529.

Lees, A.J., & Tolosa, E. (1993). Tics. In D. Retford (Ed.), *Parkinson's disease and
movement disorders.* (pp. 329–336). Baltimore: Williams and Wilkins.

Lejoyeux, M., Rouillon, F., Ades, J., & Gorwood, P. (1992). Neural symptoms induced by tricyclic antidepressants: phenomenology and pathophysiology. *Acta
Psychiatrica Scandinavica, 85*, 249–256.

Lenox, R.H., & Watson, D.G. (1994). Lithium and the brain: a psychopharmacologi-
cal strategy to a molecular basis for manic depressive illness. *Clinical Chemistry,
40*, 309–314.

Lerman, J., Robinson, S., Willis, M.M., & Gregory, G.A. (1983). Anesthetic requirements for halothane in young children 0–1 month and 1–6 months of age. *Anesthesiology, 59*, 421–424.

Levine, J.D., Gordon, N.C., & Fields, H.L. (1979). Naloxone dose dependently produces analgesia and hyperalgesia in postoperative pain. *Nature, 278*, 740–741.

Lewis, S.W., & Murray, R.M. (1987). Obstetric complications, neurodevelopmental
deviance, and risk of schizophrenia. *Journal of Psychiatric Research, 21*,
413–421.

LeWitt, P.A. (1991). Deprenyl's effect at slowing progression of parkinsonian disability: the DATATOP study. The Parkinson Study Group. *Acta Neurologica Scandinavica Supplementum, 136*, 79–86.

Ling, G.S.F., & Pasternak, G.W. (1983). Spinal and supraspinal analgesia in the
mouse: the role of subpopulations of opioid binding sites. *Brain Research, 271*,
152–156.

Lingle, C.J., & Steinbach, J.H. (1988). Neuromuscular blocking agents. *International
Anesthesiology Clinics, 26*, 288–301.

Litovitz, T.L., Schmitz, B.F., Matyunas, N., & Martin, T.G. (1988). 1987 annual report of the American Association of Poison Control Centers National Data Col-
lection System. *American Journal of Emergency Medicine, 6*, 479–515.

Lodge, D., Anis, N.A., Berry, S.C., & Burton, N.R. (1983). Arylcyclohexylamines selectively reduce excitation of mammalian neurons by asparate like amino acids.
In J.M. Kamenka, E.F. Domino, & P. Geneste (Eds.), *Phencyclidine and related
arylcyclohexylamines: present and future applications.* (pp. 595). Ann Arbor,
NPP Books.

Losher, W., & Nau, H. (1985). Pharmacological evaluation of various metabolites
and analogues of valproic acid. *Neuropharmacology, 24*, 427–435.

Losher, W., & Siemes, H. (1984). Valproic acid increases gamma-aminobutyric acid
in CSF of epileptic children. *Lancet, 2*, 225.

MacDonald, R.L., & Barker, J.L. (1979). Anticonvulsant and anesthetic barbituates:
different post-synaptic action in cultured mammalian neurons. *Neurology, 29*,
432–477.

Mackenzie, N., & Grant, I.S. (1985). Comparison of the new emulsion formulation of propofol with methohexitone and thiopentone for induction of anaesthesia in day cases. *British Journal of Anaesthesia, 57,* 725–731.

Marder, S.R. (1994). The role of dosage and plasma levels in neuroleptic relapse prevention. *Acta Psychiatrica Scandinavica, 382,* 25–27.

Marder, S.R., Ames, D., Wirshing, W.C., & Van Putten, T. (1993). Schizophrenia. *Psychiatric Clinics of North America, 16,* 567–587.

Marescaux, C., Micheletti, G., Vergnes, M., Depaulis, A., Rumbach, L., & Warter, J.M. (1984). A model of chronic and spontaneous petit mal-like seizures in the rat: comparison with pentylenetetrazole induced seizures. *Epilepsia, 25,* 326–331.

Marsden, C.D., Meldrum, B.S., Pycock, C., & Tarsy, D. (1975). Focal myoclonus produced by injection of picrotoxin into the caudate nucleus of the rat. *Journal of Physiology (London), 246,* 96P.

Martin, B.R. (1986). Cellular effects of cannabinoids. *Pharmacology Review, 38,* 45–74.

Martin, B.R. (1995). Marijuana. In F.E. Bloom & D.J. Kupfer (Eds.), *Psychopharmacology: the fourth generation of progress.* (pp. 1757–1765). New York: Raven Press.

Mayer, D.J., Price, D.D., & Rafii, A. (1977). Antagonism of acupuncture analgesia in man by the narcotic antagonist naloxone. *Brain Research, 121,* 368–372.

McCarley, R.W. (1994). Neurophysiology of sleep: basic mechanisms underlying control of wakefulness and sleep. In S. Chokrovery (Ed.), *Sleep disorders medicine: basic science, technical considerations and clinical aspects.* Boston: Butterworth-Heinemann.

McCombs, J.S., Nichol, M.B., Stimmel, G.L., Sclar, D.A., Beasley, C.M.J., & Gross, L.S. (1990). The cost of antidepressant drug therapy failure: a study of antidepressant use patterns in a Medicaid population. *Journal of Clinical Psychiatry, 51,* 60–69.

McLean, M.J., & MacDonald, R.L. (1986). Sodium valproate, but not ethosuximide, produces use- and voltage-dependent limitations of high frequency repetitive firing of action potentials of mouse central neurons in cell culture. *Journal of Pharmacological Experimental Therapy, 237,* 1001–1011.

Meldrum, B.S., & Corsellis, J.A.N. (1984). Epilepsy. In J.A.N. Corsellis & L.W. Duchen (Eds.), *Greenfield's neuropathology.* (pp. 921–950). New York: John Wiley.

Meltzer, H.Y. (1993). New drugs for the treatment of schizophrenia. *Psychiatric Clinics of North America, 16,* 365–385.

Meltzer, H.Y., & Lowy, M.T. (1987). The serotonin hypothesis of depression. In H.Y. Meltzer (Ed.), *Psychopharmacology: the third generation of progress.* (pp. 513–526). New York: Raven Press.

Melzack, R., & Wall, P.D. (1984). Acupuncture and transcutaneous electrical nerve stimulation. *Postgraduate Medical Journal, 60,* 893–896.

Merritt, H.H., & Putnam, T.J. (1938). A new series of anticonvulsant drugs tested by experiments on animals. *Archives in Neurological Psychiatry, 39,* 1003–1015.

Mersky, H. (1986). Classification of chronic pain: description of chronic pain syndromes and definitions of pain terms. *Pain, (Supplement 3),* 217.

Meyer, H.H. (1906). The theory of narcosis. In Anonymous, *Harvey Lectures.* (pp. 11–17).

Miller, K.W. (1993). Molecular mechanisms by which general anesthetics act. In S. Feldman, C.F. Scurr, & W. Paton (Eds.), *Mechanisms of drug action in anasthesia.* Boston: Edward Arnold.

Moskowitz, M.A. (1984). The neurobiology of vascular head pain. *Annals of Neurology, 16*, 157–168.

Moskowitz, M.A. (1993). The trigeminovascular system. In J. Olesen, P. Tfelt-Hansen, & K.M.A. Welch (Eds.), *The headaches*. New York: Raven Press.

Murray, T.F. (1994). Basic pharmacology of ketamine. In T.A. Bowdle, A. Horita. & E.D. Kharasch (Eds.), *The pharmacologic basis of anesthesiology*. (p. 337). New York: Churchill Livingstone.

Nebert, D.W., & Gonzalez, F.J. (1987). P450 genes: structure, evolution, and regulation. *Annual Review of Biochemistry, 56*, 945–993.

Nestler, E.J. (1994). Molecular neurobiology of drug addiction. *Neuropsychopharmacology, 11*, 77–87.

Newman, R.G. (1983). The need to redefine "addiction." *New England Journal of Medicine, 308*, 1096–1098.

Nowak, L., Bregostovski, P., Ascher, P., Herbert, A., & Prochiantz, A. (1984). Magnesium gates glutamate-activated channels in mouse central neurones. *Nature, 307*, 462–465.

Olanow, C.W.I. (1992). Protective therapy for Parkinson's disease. In C.W.I. Olanow & A. Lieberman (Eds.), *Scientific basis for the treatment of Parkinson's disease*. p. 225). New Jersey: Parthenon Publishing Group.

Olanow, C.W.I., & Lieberman, A. (1992). *Scientific basis for the treatment of Parkinson's disease*. New Jersey: Parthenon Publishing Group.

Olesen, J. (1987). The ischemic hypothesis of migraine. *Archives in Neurology, 44*, 321–322.

Olesen, J., Larsen, B., & Lauritzen, M. (1981). Focal hyperemia followed by spreading oligemia and impaired activation of rCBF in classic migraine. *Annals in Neurology, 9*, 344–352.

Olney, J.W., Labruyere, J., & Price, M.T. (1989). Pathological changes induced in cerebrocortical neurons by phencyclidine and related drugs. *Science, 244*, 1360–1362.

Olsen, R.W. (1988). Barbituates. *International Anesthesiology Clinics, 26*, 254–261.

Overton, C.E. (1990). Studies of narcosis. In R.L. Lipnick (Ed.), *Studies in narcosis*. (pp. 23–181). New York: Chapman and Hall.

Owen, R.T., & Tyrer, P. (1983). Benzodiazepine dependence: a review of the evidence. *Drugs, 25*, 385–398.

Owens, M.J., & Nemeroff, C.B. (1994). Role of serotonin in the pathophysiology of depression: focus on the serotonin transporter. *Clinical Chemistry, 40*, 288–295.

Palacios, J.M., Landwehrmeyer B., & Mengod, G. (1993). Brain dopamine receptors: characterization, distribution and alteration in disease. In D. Retford (Ed.), *Parkinson's disease and movement disorders*. (p. 35). Baltimore: Williams and Wilkins.

Pappert, E.J., Tangney, C.C., Goetz, C.G., Ling, Z.D., Lipton, J.W., Stebbins, G.T., & Carvey, P.M. (1996). Alpha-tocopherol in the ventricular cerebrospinal fluid of Parkinson's disease patients: dose-response study and correlations with plasma levels. *Neurology 47*, 1037–1042.

Pasternak, G.W. (1993). Pharmacological mechanisms of opioid analgesics. In Anonymous, *Clinical Neuropharmacology*. (pp. 1–18). New York, NY: Raven Press.

Pasternak, G.W., Childers, S.R., & Snyder, S.H. (1980). Opiate analgesia: evidence for mediation by a subpopulation of opiate receptors. *Science, 208*, 514–516.

Paterson, I.A., Juorio, A.V., & Boulton, A.A. (1990). Possible mechanism of action of deprenyl in parkinsonism [letter]. *Lancet, 336*, 183.

Paul, D., Standifer, K.M., Inturrial, C.E., & Pasternak, G.W. (1989). Pharmacological characterizations of morphine-a6β-glucuronide, a very potent morphine metabolite. *Journal of Pharmacological Experimental Therapy, 251,* 477–483.

Payne, R., & Pasternak, G.W. (1992). Pain. In M.V. Johnston, R.L. MacDonald, & A.B. Young (Eds)., *Principles of drug therapy in neurology.* (pp. 268–301). Philadelphia: F.A. Davis.

Pellow, S., & File, S.E. (1984). Multiple sites of action for anxiogenic drugs. *Psychopharmacology, 83,* 304–315.

Peroutka, S.J. (1992). Migraine. In M.V. Johnston, R.L. MacDonald, & A.B. Young (Eds.), *Principles of drug therapy in neurology.* (pp. 161–178). Philadelphia: F.A. Davis.

Pert, C.B., & Snyder, S.H. (1973). Opiate receptor: demonstrated in nervous tissue. *Science, 179,* 1101.

Perucca, E., Hebdige, S., Frigo, G.M., Gatti, G., Lecchini, S., & Crema, A. (1980). Interaction between phenytoin and valproic acid: plasma protein binding and metabolic effects. *Clinical Pharmacology and Therapeutics, 28,* 779–789.

Phillips, G.D., Robbins, T.W., & Everitt, B.J. (1994). Mesoaccumbens dopamine-opiate interactions in the control over behaviour by a conditioned reinforcer. *Psychopharmacology (Berlin), 114,* 345–359.

Phillis, J.W., & O'Reagan, M.H. (1988). The role of adenosine in the central actions of benzodiazepines. *Progress in Neuro-psychopharmacology and Biological Psychiatry, 12,* 389–404.

Plosker, G.L., & McTavish, D. (1994). Sumatriptan: A reappraisal of its pharmacology and therapeutic efficacy in the acute treatment of migraine and cluster headaches. *Drugs, 47,* 622–651.

Potter, W.Z., & Manji, H.K. (1994). Catecholamines in depression: an update. *Clinical Chemistry, 40,* 279–287.

Pratt, J.A. (1992). The neuroanatomical basis of anxiety. *Pharmacology and Therapeutics, 55,* 149–181.

Prince, D.A. (1969). Electrophysiology of "epileptic" neurons: spike generation. *Electoencephalography and Clinical Neurophysiology, 26,* 476–487.

Pritchett, D.B., Luddens, H., & Seeburg, P.H. (1989). Type I and type II GABA$_A$ benzodiazepine receptors produced in transfected cells. *Science (Washington DC), 245,* 1389–1392.

Pritchett, D.B., Sontheimer, H., Shivers, B.D., Ymer, S., Kettenmann, H., Schofield, P.R., & Seeburg, P.H. (1989). Importance of a novel GABA$_A$ receptor subunit for benzodiazepine pharmacology. *Nature (London), 338,* 582–585.

Quasha, A.L., Eger, E.I., & Tinker, J.H. (1980). Determination and applications of MAC. *Anesthesiology, 53,* 315–334.

Ragowski, M.A., & Porter, R.J. (1990). Antiepileptic drugs: pharmacological mechanisms and clinical efficacy with consideration of promising developmental stage compounds. *Pharmacological Reviews, 42,* 223.

Rainnie, D.G., Grunze, H.C., McCarley, R.W., & Greene, R.W. (1994). Adenosine inhibition of mesopontine cholinergic neurons: implications for EEG arousal [published erratum appears in Science 1994 Jul 1;265(5168):16]. *Science, 263,* 689–692.

Rapoport, J.L. (1989). The biology of obsessions and compulsions [see comments]. *Scientific American, 260,* 82–89.

Raskin, N.H. (1986). Repetitive intravenous dihydroergotamine as therapy for intractable migraine. *Neurology, 36,* 995–997.

Reich, D.L., & Silvay, G. (1989). Ketamine: an update on the first twenty-five years of clinical experience. *Canadian Journal of Anesthesia, 36,* 186–197.

Reiman, E.M., Raichle, M.E., Robins, E., Mintun, M.A., Fusselman, M.J., Fox, P.T., Price, J.L., & Hackman, K.A. (1989). Neuroanatomical correlates of a lactate-induced anxiety attack. *Archives in General Psychiatry, 46,* 493–500.

Reith, M.E.A., de Costa, B., Rice, K.C., & Jacobson, A.E. (1992). Evidence for mutually exclusive binding of cocaine, BTCP, GBR 12935, and dopamine to the dopamine transporter. *European Journal of Pharmacology, 227,* 417–425.

Reynolds, G.P. (1983). Increased concentrations and lateral asymmetry of amygdala dopamine in schizophrenia. *Nature, 305,* 527–529.

Ricaurte, G., Bryan, G., Strauss, L., Seiden, L., & Schuster, C. (1985). Hallucinogenic amphetamine selectively destroys brain serotonin nerve terminals. *Science, 229,* 986–988.

Roberts, G.W. (1990). Schizophrenia: the cellular biology of a functional psychosis. *Trends in Neuroscience, 13,* 207–211.

Robertson, B. (1989). Actions of anaesthetics and avermectin on GABAA chloride channels in mammalian dorsal root ganglion neurones. *Br J Pharmacol, 98,* 167–176.

Robertson, M.M. (1989). The Gilles de la Tourette syndrome: the current status. *British Journal of Psychiatry, 154,* 147–169.

Robinson, T.E., & Berridge, K.C. (1993). The neural basis of drug craving: an incentive-sensitization theory of addiction. *Brain Research, 18,* 247–291.

Rogawski, M.A., & Porter, R.J. (1990). Antiepileptic drugs: pharmacological mechanisms and clinical efficacy with consideration of promising developments stage compounds. *Pharmacological Reviews, 42,* 223–286.

Rogers, H.J., Spector, R.G., & Trounce, J.R. (1981). *A textbook of clinical pharmacology.* Kent: Hodder and Stoughton.

Roos, R.A.C. (1986). Neuropathology of Huntington's chorea. In P. Vinken, G. Bruyn, & H. Klawans (Eds.), *Handbook of clinical neurology: extrapyramidal disorders.* (p. 315). Amsterdam: Elsevier Science.

Rubin, A., Lemberger, L., & Dhahir, P. (1981). Physiologic disposition of pergolide. *Clinical Pharmacology and Therapeutics, 30,* 258–265.

Sakai, F., & Meyer, J.S. (1978). Regional cerebral hemodynamics during migraine and cluster headaches measured by the 133-Xe inhalation method. *Headache, 18,* 122–133.

Schiavo, G., Benfenati, F., Poulain, B., Rossetto, O., Polverino de Laureto, P., DasGupta, B.R., & Montecucco, C. (1992). Tetanus and botulinum-B neurotoxins block neurotransmitter release by proteolytic cleavage of synaptobrevin [see comments]. *Nature, 359,* 832–835.

Schildkraut, J.J. (1965). The catecholamine hypothesis of affective disorders: a review of supporting evidence. *American Journal of Psychiatry, 122,* 509–522.

Schofield, P.R., Darlison, M.G., Fujita, N., Burt, D.R., Stephenson, F.A., Rodriguez, H., Rhee, L.M., Ramachandran, J., Reale, V., Glencorse, T.A., Seeburg, P.H., & Barnard, E.A. (1987). Sequence and functional expression of the GABA$_A$ receptor shows a ligand-gated receptor super-family. *Nature, 328,* 221–227.

Schultz, R., Wuster, M., & Herz, A. (1981). Pharmacological characterization of the epsilon opiate receptor. *Journal of Pharmacological Experimental Therapy, 216,* 604–606.

Schulz, D.W., & MacDonald, R.L. (1981). Barbiturate enhancement of GABA-mediated inhibition and activation of chloride ion conductance: correlation with anticonvulsant and anesthetic actions. *Brain Research, 209,* 177–188.

Schwab, R.S., Poskanzer, D.C., England, A.C., & Young, R.R. (1972). Amantadine in Parkinson's disease. Review of more than two years of experience. *Journal of the American Medical Association, 222,* 792–795.

Schwartz, R.D., Jackson, J.A., Weigert, D., Skolnick, P., & Paul, S.M. (1985). Characterization of barbiturate-stimulated chloride efflux from rat brain synaptoneurosomes. *Journal of Neuroscience, 5,* 2963–2970.

Schwartzkroin, P.A. (1994). Cellular electrophysiology of human epilepsy. *Epilepsy Research, 17,* 185–192.

Schwarz, J.R., & Grigat, G. (1989). Phenytoin and carbamazepine: potential and frequency-dependent block of Na currents in mammalian myelinated nerve fibers. *Epilepsia, 30,* 286–294.

Seeman, P., Lee, T., Chau-Wong, M., & Wong, K. (1976). Antipsychotic drug doses and neuroleptic/dopamine receptors. *Nature, 261,* 717–719.

Shafii, M., & Shafii, S.L. (1990). *Biological rhythms, mood disorders, light therapy and the pineal gland.* Washington, D.C.: American Psychiatric Press.

Shelton, R.C., & Weinberger, D.R. (1987). Brain morphology in schizophrenia. In H.Y. Meltzer (Ed.), *Psychopharmacology: the third generation of progress.* (pp. 773–781). New York: Raven Press.

Simpson, G.M., & de Leon, J. (1989). Tyramine and new monoamine oxidase inhibitor drugs. *British Journal of Psychiatry Supplement,* 32–37.

Smith, D.J., Bouchal, R.L., deSanctis, C.A., Monroe, P.J., Amedro, J.B., Perrotti, J.M., & Crisp, T. (1987). Properties of the interaction between ketamine and opiate binding sites *in vivo* and *in vitro. Neuropharmacology, 26,* 1253–1260.

Smith, G.P., Gibbs, J., Pi-Sunyer, F.X., Kissileff, H.R., & Thornton, J. (1981). The satiety effect of cholecystokinin: a progress report. *Peptides, 2,* 57–59.

Smith, M.C., & Riskin, B.T. (1991). The clinical use of barbituates in neurological disorders. *Drugs, 42,* 365–378.

Snell, L.D., & Johnson, K.M. (1985). Antagonism of N-methyl-D-aspartate induced transmitter release in the rat striatum by phencyclidine-like drugs and its relationship to turning behavior. *Journal of Pharmacological Experimental Therapy,* 50–57.

Spector, R., & Johanson, C.E. (1989). The mammalian choroid plexus. *Scientific American, 261,* 68–74.

Speth, R.C., Guidotti, A., & Yamamura, M. (1980). The pharmacology of the benzodiazepines. In G.C. Palmer (Ed.), *Neuropharmacology of central nervous system and behavioural disorders.* (pp. 243–283). New York: Academic Press.

Spiegel, K., Kourides, I.A., & Pasternak, G.W. (1983). Analgesic activity of tricyclic antidepressants. *Annals of Neurology, 13,* 462–465.

Srivastava, E.D., Russell, M.A.H., Feyerabend, C., Masterson, J.G., & Rhodes, J. (1991). Sensitivity and tolerance to nicotine in smokers and nonsmokers. *Psychopharmacology, 105,* 63–68.

Steriade, M. (1992). Basic mechanisms of sleep. *Neurology, 42,* 9–18.

Steriade, M, Jones, E.G., & Llinas, R.R. (1990). *Thalamic oscillations and signalling.* New York: Wiley-Interscience.

Stevens, J.R. (1973). An anatomy of schizophrenia? *Archives of General Psychiatry, 29,* 177–189.

Stevenson, R.D., & Wolraich, M.L. (1989). Stimulant medication therapy in the treatment of children with attention deficit hyperactivity disorder. *Pediatric Clinics of North America, 36,* 1183–1197.

Stewart, J., de Wit, H., & Eikelboom, R. (1984). Role of unconditioned and conditioned drug effects in the self-administration of opiates and stimulants. *Psychological Review, 91,* 251–268.

Stimson, G.V., & Oppenheimer, E. (1982). *Heroin addiction: treatment and control in Britain.* London: Tavistock.

Stoetter, B., Braun, A.R., Randolph, C., Gernert, J., Carson, R.E., Herscovitch, P., & Chase, T.N. (1992). Functional neuroanatomy of Tourette syndrome limbic-motor interactions studied with FDG PET. In T.N. Chase, A.J. Friedhoff, & D.J. Cohen (Eds.), *Advances in neurology.* New York: Raven Press.

Stokes, P.E. (1993). Fluxotine: a five-year review. *Clinical Therapeutics, 15,* 216–43; discussion 215.

Strange, P.G. (1992). *Brain biochemistry and brain disorders.* New York: Oxford University Press.

Strauss, J.S., Carpenter, W.T.J., & Bartko, J.J. (1974). The diagnosis and understanding of schizophrenia. Part III. Speculations on the processes that underlie schizophrenic symptoms and signs. *Schizophrenic Bulletin, 11,* 61–69.

Strichartz, G.R. (1973). The inhibition of sodium currents in myelinated nerve by quaternary derivatives of lidocaine. *Journal of General Physiology, 62,* 37–57.

Swanson, J.M., Cantwell, D., Lerner, M., McBurnett, K., & Hanna, G. (1991). Effects of stimulant medication on learning in children with ADHD. *Journal of Learning Disabilities, 24,* 219–230.

Swerdlow, M. (1984). Anticonvulsant drugs and chronic pain. *Clinical Neuropharmacology,* 7:51–82.

Tabakoff, B., & Hoffman, P.L. (1987). Biochemical pharmacology of alcohol. In H.Y. Meltzer (Ed.), *Psychopharmacology: the third generation of progress.* (pp. 1521–1526). New York: Raven Press.

Taylor, D.P. (1990). Serotonin agents in anxiety. *Annals of the N Y Academy of Sciences, 600,* 545–556; discussion 556–557.

Tetrud, J.W., & Langston, J.W. (1989). The effect of deprenyl (selegiline) on the natural history of Parkinson's disease [see comments]. *Science, 245,* 519–522.

Tfelt-Hansen, P., & Johnson, E.S. (1987). Nonsteroidal anti-inflammatory drugs in the treatment of acute migraine attack. In S. Olesen, P. Tfelt-Hansen, & K.M.A. Welch (Eds.), *The headaches.* New York: Raven Press.

Tollefson, G.D. (1983). Monoamine oxidase inhibitors: a review. *Journal of Clinical Psychiatry, 44,* 280–288.

Torebjork, H.E., & Hallin, R.G. (1979). Microneurographic studies of peripheral pain mechanisms in man. In J.J. Bonica (Ed.), *Advances in pain research and therapy.* (pp. 121–131). New York: Raven Press.

Tucker, G.T., & Mather, L.E. (1975). Pharmacology of local anaesthetic agents. Pharmacokinetics of local anaesthetic agents. *British Journal of Anaesthesiology, 47 supplement,* 213–224.

Twombly, D.A., Yoshii, M., & Narahashi, T. (1988). Mechanisms of calcium channel block by phenytoin. *Journal of Pharmacological Experimental Therapy, 246,* 189–195.

Twyman, R.E., Rogers, C.J., & MacDonald, R.L. (1989). Differential regulation of GABA$_A$ receptor channels by diazepam and phenobarbital. *Annals of Neurology, 25,* 213–220.

Uhde, T.A., & Taner, M.E. (1989). Chemical models of panic: a review and critique. In P. Tyrer (Ed.), *Psychopharmacology of anxiety.* (pp. 108–131). Oxford: Oxford University Press.

Van Putten, T. (1975). The many faces of akathisia. *Comprehensive Psychiatry, 16,* 43–47.

Vergnes, M., Marescaux, C., Depaulis, A., Micheletti, G., & Warter, J.M. (1987). Spontaneous spike and wave discharges in thalamus and cortex in a rat model of genetic petit mal-like seizures. *Experimental Neurology, 96,* 127–136.

Vermeij, P., Ferrari, M.D., Buruma, O.J., Veenema, H., & de Wolff, F.A. (1988). Inheritance of poor phenytoin parahydroxylation capacity in a Dutch family. *Clinical Pharmacology and Therapeutics, 44,* 588–593.

Von Voigtlander, P.F., & Moore, K.E. (1971). Dopamine: release from the brain in vivo by amantadine. *Science, 174,* 408–410.

Waddington, J.L. (1989). Functional interactions between D-1 and D-2 dopamine receptor systems: their role in the regulation of psychomotor behaviour, putative mechanisms, and clinical relevance. *Journal of Psychopharmacology, 3,* 54–63.

Watkins, L.R., Kinscheck, I.B., & Mayer, D.J. (1984). Potentiation of opiate and analgesia and apparent reversal of morphine tolerance by proglumide. *Science, 224,* 395–396.

Watts, A. (1991). Magnetic resonance studies of lipid-protein interfaces and lipophilic molecule partioning. *New York Academy of Sciences, 625,* 653–667.

Waud, B.E., & Waud, D.R. (1970). On dose-response curves and anesthetics. *Anesthesiology, 33,* 1–4.

Weerasuriya, K., Patel, L., & Turner, P. (1982). β-adrenoceptor blockade and migraine. *Cephalalgia, 2,* 33–45.

Weinberger, D.R. (1988). Schizophrenia and the frontal lobe. *Trends in Neuroscience, 11,* 367–370.

Weinberger, D.R., Berman, K.F., & Zec, R.F. (1986). Physiologic dysfunction of dorsolateral prefrontal cortex in schizophrenia. I. Regional cerebral blood flow evidence. *Archives of General Psychiatry, 43,* 114–124.

Weiner, D.M., Levey, A.I., Sunahara, R.K., Niznik, H.B., O'Dowd, B.F., Seeman, P., & Brann, M.R. (1991). D1 and D2 dopamine receptor mRNA in rat brain. *Proceedings of the National Academy of Sciences of the United States of America, 88,* 1859–1863.

Weiss, S.R.B., Post, R.M., Patel, J., & Marangos, P.J. (1985). Differential mediation of the anticonvulsant effects of carbamezepam. *Life Science, 36,* 2413–2419.

Welch, K.M.A. (1987). Migraine: a biobehavioral disorder. *Archives of Neurology, 44,* 323.

Wells, P.G., Nagai, M.K., & Greco, G.S. (1989). Inhibition of trimethadione and dimethadione teratogenicity by the cyclooxygenase inhibitor acetylsalicylic acid: a unifying hypothesis for the teratologic effect of hydantoin anticonvulsants and structurally related compounds. *Toxicology and Applied Pharmacology, 97,* 406–414.

Westerink, B.H.C. (1985). Sequence and significance of dopamine metabolism in the rat brain. *Neurochemistry International, 7,* 221–227.

White, F.J., & Wang, R.Y. (1983). Comparison of the effects of chronic haloperidol treatment on A9 and A10 dopamine neurons in the rat. *Life Sciences, 32,* 983–993.

Williams, R.L., Karacan, I., & Hursch, C.J. (1974). *Electroencephalogrpahy (EEG) of human sleep: clinical applications.* New York: John Wiley.

Willow, M., Gonoi, T., & Catterall, W.A. (1985). Voltage clamp analysis of the inhibitory actions of diphenylhydantoin and carbamazepine on voltage-sensitive sodium channels in neuroblastoma cells. *Molecular Pharmacology, 27,* 549–558.

Wilson, S.A.K. (1912). Progressive lenticular degeneration: a familial nervous disease associated with cirrhosis of the liver. *Brain, 34,* 295–509.

Winn, P. (1994). Schizophrenia research moves to the prefrontal cortex. *Trends in Neuroscience, 17,* 265–268.

Wirz-Justice, A., Graw, P., Krauchi, K., Sarrafzadeh, A., English, J., Arendt, J., & Sand, L. (1996). 'Natural' light treatment of seasonal affective disorder. *Journal of Affective Disorders, 37,* 109–120.

Wise, R.A., & Bozarth, M.A. (1987). A psychomotor stimulant theory of addiction. *Psychological Review, 94,* 469–492.

Wolff, H.G. (1963). *Headache and other head pain.* New York: Oxford University Press.

Wood, A., Tollefson, G.D., & Birkett, M. (1993). Pharmacotherapy of obsessive compulsive-disorder—experience with fluoxetine. *International Clinical Psychopharmacology, 8,* 301–306.

Wykes, P. (1968). The treatment of angine pectoris with coexistent migraine. *Practitioner, 200,* 702–704.

Yaari, Y., Konnerth, A., & Heinemann, U. (1986). Nonsynaptic epileptogenesis in the mammalian hippocampus in vitro. II. Role of extracellular potassium. *Journal of Neurophysiology, 56,* 424–438.

Yaari, Y., Selzer, M.E., & Pincus, J.H. (1986). Phenytoin: mechanisms of its anticonvulsant action. *Annals of Neurology, 20,* 171–184.

Yebenes, J.G., & Gomez, M.A.M. (1993). Dopamine systems in the mammalian brain. In D. Retford (Ed.), *Parkinson's disease and movement disorders.* (pp. 13–28). Baltimore: Williams and Wilkins.

Young, A.B., Shoulson, J., Penney, J.B., Starosta, S., Gomez, F., Travers, H., Ramos-Arroya, M.A., Snodgrass, S.R., Bonilla, E., Moreno, H., & Wexler, N.S. (1986). Huntington's disease in Venezuela neurologic features and functional decline. *Neurology, 36,* 244–249.

Yu, O., Chiu, T.H., & Rosenburg, H.C. (1988). Modulation of GABA-gated chloride ion flux in rat brain by acute and chronic benzodiazepine administration. *Journal of Pharmacological Experimental Therapy, 246,* 107–113.

Zametkin, A.J., Liebenauer, L.L., Fitzgerald, G.A., King, A.C., Minkunas, D.V., Herscovitch, P., Yamada, E.M., & Cohen, R.M. (1993). Brain metabolism in teenagers with attention-deficit hyperactivity disorder. *Archives of General Psychiatry, 50,* 333–340.

Ziegler, D.K. (1981). Prolonged relief of dystonic movements with diazepam. *Neurology, 31,* 1457–1458.

Zigmond, R.E., Schwarzchild, M.A., & Rittenhouse, A.R. (1989). Acute regulation of tyrosine hydroxylase by nerve activity and by neurotransmitters via phosphorylation. *Annual Review of Neuroscience, 12,* 415–461.

Zivin, J.A., & Choi, D.W. (1991). Stroke therapy. *Scientific American, 265,* 56–63.

Questions

Chapter 1

1. What are the major functional regions of a neuron?

2. How are small- and large-molecule neurotransmitters, centrally acting gases, and neurotrophic substances similar and how do they differ?

3. What are the major structures of the brain and what are their functions?

4. What are the major subdivisions of the cerebral cortex and what are their functions?

5. What is implied when the terms motor, sensory, memory, limbic, and cognitive processing are used?

6. What is the general structure of the autonomic nervous system and which organs and tissues are innervated by the parasympathetic and sympathetic nervous systems?

7. What are the primary actions of the SANS and the PANS at each of the following organ systems: heart, gastrointestinal tract, pupil, peripheral vascular beds, muscular vascular beds, sweat glands, and salivary glands?

8. What are the effects of the following drug classes at each of the systems described in question 8: an alpha-adrenergic receptor agonist, a beta-adrenergic receptor agonist, a muscarinic receptor agonist, and a nicotinic receptor agonist?

9. What is the significance of the amplification of signal that is an inherent part of the sympathetic nervous system? Be sure you consider the role of the adrenal medulla in this discussion.

Chapter 2

1. What are the different routes of drug absorption and how can they influence the actions of centrally acting drugs?

2. What effect does an acidic or basic pKa have on the absorption and distribution of a centrally acting drug assuming a pH of 4.4 in the gut and 7.4 in the brain?

3. Why is the blood brain barrier (BBB) important to the action of centrally acting drugs and what happens to a drug after it passes the BBB?

4. How readily does a drug diffuse through the parenchyma of brain and what are some of the barriers to diffusion?

5. How predictive are plasma drug levels of brain and CSF levels of drugs? Why is protein binding in plasma an important consideration in this process?

6. What is the role of brain perfusion in drug action and redistribution?

7. What is similar and what is different about pharmacokinetic, physiological, pharmacodynamic, and reverse tolerance?

Chapter 3

1. How many kinds of receptor are there and what distinguishes them?

2. Why are the terms target and receptor specific and target and receptor nonspecific important and how do they relate to the specificity of drug action and to side effects?

3. How are ionotropic and metabotropic receptors similar and how are they different?

4. What is the role of the G protein in initiating neuronal signals?

5. What are the basic components of the cyclic nucleotide, PLA_2, and phosphoinositide cascades?

6. How can a drug alter the production of proteins by influencing transcription rates?

7. What are the adaptive advantages of a system comprised of multiple receptor subtypes over a system which has only one receptor subtype?

8. Any drug can be classified as a direct- or indirect-acting agonist or antagonist. In terms of anticipated side effects, which of these modes of drug action will usually have fewer side effects?

9. When does receptor-site up-regulation occur? When does down-regulation occur? What effect does each have on the actions of an agonist? What effect on an antagonist?

10. What is the difference between an autoreceptor and a heteroreceptor? What are the anticipated effects of agonism at receptors located on the proximal or distal ends of dendrites, the cell body, and the terminal bouton when Na^+ channels are opened? When Cl^- channels are opened?

11. How does a dose-response curve help in understanding the receptor binding kinetics of a drug?

12. What is the meaning of ED_{75}?

13. How does the slope of a dose-response curve affect your ability to carefully titrate drug delivery (concept of "wiggle room")?

14. What is the difference between a therapeutic index and a therapeutic range?

15. What is implied by left or right lateral shifts in a dose-response curve?

Chapter 4

1. What are the two facets of pain and what pathways do they follow into the brain?

2. What chemicals, substances, and actions will stimulate the terminals of primary sensory pain afferents?

3. What is the role of the PAG, the limbic system, the spinal cord, and the cortex in pain appreciation?

4. How does the action of an opioid drug at the Sub P terminal conform to the notion of the pain-gate theory?

5. What are the different opioid receptor subtypes? What receptor affinity profile would the perfect opioid analgesic have?

6. What is the mechanism through which morphine induces: 1—euphoria; 2—respiratory depression; 3—nausea/vomiting; 4—oliguria; 5—hypotension; 6—constipation; 7—right upper quadrant pain? Based on the principle of counteradaptation, what syndrome involving the seven effects described above would be expected following morphine withdrawal?

7. What is the pathognomonic triad of morphine overdose? Why is it considered standard ER procedure to administer naloxone indiscriminately to patients in respiratory depression? Why is it considered standard ER practice to not administer O_2 to a patient in respiratory depression from drug overdose until that patient's response to naloxone has been established?

8. How do the commonly used opioid agonists differ from the primary effects of morphine?

9. What is the rationale for the use of a partial opioid agonist in a patient with minor pain?

10. What arguments would you provide to a physician who is reluctant, out of fear of inducing dependence, to administer a full opioid agonist to a patient in severe pain?

11. What are three pharmacologic strategies for controlling very severe pain? For controlling chronic pain?

Chapter 5

1. How can the ischemic hypothesis, the sterile inflammatory hypothesis, and the biobehavioral hypothesis explain migraine headache with and without aura?

2. What are the mechanisms of action of aspirin and acetaminophen and how do they relate to the treatment of migraine headache? What is the basis for the statement that OTC headache medication should be taken as early as possible in the pain phase of a headache?

3. What is the mechanism(s) responsible for aspirin-induced GI upset?

4. How do the proposed mechanisms of action for the ergot alkaloids relate to the vascular hypothesis of Woolf and the sterile inflammatory hypothesis?

5. What are the signs and symptoms of acute and chronic ergotism?

6. Why are adjunctive medications often needed in the acute treatment of migraine headache?

7. What is the theoretical rationale for the mechanism through which migraine attacks could be prevented pharmacologically?

8. What is the role of $5HT_{1D}$ receptors in the regulation of CGRP release and how does sumatriptan reduce the pain of migraine headache?

9. What are the common side effects of sumatriptan and what is their impact on the patient's perception of the safety of the drug?

10. How are methysergide, amitriptyline, propranolol, and Ca^{2+} channel antagonists thought to prevent the development of migraine headache?

11. What are the various treatment strategies for ER patients in an acute pain phase of migraine?

12. What role do benzodiazepines and other muscle-relaxing drugs play in the management of headache?

Chapter 6

1. What is the relationship between the dosage of sedative-hypnotic administered and the subsequent levels of consciousness? What are the advantages of viewing consciousness as existing along a continuum?

2. What is the disinhibition release phenomenon? Provide an argument to support the notion that these drugs are CNS depressants despite the lay assumption that they elevate mood.

3. Why do most CNS depressants induce dose-dependent respiratory depression while benzodiazepines do not? What other side effects are shared by the CNS depressants?

4. What effects do CNS depressants have on the different forms of memory? (Is this effect on memory considered useful or is it a side effect?)

5. Why should "sleeping pills" not be used for the chronic management of insomnia?

6. What contributes to the long half-life of the benzodiazepines? Why, despite their long half-lives, do they not induce a sedation lasting 50 hours? Which benzodiazepines are metabolized extrahepatically?

7. How are the cellular mechanisms of the benzodiazepines and other sedative-hypnotic drug classes similar and how are they different?

8. What four brain regions participate in the regulation of the sleep state? What are the major functions of those regions?

9. How is sleep architecture normally described?

10. How is anxiety thought to arise in the CNS? How can activation of one central nucleus give rise to the myriad of behaviors that characterize anxiety?

11. From a neurobiological perspective, why do some individuals experience anxiety easier than others?

12. Why do some benzodiazepines possess anxiolytic action while others do not?

13. How do buspirone, benzodiazepines, and propranolol attenuate anxiety?

Chapter 7

1. How does an anesthetic apparatus regulate anesthesia and what is meant by the notion that anesthetics act within a closed system?

2. What relationship exists between lipid solubility and anesthetic induction rate? Why is this relationship critical to understanding the mechanisms of action of volatile anesthetics? Based on these principles, explain the "bucket theory."

3. If volatile anesthetics act in a stereoselective fashion, how can their action still conform to the Overton-Meyer hypothesis?

4. Define and provide practical applications for the terms MAC, and catecholamine sensitization.

5. How is it possible that a volatile anesthetic can induce anesthetic plane without necessarily blocking neuronal conduction down an axon?

6. What are the common actions, side effects, and major benefits of each of the commonly used volatile anesthetic agents? Which anesthetic agents are significantly biotransformed (>10%)?

7. What are the classes of the major adjuvant agents used in gas anesthesia? How and why do they reduce morbidity? How are depolarization and desensitization blockade similar and how are they different?

8. What are the advantages and disadvantages of the various intravenous anesthetic agents commonly used? What are the advantages and disadvantages of neurolept-anesthesia, neurolept-analgesia, and dissociative anesthesia?

9. What characteristics describe an ideal general anesthetic agent?

10. Identify the salt, free-base, and ionized forms of local anesthetics. Given two equipotent local anesthetics with pKa's of 8.4 and 9.4, which agent will produce anesthesia first when injected into an inflamed area (pH = 4.4)?

11. What is the basis for the sequence of functional neuronal dropout in a compound nerve following local anesthetic administration?

12. How do amide and ester local anesthetics differ in their biotransformation and how do these differences influence the distribution and side effects of these drugs?

13. How are the local anesthetics formulated to maintain stability during storage and how do these formulations impact local anesthetic action?

14. What are the major systemic side effects that might occur when using a local anesthetic? Even though these drugs are referred to as local anesthetics, how, and through what mechanisms are systemic side effects induced?

Chapter 8

1. Define focus, mirror focus, generalization, ictus, interictus, and status epilepticus. List the various seizure types and define them.

2. What is the potential relationship between the PDS, memory, and epilepsy? Based on these relationships what are three potential treatments for epilepsy?

3. Diagram the structure of barbiturate and hydantoin. What are the consequences of substituting alkyl and cyclic groups on the 5'carbon of the barbiturate molecule?

4. What side effects are common to the administration of all AEDs? What side effects are unique to phenytoin and phenobarbital? What are the two most significant side effects attending the use of the other AEDs?

5. What are the major categories of AEDs, and based on their respective mechanisms of action, how would each be expected to influence the focus and spread of epileptic activity?

6. What are the implications of use dependency for antiseizure activity involving Na^+ channel blockers in antiepileptic therapy? How could this explain the discrepancy between plasma level and drug efficacy?

7. Various actions of phenobarbital exhibit variable rates of tolerance. Why is this important to understanding chronic antiseizure management?

8. What are the mechanisms of action of the new AEDs?

9. What treatment considerations are relevant when a patient is in status epilepticus?

Chapter 9

1. How is DA synthesized and biotransformed? What are the major CNS DA pathways and their origins and target structures? What are the peripheral actions of DA?

2. What are the five DA receptor subtypes and how are they linked to the synthesis of adenylate cyclase?

3. Which dopaminergic agonists act directly and which act indirectly?

4. What are the LADME characteristics of levodopa and how are they related to large neutral amino acids, pyridoxine, and methionine?

5. What are the central and peripheral consequences of adding carbidopa to levodopa?

6. What is the balance hypothesis of striatal function and how does it relate to drug therapy for hyperkinetic and hypokinetic movement disorders?

7. Which antiparkinsonian drugs are used during the various stages of PD and what is the rationale for their use?

8. What are the major side effects of the antimuscarinic agents and the DA agonists? What complications to levodopa therapy attend the use of levodopa in mid- to late-stage PD?

9. What are the basic pathologies underlying Wilson's disease and Huntington's disease and how are they treated?

10. What are the four characteristics of multifocal tic and how are tics treated?

11. What controversies surround the drug treatment of AD/HD? What dosage considerations surround the treatment of school-aged children with AD/HD based on drug half-life and body growth?

12. What are the three different types of tremor and how are they treated?

13. What is the mechanism through which botulinum toxin reduces focal dystonias?

Chapter 10

1. What are the positive and negative symptoms of schizophrenia and what can induce psychotic behavior? What is meant by a psychotic break?

2. What is the DA theory of schizophrenia and what data supports it or is inconsistent with it? What pathology and pathophysiology are thought to underlie schizophrenia?

3. How long does antipsychotic efficacy normally take to develop and state two theories for this efficacy delay?

4. What are the various types of acute extrapyramidal side effects and when do they tend to emerge? How does depolarization blockade produce EPSEs and how does antimuscarinic activity influence this phenomenon? What is meant by the terms typical and atypical antipsychotic?

5. What is thought to be the relationship between DA-receptor proliferation and TD? What inconsistencies exist to suggest that this hypothesis may not be true? Based on this hypothesis, how do breakthrough and withdrawal TD emerge?

6. What is the phenothiazine structural nomenclature (aliphatic, piperidine, and piperazine)? Based on their antimuscarinic potencies, what are the propensities of the three classes of phenothiazines for producing EPSEs?

7. What is the relationship between DA antagonism and antipsychotic drug side effects? What are the common side effects of the antipsychotic drug class and which agent is most/least likely to produce it?

8. Why is clozapine so atypical as an antipsychotic? Based on its mechanism of action, why doesn't it produce EPSEs or TD?

9. What is the major limitation to the use of clozapine and how does this important side effect develop?

10. Why is risperidone classified as an atypical antipsychotic agent even though it can produce EPSEs?

Chapter 11

1. What are the catecholamine and indoleamine hypotheses of depression? What data supports and what data refutes each?

2. Based on the Foote and Morrison hypothesis, how can 5HT and/or NE deficiencies lead to depressive symptoms?

3. What circadian rhythm disturbances underlie depressive symptoms and what role, if any, is melatonin thought to play in depression?

4. What are the four major classes of antidepressant medication and how is the action of each drug class consistent with the biogenic amine hypotheses of depression?

5. How do the TCA and SSRI antidepressants alter neuron firing rates and what receptor changes are associated with the chronic use of each drug class?

6. How do MAOIs produce the tyramine effect and why don't the RIMAs?

7. Classify each antidepressant agent as to its relative NE and 5HT specificity (i.e., low, medium, or high)?

8. What are the major side effects of the antidepressant drug classes?

9. Why have the SSRIs revolutionized antidepressant therapy despite their lack of better efficacy?

10. What are the characteristic signs and symptoms of toxicity following TCA, SSRI, and MAOI overdose?

11. What is the proposed mechanism of action of lithium?

12. What are the signs and symptoms of lithium toxicity and how do exercise and diuretic agents influence that toxicity?

13. What role does carbamazepine and valproate play in the management of bipolar disorder?

Chapter 12

1. What do the terms dependence, drug abuse, recreational use, situational use and addiction mean?

2. What is the incentive-salience hypothesis of dependence and how can this hypothesis be explained by sensitization in the n. accumbens? Why do different drugs produce differing forms of withdrawal syndromes and exhibit differing rates of tolerance?

3. How is DA related to dependence liability and through what mechanisms do the various drugs of abuse influence DA in the brain?

4. What are the differences and similarities in the actions of psychostimulants and how does Ca^{2+}-independent release occur?

5. What general actions are shared by psychostimulants and how is the toxic profile for cocaine different from that for amphetamine?

6. What is the significance of the inverted U-shaped self-administration pattern associated with caffeine?

7. What are the general actions of alcohol and the mechanisms through which it is thought to induce its effects?

8. How are alcohol and methanol biotransformed and how is their metabolism influenced by disulfiram and chloral hydrate?

9. What are the mechanisms of action of disulfiram and how does it produce its effects in the presence of alcohol?

10. How is cyclic coma produced by PCP?

11. What are the general effects of THC and what effects make it unique relative to other drugs of abuse?

12. What is a gateway drug and which drugs are generally considered members of this drug group?

13. How is LSD thought to induce hallucinations and what are the common actions of its drug class?

14. How are designer drugs similar to and how are they different from the hallucinogens?

15. What is HPPD and how is it related to prior LSD ingestion?

16. Why are the hallucinogens not associated with significant dependence liability?

17. What characterizes the anticholinergic syndrome?

18. What are the most common forms of self-administration of the anabolic steroids?

Index